Medically Unexplained Illness

Medically Unexplained Illness

Gender and Biopsychosocial Implications

SUSAN K. JOHNSON

American Psychological Association
Washington, DC

Published by
American Psychological Association
750 First Street, NE
Washington, DC 20002
www.apa.org

To order
APA Order Department
P.O. Box 92984
Washington, DC 20090-2984
Tel: (800) 374-2721; Direct: (202) 336-5510
Fax: (202) 336-5502; TDD/TTY: (202) 336-6123
Online: www.apa.org/books/
E-mail: order@apa.org

In the U.K., Europe, Africa, and the Middle East, copies may be ordered from
American Psychological Association
3 Henrietta Street
Covent Garden, London
WC2E 8LU England

Typeset in Goudy by Stephen McDougal, Mechanicsville, MD

Printer: Maple-Vail Book Manufacturing, Binghamton, NY
Cover Designer: Scribe Typography, Port Townsend, WA
Technical/Production Editor: Harriet Kaplan

The opinions and statements published are the responsibility of the authors, and such opinions and statements do not necessarily represent the policies of the American Psychological Association.

Library of Congress Cataloging-in-Publication Data

Johnson, Susan K.
    Medically unexplained illness : gender and biopsychosocial implications / by Susan K. Johnson. — 1st ed.
        p. cm.
    Includes bibliographical references.
    ISBN-13: 978-0-9792125-8-1
    ISBN-10: 0-9792125-8-8
    1. Somatoform disorders. 2. Chronic fatigue syndrome—Etiology. 3. Multiple chemical sensitivity—Etiology. 4. Fibromyalgia—Etiology. 5. Sex differences (Psychology)
I. American Psychological Association. II. Title.
    [DNLM: 1. Psychophysiologic Disorders—psychology. 2. Psychophysiologic Disorders—therapy. 3. Fatigue Syndrome, Chronic. 4. Fibromyalgia. 5. Irritable Bowel Syndrome.
6. Sex Factors. WM 90 J69m 2007]
    RB113.J6448 2007
    616'.0478—dc22   2007010292

British Library Cataloguing-in-Publication Data
A CIP record is available from the British Library.

Printed in the United States of America
First Edition

For Dennis, Elise, and Caroline

CONTENTS

FOREWORD

Medical practitioners are taught fact-based medicine. They are taught to use a patient's story of his or her illness as a path to suggest various diagnoses confirmed in part by the physical examination and then more definitively by appropriate laboratory testing. Unfortunately, the fact-based approach often is not sufficient. This is because many patients seen in the outpatient setting have complaints or symptoms with no detectable abnormality. The most common of these are fatigue, pain, or achiness—either in localized parts of the body such as the head or abdomen or throughout the body, problems with sleep, or feeling as if it is hard to concentrate (a complaint that patients will often call "brain fog"). The practitioner has no barometer with which to gauge fatigue and has to turn to the neuropsychologist for help in gauging brain fog. With patients who complain of pain, the practitioner can often find tenderness on palpation but no hint as to why it exists. So even if the examination can elicit abnormal signs such as tenderness or abnormalities on cognitive testing, the results often do not point to a definitive diagnosis, which leaves the practitioner without an explanation. This can lead to a disconnect between what the patient is expecting to happen and what actually does happen in the doctor's office. When the medical model fails, practitioners turn to psychogenic mechanisms. If they cannot find a physiological cause for symptoms, they believe that none exists. This leads to the conclusion that patients are either making up their pain or that it is "all in their heads." Some doctors actually say as much; others prefer to tell their patients that "nothing is wrong." Patients leave the doctor's office feeling dissatisfied and still ill. They have fallen between the cracks of classical medicine and are on their own. This is probably the biggest reason that vitamins and health-related foods are now a billion-dollar industry in America.

Of course, this scenario represents a failure of the medical profession to care for the patient. If a diagnosis doesn't fit, reject the patient! However, this is the antithesis of what a doctor should be doing, and that is whatever helps the patient feel better. Somehow, the fact-based approach to medicine, with its need to solve the medical puzzle, has trumped the original reason for the existence of the medical profession. In the high-tech world of modern medicine, the patient with disabling symptoms but no definite illness is left on his or her own. George Engel's[1] biopsychosocial approach to illness has fallen to the wayside.

The consequences of this shift are just now hitting the American medical educational system with the following questions for the near future. Who is going to take care of all these patients? How can we increase this number by shifting the focus from the machine back to the patient? How can we teach doctors to deal with uncertainty when they are trained to be comfortable only when they know all the answers?

Answering these questions constitutes a process in education. Susan K. Johnson's book is a clear step in this process. The book is a rarity in that it provides one scholar's synthesis, integration, and conclusions from many complex and often contradictory studies. To the inquisitive, the book opens many research questions. To the practitioner, the book provides an up-to-date review of what is known and how to apply it to the patient, and it does this in a way in which the clinician, whether a psychologist or a physician, can learn the biological bases for these medical problems. Thus, the person who reads this book can understand the pathophysiological bases for the problems seen in the office. This broad background is critical for the future research that is needed to improve the therapeutic armamentarium available to the practitioner. However, the biopsychosocial component reviewed in depth herein is also a critical factor, because it makes the point that the practitioner can develop a prescription hand tailored to each patient that can lead to reduced symptoms and thus better health. A careful reading of this book plus a bit of thought will make you a better caregiver. Patients will leave your office feeling better rather than feeling lost or rejected, as is too often the case with classical medicine today.

Benjamin Natelson, MD

---

[1]Engel, G. (1977, April 8). The need for a new medical model: A challenge for biomedicine. *Science, 196,* 129–136.

Medically Unexplained Illness

INTRODUCTION

Interest in medically unexplained illnesses (MUIs) is on the rise, not surprising considering that they constitute the most common disorders seen in primary care (Kroenke et al., 1997). MUIs are syndromes characterized by multiple symptoms, significant suffering, and disability that fail to show consistent pathophysiology (Barsky & Borus, 1999). MUIs present a conundrum for conventional biomedical approaches. Their high degree of prevalence, together with chronicity, attendant disability, and skyrocketing costs to the health care system, have fed this interest. Undoubtedly, some of the recent fascination with MUIs is related to the clues they offer to the mind–body relationship. Research in the physiology of these illnesses in an attempt to fit them into the biomedical model has illuminated both the inadequacy of the biomedical model and the bidirectional nature of the biobehavioral transaction. This volume tackles the complex nature of the mind–brain–behavior relationship.

The guiding purpose of this book is to present a balanced, biopsychosocial approach to exploring the role of gender in several representative MUIs. An inclusive classification of MUIs would include such illnesses as chronic fatigue syndrome (CFS), fibromyalgia (FMS), premenstrual syndrome, chronic pelvic pain, irritable bowel syndrome (IBS), multiple chemical sensitivities (MCS), Gulf War syndrome, temporomandibular joint dysfunction (TMD), noncardiac chest pain, hyperventilation syndrome, and tension headaches (Manu, 2004; Wessely, Nimnuan, & Sharpe, 1999). Common factors among all the MUIs are a lack of sufficient medical explanation, significant impairment in functioning, and female predominance. Many labels have been used in the literature to describe these conditions, such as *medically unexplained symptoms, functional somatic syndromes, chronic dysfunctional illnesses, functional stress syndromes, chronic multisymptom illnesses, affective spectrum disorders, multisomatoform disorders, antidepressant responsive disorders,* and *unexplained illnesses.* Although the literature often notes that these syndromes are poorly understood and underresearched, there is actually an abundance of research in a wide variety of disciplines, ranging from physiology, medicine, psychology, sociology, and epidemiology to public health, but these disparate reports do not always acknowledge the contributions from other areas. The research from these myriad fields can contribute to a further biopsychosocial understanding of MUIs and their preponderance in women.

Female predominance is well documented and established in MUIs, but the reasons for this gender disparity are still unclear (Jason, Taylor, Song, Kennedy, & Johnson, 1999; Toner, 1995; Wessely et al., 1999; Whitehead, Palsson, & Jones, 2002; Wool & Barsky, 1994). Relatively few investigators have broached this topic other than to note the prevalence of disparities between genders. The ratio of women to men is generally reported to 2:1 for irritable bowel syndrome (IBS; Mayer, Naliboff, Lee, Munakata, & Chang, 1999) and CFS (Evengard, Jacks, Pedersen, & Sullivan, 2005; Lindal, Stefansson, & Bergmann, 2002), 9:1 for FMS (Gran, 2003; Yunus, 2001), and 4:1 for MCS (Fiedler & Kipen, 1997). Since vital health statistics have been recorded in the United States, mortality rates have been higher among men, whereas morbidity from acute and chronic conditions, short-term disability, health care use, and medical drug use have been higher among women. Men suffer more than women do from life-threatening diseases that cause earlier death. Women live longer than men, but they also live "sicker," restricting their activity and spending more days in bed. The differences are largest during the reproductive years for women, yet even when reproductive conditions are excluded, differences in morbidity remain (Verbrugge, 1985). The reproductive age is also the prime age for the development of MUIs, although these illnesses (with the exception of premenstrual syndrome) are not closely related to women's reproductive physiology. Because they are so prevalent and disabling, MUIs account for a great deal of women's morbidity (Wessely et al., 1999).

This book is based on the premise that there is an interaction of physiological, psychological, and sociocultural variables that contribute to female predominance in MUIs. The relative influence of these three factors varies among individuals. The trauma of childhood sexual abuse may be strongly salient for one individual with FMS or IBS, whereas another may be psychologically unscathed yet have neuroendocrine dysfunction expressed as hypocortisolism and resulting in fatigue, sleep difficulties, pain symptoms, and reduced coping abilities.

Accordingly, the approach to understanding the relationship between gender and MUIs must be interdisciplinary. This book presents a biopsychosocial model for several representative MUI syndromes: IBS, FMS, CFS, and MCS. These four syndromes are explored in depth because they represent a broad spectrum of body systems. They range in terms of medical legitimacy from IBS (less controversial and more accepted) to MCS (more controversial and less clearly defined). These syndromes challenge traditional perspectives on illness and demand innovative paradigms to advance our understanding. By examining the empirical evidence through the lens of gender, this book shows that MUIs result from an interaction of physiological, psychological, interpersonal, and sociocultural factors that affect symptom expression differently in men and women.

A brief history of MUIs is presented in chapter 1. Chapter 2 addresses the issue of comorbidity of somatization, depression, and anxiety in MUIs as well as the high co-occurrence of somatization with other psychiatric disorders and the high rates of health care use by people with somatizing tendencies. Bidirectional processes in MUIs (the psychosocial factors discussed in chap. 3) influence physiological processes presented in chapter 4, and physiological processes impact the psychosocial experience of the patient. Chapter 3 highlights the explanations for gender differences in symptom reporting, sensation thresholds, stressful life events, and health care seeking. Additionally, chapter 3 explores the problem faced by people with MUIs of having to prove the legitimacy of their illnesses when the medical system does not validate their illness experiences. Because patients recognize the stigma of psychiatric diagnosis, much patient activism is directed toward achieving a medical diagnosis. The evidence for hypothalamic–pituitary–adrenocortical axis, autonomic, and neuromuscular dysregulation in patients with medically unexplained syndromes, such as cortisol and serotonin deficiencies, smooth muscle contractions, and central nervous system and visceral hypersensitivity, are presented in chapter 4. These biological alterations may be experienced as symptoms by the patient. The influences on this process are cognitions (beliefs, interpretations, attributions, expectancies), mood factors (depression, anxiety), and sociocultural expectancies, which differ for men and women. These psychosocial differences influence MUIs through biological systems that mediate sensation and function and through the development of illness behavior.

Part II considers the arguments for approaching MUI as one syndrome or as distinct syndromes. Chapters 5 through 8 present a detailed analysis of the state of current research on IBS, FMS, CFS, and MCS. Approaches to epidemiology, classification criteria, biopsychosocial etiology, gender influences, course of illness, and outcomes for these MUIs are discussed.

General treatment issues in MUIs are addressed in Part III. The efficacy of approaches such as pharmacology, cognitive–behavioral treatments, stress management, hypnotherapy, and graded exercise are presented. Treatment for women with MUIs should take into consideration the unique therapeutic needs of women in relation to socialization around issues of self-esteem, assertiveness, role strain, and dependency. Sex-specific triggers such as history of sexual abuse, battering, stressful life events, and the relation of symptoms to menstrual cycle or hormonal events should all be addressed as part of an individualized treatment approach. The experience of some patients who engage in endless rounds of "doctor shopping," in fruitless attempts to legitimate their illness experiences, results in frustration in patients and physicians alike. Doctor shopping can also result in excessive medical testing and overprescribing of pharmaceuticals, which can result in iatrogenic symptoms. Physicians often view unexplained symptoms as a threat to medical competence and dismiss such symptoms as psychogenic. This does not satisfy the patient whose physical body is suffering and who views psychological explanations as inadequate and stigmatizing.

A helpful approach discussed in Part III is the framing of MUIs as stress disorders, thereby providing an entry intro framing the biopsychosocial approach for the patient and emphasizing the importance of stress management. In chapters 9 through 12, treatment approaches are highlighted for each MUI, which emphasize identifying and managing stressors in the patient's life. This is crucial, because chronic life stress is a powerful predictor of symptom intensity in MUIs.

The paradigmatic model in health psychology is the biopsychosocial model. Although universally accepted as the cornerstone for theory and research, a reflexive Cartesian dualism still seeps into much of the discourse on MUIs. The approach herein attempts to move beyond "either–or" mind–body labeling and synthesize contemporary theory and research into a better understanding of the mechanisms through which MUI symptoms occur. This understanding can then be translated into more effective treatment approaches for individuals disabled by MUIs.

This volume is intended for health psychologists, clinical psychologists, gender researchers, physiological psychologists, public health officials, and medical sociologists. Physicians, nurses, physical therapists, and other medical personnel, as well as lay people who are affected by these very prevalent syndromes, can also gain insight into a broader theoretical understanding of MUI.

MUIs exist in a gray zone between psychiatry and medicine. MUIs tend to defy efforts to be simplified, just as individuals with MUIs cannot be lumped into a single category. Early diagnosis and management can help reduce disability, and integrating psychological treatment into general medical care will improve the care of patients with MUIs. The treatment evidence presented in this volume indicates that psychological approaches are generally more efficacious than biomedical treatments for MUI. The evidence in this volume should help psychologists and health care practitioners advocate for a biopsychosocial approach to patients with MUIs rather than for treatments guided by dualistic explanations.

Researchers must avoid biological reductionism and examine the contributions of interdependent mechanisms. The complexity of understanding MUIs calls for more dynamic models to better apportion variance among multiple factors (Hamilton & Gallant, 1993; Van Houdenhove, Egle, & Luyten, 2005). This volume presents the evidence for multiple factors and for the complex and dynamic interaction of biopsychosocial factors that underlie MUIs.

I

OVERVIEW OF MEDICALLY UNEXPLAINED ILLNESS

The chronic and disabling medically unexplained illnesses (MUIs) represent a confluence of multifactorial mechanisms. A complex interaction of psychological, biological, and socio–environmental factors contribute to a varied symptom complex. One of the perennial debates surrounding MUIs is the extent to which they have always been with us. As Simon Wessely (1990) has asked, are the MUIs "old wine in new bottles"—age-old symptom patterns dressed up with new diagnostic criteria? Certainly there is evidence for this thesis as explicated in the brief history of MUIs presented in chapter 1. The labels for MUI vary with the zeitgeist, but irritable bowel syndrome (IBS), fibromylagia (FMS), and chronic fatigue syndrome (CFS) have a long history, whereas a diagnosis of multiple chemical sensitivities (MCS) is more dependent on exposure to modern chemicals and toxins and thus has a shorter history. It is important to emphasize the "new bottles" aspect of Wessely's observation, however. New research presented in this volume suggests that investigators are gaining more sophisticated understanding of MUIs using broader conceptual models that include biopsychosocial and person-centered approaches to MUIs (Masi, White, & Pilcher, 2002).

The question of whether MUIs are somatically disguised psychiatric disorders is discussed in chapter 2. This chapter connects the high prevalence of psychiatric disorders with the etiology of MUIs. Higher symptom

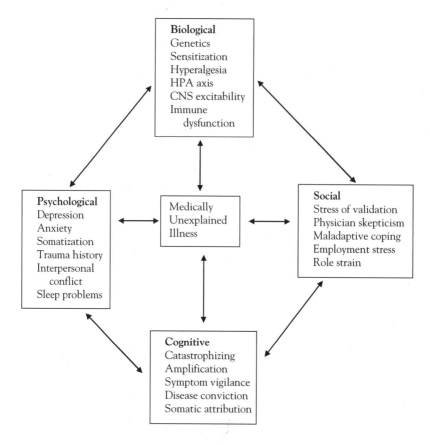

Figure 1. Integrated biopsychosocial model of mutually influential factors of medically unexplained illness. HPA = hypothalamic–pituitary–adrenocortical; CNS = central nervous system.

reporting among women is linked to higher rates of depression and anxiety, and thus an increased likelihood of symptom somatization. Currently, the MUIs do not fit comfortably into a *Diagnostic and Statistical Manual of Mental Disorders* (DSM; American Psychiatric Association, 1952, 1968, 1980, 1994, 2000) framework, although the overlap in symptoms with depression, anxiety, and somatoform disorders is substantial. *DSM* scholars have been debating the limitations of the categorical classification system that is the hallmark of the *DSM* (Widiger & Samuel, 2005). It is interesting to note that criticism of the *DSM*'s approach—that psychiatric syndromes do not represent distinct categorical etiologies, do not have laboratory markers, and have high rates of co-occurrence—echo the controversies surrounding classification of MUIs. A dimensional framework has been proposed for the not-yet-published fifth edition of the *DSM* (Widiger & Samuel, 2005), and it is possible that MUIs would fit into new dimensional classification systems. MUIs may represent the extreme end of a continuum of somatic complaints. It is debatable whether this advances understanding or just creates a more accessible box into which MUIs can be wedged. What is not debatable is the interaction of social and cognitive factors with biological sensitivities that influence symptom perception. The contributions of these factors are addressed in chapters 3 and 4, with an emphasis on the role of gender.

Chapter 3 makes an argument for sociocultural and cognitive factors as mediators of MUIs. The key psychosocial explanations include gender stereotypes, role strain, and history of abuse; cognitive explanations include negative affect, catastrophizing, symptom reporting style, and symptom perception. The biological factors that appear to play an important role in MUIs include genetic explanations, physiological sensitization, and neuroendocrine influences on immune system functioning. Past research has primarily described gender as a demographic variable rather than a variable that may directly influence other risk factors. Further research is needed to look more explicitly at how gender informs the biopsychosocial model.

Figure 1 presents an integrated biopsychosocial model of factors mutually influencing MUIs that are discussed in great detail in chapters 2, 3, and 4. The relative influence and interaction of these factors varies across individuals and across different MUIs. Future research is required to address questions generated by this model: How does gender influence physician skepticism to increase symptom vigilance and disease conviction in MUIs? Biological sensitization has been shown to be a factor in FMS and IBS; is a similar sensitization operating in CFS? Is there an underlying factor in autoimmune disease that would help explain female predominance in MUIs? Does the stress of working to validate MUIs contribute to interpersonal conflict and stronger somatic attribution? How can multimodal treatment be effectively delivered in primary care settings? How can health care providers deliver the message of the biopsychosocial model effectively to patients to reduce doctor shopping? Would feminist therapy be more effective than cognitive–behavioral therapy? Would disease conviction, somatic attribution, and its role in doctor shopping be reduced if complementary and alternative medicine approaches were tried? The model outlined in Figure 1 should generate many more similar questions for researchers and clinicians. The research that lays the foundation for these questions is presented in this volume.

1

A BRIEF HISTORY OF GENDER IN
MEDICALLY UNEXPLAINED ILLNESS

Mysterious symptoms that confound physicians have been reported for centuries in various cultures. Any discussion of the history of medically unexplained illness (MUI) must begin with hysteria. Hysteria was recognized as a medical condition by early Egyptian and Greek cultures, and references to it were made in the writings of Hippocrates and Galen. Hysteria has traditionally been viewed as a women's disease; its literal translation from the Greek is "'wandering womb." Trimble (2004) noted that symptoms similar to those reported in MUI today, and with a gender-specific etiology, were documented more than 2,000 years ago in at least two different cultures. The term *hysterical* became almost "interchangeable with 'feminine' in literature, where it stood for all extremes of emotionality" (Showalter, 1985, p. 129). Showalter (1985) argued that the vast repertoire of emotional and physical symptoms ranging from fits, fainting, vomiting, choking, sobbing, laughing, paralysis, and the rapid passage from one symptom to another was consistent with the perception of the lability and capriciousness associated with feminine nature.

Neurotic hysteria has been viewed as either a heroic protest against Victorian repression or as a pathetic collapse into maladaptive illness (Micale 1995; Smith-Rosenberg, 1985). The Freudian perspective was extremely influential in establishing hysteria as an expression of unconscious conflicts displayed through bodily symptoms (Breuer & Freud, 1895/1987). Symptoms served a symbolic function in the world of the Victorian woman. Freud's female patients became the prototype for the hysterical neurotic, and psychoanalysis has even been called the child of the hysterical woman. Because Freud viewed the repression of sexual impulses to be the source of all neurosis, psychoanalytic treatment was aimed at unearthing this unconscious repression in the hysterical patient. Her bodily symptoms were then expected to dissipate as she gained insight into her unconscious conflicts.

By the late 19th century, hysteria was often confounded with neurasthenia; together they were referred to as the "nervous" disorders. Their symptoms could certainly overlap, and both resulted in profound disability. Hysteria tended to consist of more dramatic, colorful symptoms, whereas neurasthenia was characterized by fatigue (Micale, 1995; Oppenheim, 1991). Becker (2005) argued that the pairing of "nerves" and distress in hysteria, the "female" disease, preceded the appearance of neurasthenia, the "American" nervous disease. Showalter (1985) contended that neurasthenia was a more attractive form of female nervousness than hysteria, although the two were not always distinguishable.

Fatigue as a debilitating symptom, first reported in the mid-1800s, was believed to afflict primarily upper-class women (Shorter, 1993; Wessely, 1991). These women complained mainly of fatigue and muscle weakness, but pain was also often a prominent symptom. George Beard, an American physician, was the first to describe neurasthenia as a distinct clinical category (Beard, 1880). The symptoms of neurasthenia included general malaise, disability, weakness, poor appetite, neuralgic pains, hysteria, hypochondriasis, avoidance of mental labor, and headaches (Macmillan, 1976). By 1900, neurasthenia had become an extremely common diagnosis, although it appeared to be a "catch-all" category (Shorter, 1993). *Neurasthenia* was used alternately as a synonym for general nervousness and evolving psychosis, as the "male" equivalent of hysteria, as a synonym for minor depression, and as a diagnosis for unexplained fatigue states (Shorter, 1993; Torres-Harding & Jason, 2005).

Showalter (1985) described neurasthenia patients as women who languished with fatigue and who were often incapable of any purposeful activity or of even rising from bed. Although she acknowledged the occurrence of the illness in men, the main thrust of her argument was that it arose in women as a form of protest against their empty and unfulfilled lives. Primary sources reveal contradictory views on the gender distribution of neurasthenia. Some writers saw it as a disease of professional and intellectual men, leaders, and captains of industry (Pritchard, 1905). However, some believed that women were more vulnerable owing to their "weaker nervous systems." Medical texts of the late 1800s contained comments indicating that young women were much more prone than young men to nervous complaints. They also voiced the common concern that educating women could contribute to nervous symptoms and damage women's reproductive capacities (Oppenheim, 1991).

Although neurasthenia was diagnosed in both men and women, physicians perceived numerous differences related to symptoms, causes, and treatments (Becker, 2005). Beard (1880) made the distinction between male "cerebrasthenia" brought on by mental overwork and female "myelasthenia" brought on by physical or emotional shocks. The rest cure was more often applied to women, whereas men were more likely to be instructed to build up their energy reserves through vigorous exercise. Gender was an important factor in diagnosis; physicians were loathe to diagnose hysteria in men because it was considered a "feminizing'" label, implying weakness and vulnerability.

Over time, diagnoses of hysteria and neurasthenia declined as they came to be redefined as psychiatric because of the stigma of psychiatric labels (Wessely, 1991). Within the medical profession, the development of psychoanalysis and the increase in psychological treatments all but eliminated the diagnosis of disorders that were a physical expression of distress (Swartz, Blazer, George, & Landerman, 1986). Shorter (1992) argued that the decreased prevalence of neurasthenia was due to a paradigm shift in medicine in which neurasthenic symptoms came to be regarded as psychological. Somatizing patients therefore selected symptoms that were more likely to be construed as organic from the "symptom pool." As people became more psychologically literate, they understood the psychodynamics behind "nervous" symptoms. Then, as now, psychological symptoms were seen as less legitimate than organically based ones.

Micale (1995) argued that as society progressed away from Victorian strictures on women, escape into illness became less necessary. It has been acknowledged that hysteria and neurasthenia may have acted as symbols for women's restricted opportunities (Showalter, 1985; Smith-Rosenberg, 1985). The emancipation of women and the liberation of sexual attitudes were important in decreasing women's need to express themselves somatically (Showalter, 1985; Smith-Rosenberg, 1985). It is interesting that today's discussions of MUI rarely link women's current role requirements to burgeoning rates of MUIs.

Neurasthenia and hysteria were diagnosed less frequently as more working class people began to suffer from them. New research has indicated that symptoms of hysteria and neurasthenia were not rare among the working classes but that the conditions were unrecognized, untreated, and underreported (Micale, 1995; R. Taylor, 2001). This is similar to the case of chronic fatigue syndrome (CFS), which was originally labeled "yuppie flu" until several community-based epidemiological studies showed that higher levels of fatigue were found among non-White minority groups (Song, Taylor, & Jason, 1999; Steele et al., 1998), and the yuppie label became obsolete.

The first *Diagnostic and Statistical Manual of Mental Disorders* (*DSM*; American Psychiatric Association, 1952) had several categories for Hysteria: by symptom, conversion disorder, and personality trait ("Emotionally Unstable Personality"). The second edition of the *DSM* (*DSM–II*; American Psychiatric Association, 1968) further categorized hysteria as "Hysterical Neurosis" (conversion reaction and dissociative reaction) and "Hysterical Personality." In the third edition of the *DSM* (*DSM–III*; American Psychiatric Association, 1980), the term *Hysterical Personality* was replaced with *Histrionic Personality Disorder* to emphasize the histrionic behavior pattern and to reduce the confusion caused by the historical links of hysteria to conversion symptoms. *Hysterical Neurosis, Conversion Type* became *Conversion Disorder*. The third revised edition of the *DSM* (*DSM–III–R*; American Psychiatric Association, 1987) retained the term *Histrionic Personality Disorder*, but the criteria for it were revised. The fourth edition of the *DSM* (*DSM–IV*; American Psychiatric Association, 1994) includes the classification Somatoform Disorders, which includes Conversion Disorder, and it still retains Histrionic Personality Disorder.

The history of neurasthenia in the *DSM* is equally convoluted. Neurasthenia did not appear in the original *DSM*; it appeared in *DSM–II*, but it was summarily dropped in *DSM–III*. It reappeared in *DSM–IV* in the appendices as a culture-bound syndrome. The core symptoms of neurasthenia were described in *DSM–IV* as persistent mental or physical fatigue accompanied by at least two of seven symptoms: dizziness, dyspepsia, muscular aches or pains, tension headaches, inability to relax, irritability, and sleep disturbance. Exclusion criteria were described as mood or anxiety disorders.

Some have argued that neurasthenia has not disappeared but that the symptom complex was first subdivided into various neuroses, including obsessive–compulsive disorders, anxiety neuroses, and hysterical personality (Shorter, 1992), and more recently as CFS, fibromyalgia (FMS), multiple chemical sensitivities (MCS), and various other MUIs (Ford, 1997; Micale, 1995; Wessely, 1996). Neurasthenia is still included in the latest revision of the *International Classification of Diseases, 10th Revision* (World Health Organization, 1992), and it is still diagnosed in parts of Europe, Russia, and Asia, where it is seen as a physical disorder (P. Y. Schwartz, 2002; Wessely, 1991).

In the 1970s, a variant of hysteria apparently began to be diagnosed as a psychiatric disorder called *Briquet's syndrome*. First described by a French psychiatrist in 1859, Briquet's syndrome was formally defined by Guze, Woodruff, and Clayton (1971) as a subtype of hysteria occurring predominantly in women with a complicated and dramatic medical history beginning before age 30. Briquet's syndrome consists of the presence of a minimum of 25 medically unexplained symptoms in at least 9 of 10 symptom groups (Guze, 1975); it is found to be a reliable and valid diagnosis (Guze, Cloninger, Martin, & Clayton, 1986). Briquet's syndrome is associated with familial aggregation in women but not in men (Cloninger, Martin, Guze, & Clayton, 1986).

Liskow, Othmer, Penick, DeSouza, and Gabrielli (1986) found that female psychiatric outpatients with Briquet's syndrome had an average of 4.3 other psychiatric syndromes. These disorders include depression, panic, phobia, obsessive–compulsive disorder, antisocial personality disorder, and substance abuse. Liskow et al. suggested that Briquet's syndrome patients have a response bias and answer yes to many questions regarding psychopathology just as they do to questions relating to medical symptoms. Support for the sheer multiplicity of complaints in Briquet's was also found by Wetzel, Guze, Cloninger, Martin, and Clayton (1994). They compared women with primary affective disorder with women with Briquet's syndrome on the Minnesota Multiphasic Personality Inventory. The women with Briquet's syndrome reported more complaints of all types in all areas than depressed women, even after controlling for response bias. Wetzel et al. concluded that women with Briquet's syndrome present with multiple somatic and psychological symptoms. Orenstein (1989) proposed that Briquet's syndrome represents the most extreme expression of a tendency for the aggregation of physical symptom reporting, depression, panic disorder, and agoraphobia.

In *DSM–III*, Briquet's syndrome surfaced as somatization disorder; the criteria for identifying it were simplified and fewer symptoms were required for diagnosis. Thus, one could argue that hysteria has evolved into the somatoform disorders. Rief and Sharpe (2004) observed that the medical community rarely uses the term *somatoform disorder*. Rather, every medical specialty has its own MUI syndrome: gastroenterology has irritable bowel syndrome, rheumatology has FMS, gynecology has pelvic pain syndrome, and so on. Rief and Sharpe argued that a general label such as *medically unexplained symptoms* or *functional somatic syndromes*, although not ideal, is required, because separate MUI categories are not sufficiently distinct, and their similarities outweigh their differences.

The symptom of fatigue is a good example of a commonly occurring symptom in MUIs that has garnered different taxonomy throughout history. Shorter (2005) charted the rise and fall of fatigue as a psychiatric symptom. In the first edition of the *DSM*, which appeared in 1952, general fatigue was listed as the chief symptom in the condition "psychophysiologic nervous system reaction." In *DSM–II*, published in 1968, the term *neurasthenic neurosis (neurasthenia)* was introduced as an official diagnosis. Also added was a seldom-used diagnosis, *asthenic personality*, characterized by easy fatigability. In *DSM–III*, American psychiatry thus relegated fatigue to the level of one of many symptoms required to meet criteria for various affective disorders. The former asthenic personality was collapsed into "dependent personality disorder."

As fatigue faded from psychiatric taxonomy, it started to become epidemic in physicians' offices (Shorter, 2005), perhaps because it was perceived as a physical symptom without the stigma associated with asthenia. In the 1980s, patients began attributing feelings of chronic weariness and chronic pain to infection by Epstein–Barr virus. Shorter (2005) contended that this epidemic differed from other similar epidemics across the ages by the tenacity of patients' belief in a particular pathogen. Although Epstein–Barr virus was soon discredited scientifically as the cause of fatigue symptoms, the diagnosis of CFS or myalgic encephalitis took hold, purported to be the consequence of a breakdown in the immune system or a viral infestation (Shorter, 1992, 2005; Wessely, 1990).

Torres-Harding and Jason (2005) summarized the view of many mid 20th century physicians who espoused a holistic approach to fatigue and emphasized the need to take into account physical factors, such as infection or overwork, in addition to psychogenic or personality factors. Several outbreaks of illnesses with fatigue as a chief or principal symptom and with unknown etiology were also reported (Levine, 1994; Wessely, 1991). These unexplained fatigue illnesses were given multiple labels, including *epidemic neuromyasthenia, myalgic encephalomyelitis, Iceland disease,* and *atypical poliomyelitis.*

In addition to neurasthenia, other unexplained illnesses were reported in the late 19th and early 20th century. Some of these illnesses were called *effort syndrome, disordered action of the heart,* and *neurocirculatory asthenia.* T. Lewis (1940) first described effort syndrome, the symptoms of which included breathlessness, pain, palpitation, fainting, giddiness, headaches (especially after exertion), and complaints of fatigue (summarized by Torres-Harding & Jason, 2005). Initially, these disorders were regarded as arising from anomalies of cardiac function. Over time, however, as efforts to find underlying physiological abnormalities were not successful, these illnesses began to be regarded as primarily psychosomatic in nature.

Feinstein (2001) described a number of syndromes that have affected soldiers since the Crimean War. Among the names given to these syndromes were *DaCosta syndrome* (DaCosta, 1871); *soldier's heart; shell shock; combat stress; neuocirculatory neurasthenia;* and most recently, *Gulf War syndrome.* A syndrome akin to fibromyalgia was described by Gowers (1904) as *fibrositis,* marked by tenderness in a number of body regions that was not accompanied by tissue inflammation. Later, disturbed sleep, particularly a deficit in deep sleep, and exhaustion were part of the syndrome (Smythe, 1989). The term *fibrositis* was widely used until the American College of Rheumatology developed the criteria for FMS in 1990.

Multiple chemical sensitivity emerged as a descendant of food allergy problems, which were described in the 1920s and 1930s, when theorizing about sensitization to low levels of chemicals was set in the framework of allergy. Concerns about food allergies were transferred to the environment more broadly by the 1960s, when the term *chemical sensitivity* began to be used, and the clinical definition was developed in the 1980s (Shorter, 1992, 1997).

Many individuals report a complex mix of somatic and psychological symptoms that belie discrete categorization (Hickie, Hadzi-Pavlovic, & Ricci,

1997). MUIs have always challenged traditional perspectives on illness. Although the lack of definitive pathophysiology is frustrating, there do appear to be subtle physiological abnormalities in most MUIs (S. K. Johnson, DeLuca, & Natelson, 1999). Some have argued that many of Freud's classic "hysteria" cases were likely suffering from undiagnosed neurological disorders (Webster, 1995). Slater and Glithero (1965) asserted that in a group of patients diagnosed with hysteria in the 1950s, 33% actually suffered from serious organic disease. Increases in medical sophistication have significantly reduced the number of inaccurate hysteria diagnoses, but prognosis for chronic symptoms remains poor (Mace & Trimble, 1996). Stone et al. (2005) systematically reviewed 27 studies done since 1965 that had median follow-up durations of 5 years and included a total of 1,466 patients. Misdiagnosis was considered to have occurred when investigators concluded that most of a patient's original symptoms or signs were subsequently explained by disease. The average rate of misdiagnosis in these later studies was only 4%, which led the researchers to conclude that most medically unexplained symptoms were rarely misdiagnosed in contemporary investigations.

R. Taylor (2001) noted that a core cluster of nonspecific unexplained symptoms can be identified in historical case records and have continued to be reported by a significant proportion of individuals seeking medical treatment over the past 2 centuries. The diagnostic categories for these unexplained symptoms have fluctuated over time, with a shift in the 20th century to psychological diagnoses. Patients with unexplained physical symptoms have suffered considerably and have been passed to and fro between medical doctors and psychiatrists (Shorter, 2005).

This brief history conveys some of the similarities among hysteria, neurasthenia, and contemporary MUI. A number of theorists (Barsky & Borus, 1999; Feinstein, 2001; Shorter, 1992; Showalter, 1997; Wessely, 1991) have argued that MUIs are modern, media-driven forms of hysteria resulting from a stressed-out, exhausted populace unwilling to accept their symptoms as emotionally caused. They contend that the zeitgeist of the times and a quest for organicity determines the pattern of symptoms displayed. Ford (1997) went so far as to call MUIs "nondiseases" and stated that "hysteria is alive and well, and one contemporary hiding place is fashionable illness" (p. 7). Ford claimed that certain diagnoses were fashionable, namely MCS, FMS, reactive hypoglycemia, repetitive strain injury, and CFS. This skeptical view was echoed by Shorter (1997), who contended that MCS was the latest in a line of "pseudodiseases" that started with hypoglycemia in the 1960s and 1970s and was replaced by CFS and fibrositis in the 1980s and repetitive strain injury and sick building syndrome in the 1990s.

The view of MUI as shaped by the media zeitgeist, the Internet, and peer groups is somewhat overstated. Furthermore, such arguments can heighten the divisions between MUI advocates and the medical community. There is no doubt that the culture plays a role in shaping symptoms and labeling syndromes (Gureje, 2004). Additionally, economic factors may motivate patients to be more inclined to present with physical symptoms, because insurance reimbursement for psychiatric treatment is substantially lower than for physical illness treatment. Some would argue that MCS is an entirely socially constructed illness because it exists only in certain countries (Zavestoski et al., 2004). Yet, there are several important distinctions between 19th-century interpretations and contemporary ones. Today's level of medical sophistication makes medical diagnosis more accurate and efficient, which means that fewer symptoms are unexplained. Moreover, technological advancement and knowledge of molecular biology, biochemistry, infectious microbiology, and neurophysiology has helped advance the understanding of interactions between mind and body such as the stress/hypothalamic–pituitary–adrenal axis connection.

A biopsychosocial model posits that culture may influence symptom reporting and that there is also a bidirectional influence between brain physiology and symptoms. Katon, Sullivan, and Walker (2001) gave the example of irritable bowel syndrome, in which changes in brain physiology secondary to stressful events can cause abnormalities in smooth muscle tone in the gut and that these gut abnormalities are also associated with changes in brain physiology. Thus, cultural, psychosocial, and cognitive processes can become dominant in a vulnerable biological system.

2

PSYCHIATRIC DISORDER IN
MEDICALLY UNEXPLAINED ILLNESS

Many symptoms people experience cannot be explained by an established medical condition. Seventy percent of people with symptoms who visit primary care doctors leave without a diagnosis or treatment plan (Kroenke & Harris, 2001). This implies that a huge number of symptoms that bring people to physicians' offices are unexplained. Although many somatic symptoms are self-limited and have a favorable prognosis, about 25% of patients report persistent, chronic symptoms such as pain, fatigue, and headache (Kroenke, 2001a, 2001b; Kroenke et al., 1997; Kroenke & Harris, 2001; Verhaak, Meijer, Visser, & Wolters, 2006). In up to 50% of primary care visits, no organic cause is found for the presenting symptom, and most patients do not receive a definite diagnosis (Barsky & Borus, 1995; Kroenke & Mangelsdorff, 1989). Fink, Rosendal, and Toft (2002) summarized this situation by stating that it is "the exception rather than the rule in primary care for physical symptoms to be caused by organ pathology or pathophysiological disturbances" (p. 99). Many medically unexplained symptoms (MUS) fall into clusters and have evolved into syndromes. Irritable bowel syndrome (IBS), chronic fatigue syndrome (CFS), fibromyalgia (FMS), and multiple chemical sensitivity (MCS), the medically unexplained illnesses (MUIs) examined in this volume, are among the most common.

A perennial topic in the MUI literature is the high prevalence of lifetime and comorbid psychiatric disorders. The most commonly reported of such disorders are depression, anxiety, and somatization disorder (SD). (*Somatization* has a number of definitions, but its core characteristic is presentation of physical symptoms that are not sufficiently explained by medical, organic findings.) This high prevalence may mean that psychiatric disorders are a crucial part of the etiology of MUI and that there are many overlapping symptoms, which suggests a common pathophysiology. Alternately, common symptoms may be amplified because of psychiatric distress, because a person with MUI may experience reactive depression to the disability imposed by MUI, or because physicians may have a tendency toward "psychologizing" women's symptoms. What is not in dispute is that numerous research studies have shown high rates of lifetime and current diagnoses of somatoform, mood, and anxiety disorders among MUIs. The relationship between these psychiatric disorders and MUIs and the role of gender is discussed in this chapter.

Strong epidemiological evidence suggests female preponderance in all of the MUIs (Barsky & Borus, 1999; Kroenke & Spitzer, 1998). All of the MUIs are diagnosed on the basis of subjective symptom report. Women have consistently been shown to report higher numbers of symptoms than men. Most physical symptoms are reported at least 50% more often by women than by men, and this is not completely explained by higher levels of mental disorders in women (Kroenke & Spitzer, 1998). Although many studies have shown higher levels of somatization in women than in men, levels of hypochondriacal concerns are not different between men and women. Women also do not worry about serious illness more than men do (Barsky & Wyshak, 1990; Creed & Barsky, 2004).

There is no sharp delineation between symptoms of psychiatric disorder in MUIs that are clearly psychological and those that are clearly organically based. Numerous symptoms, such as fatigue, cognitive difficulties, sensitivity to pain, and sleep problems, occur commonly in both psychiatric and organic conditions. Thus, it is often the health care professional who must make the distinction between psychological symptoms and organic symptoms. S. K. Johnson, DeLuca, and Natelson (1996a) found that designation of CFS symptoms as organic strongly affects the diagnosis of SD within the CFS population; if the examiner attributes the patient's CFS symptoms to physical illness, diagnosis of SD is unlikely. Kirmayer, Robbins, and Paris (1994) also make the point that the designation of symptoms as unexplained vacillates, depending on current medical explanations of symptoms.

Although discussing MUIs in the context of SDs is controversial, somatizing tendencies must be considered when organic findings are insufficient to explain high levels of disability. MUIs often share a number of characteristics with somatoform disorders in addition to multiple unexplained symptoms in a variety of body systems: Doctor shopping, disease conviction, aversion to psychogenic explanations, and comorbidity with other psychiatric disorders are some of the most common (Bornschein, Hausteiner, Konrad, Forstl, & Zilker, 2006).

Fink (1996) suggested that MUIs such as CFS and FMS may be artifacts of suggestibility in somatizing patients; for example, individuals with somatizing tendencies grasp onto publicized syndrome criteria to shape their symptom presentation. Similarly, Barsky and Borus (1995) viewed the increase in MUIs as influenced by sociocultural trends that reduce people's tolerance for mild symptoms and lower the threshold for seeking medical care. People amplify and misattribute discomforts to disease, a process that may be abetted by medical professionals and the media. They call for recognition of the normative presence of symptoms and distress that do not require medical intervention. In this context, it is interesting to note that men are more likely than women to make normalizing attributions for somatic symptoms (see chap. 3, Somatic Attribution section, this volume).

SOMATOFORM DISORDERS AND SOMATIZATION

The behavioral tendency to note and report physical symptoms is thought to be related to three cognitive traits: selective attention and amplification of somatic symptoms, a belief that these symptoms are caused by physical disease, and attempts to seek medical care for symptom relief (Barsky & Wyshak, 1990; Lipowski, 1988; Whitehead & Palsson, 1998). Kirmayer et al. (1994) summarized a number of processes that contribute to somatic distress: neuroticism, individual differences in physiological reactivity, symptom perception, symptom thresholds, somatic attention, coping resources, and tendencies toward help seeking. Trait anxiety and trait negative affect, both higher in women, appear to be associated with a cognitive style of heightened vigilance toward body sensations (Pennebaker, 1994). Numerous investigators (Barsky & Borus, 1999; Kirmayer et al., 1994; Kroenke et al., 1997; Manu, 2004) have made persuasive arguments that somatizing processes pervade the MUI, especially in those who seek medical care and medical validation and are very disabled by MUIs. Gleason and Yates (2002) have noted that "female gender stands out as the most important risk factor for somatization" (p. 309). They explained this in terms of the five mechanisms proposed by Wool and Barsky (1994): (a) Somatic symptom reporting is more culturally approved in women compared with men; (b) women more readily seek medical care for symptoms than men do; (c) psychiatric disorders that include somatizing tendencies are more common in women than in men; (d) women have higher rates of childhood trauma than men; and (e) women have greater sensitivity to bodily sensations than men.

Because so many terms are used to label SD, and because somatization is often described as a behavior or a process, it is important to remember that somatization does exist as a *Diagnostic and Statistical Manual of Mental Disorders* (DSM) classification, albeit a problematic one. According to the fourth edition of the *DSM* (*DSM–IV*; American Psychiatric Association, 1994), SD is characterized by a lifetime history of multiple medically unexplained physical symptoms, including at least four unexplained pain symptoms, two unexplained nonpain gastrointestinal symptoms, one unexplained sexual symptom, and one pseudoneurological symptom. SD is rarely diagnosed in men. Most men with somatic complaints have disorders with prominent anxiety symptoms (Cloninger, Martin, Guze, & Clayton, 1986).

Many patients with SD meet criteria for other psychiatric disorders (Robins et al., 1984; Swartz, Blazer, George, & Landerman, 1986) and incur very high rates of recurring health care utilization (Barsky & Borus, 1995; Hiller & Fichter, 2004; Kolk, Schagen, & Hanewald, 2004; G. R. Smith, Monson, & Ray, 1986). SD seems to represent the extreme end of a somatization continuum (Allen & Escobar, 2005; Escobar, Burnam, Karno, Forsythe, & Golding, 1987; Katon et al., 1991; Melville, 1987). To describe individuals who do not meet SD criteria, Escobar et al. (1987) introduced the label *abridged somatization* for men complaining of at least four unexplained physical symptoms and women complaining of at least six unexplained physical symptoms. Abridged somatization is also associated with increased use of medical services and elevated levels of disability and psychopathology (Escobar et al., 1987; Katon et al., 1991). Moderate levels of somatization appear to be widespread in primary care, with the prevalence of abridged somatization in the population estimated to be 22% (Escobar, Waitzkin, Silver, Gara, & Holman, 1998).

Fink, Hansen, and Oxhoj (2004) examined prevalence of full-blown SD in a sample of 294 consecutively admitted general medical inpatients in Denmark. They found that 18.1% of individuals met *International Classification of Diseases* (World Health Organization, 1992) criteria for a diagnosis of SD, whereas 20.2% met *DSM–IV* criteria for SD. SDs were much more prevalent among women, and there was a significant trend for female prevalence to decrease with increasing age.

Other *DSM–IV* SDs include undifferentiated SD (which would include most unexplained illnesses), conversion disorder, pain disorder, hypochondriasis, and SD not otherwise specified. Creed and Barsky (2004) reviewed the epidemiology of SD and hypochondriasis in primary care and population-based samples. They searched MEDLINE and PsycLIT from 1966 to 2002 and found that only 47 studies fulfilled the inclusion criteria of calculating a prevalence figure using a standardized definition. They concluded that population studies do not support the assumption that SD and hypochondriasis are discrete psychiatric disorders. Rather, there is considerable evidence that these disorders are very closely allied with anxiety and depressive disorders. They also noted that there was a predominance of women with SD in population and primary care samples. When abridged somatization definitions are used, female predominance drops, underlining the connection between multiple symptom reporting and female gender. Hypochondriasis, however, did not seem to show a gender bias. A preponderance of evidence indicates that women somatize more than men, and women are diagnosed significantly more frequently with SD (Gijsbers van Wijk & Kolk, 1997; Gleason & Yates, 2002).

Research has consistently shown that the number of unexplained symptoms is linearly associated with psychological dysfunction. Hotopf, Wadsworth, and Wessely (2001) addressed this issue directly in a case control study using a national birth cohort sample. They found that 955 out of a sample of 3,262 people were identified as having probable psychiatric disorder. On a separate question, 43% of these people acknowledged the presence of psychiatric disorder; compared with the nonacknowledging group, acknowledgers were found to be more likely to be female, more educated, have more severe psychiatric disorder, and report more physical symptoms. Thus, reporting multiple physical symptoms does not appear to act as a defense against psychiatric disorder diagnosis or acknowledging psychiatric disorder. Yet it is clearly related to psychiatric disorder.

Dualism and Somatization

Does labeling behavior as somatizing set up a false dualism wherein somatization is not a useful concept? The myriad problems and contradictions inherent in the SD classification of the DSM have been cogently addressed by Mayou, Kirmayer, Simon, Kroenke, and Sharpe (2005), who call for an abolition of the SD category from the DSM–IV. MUIs are the epitome of what is wrong with the SD diagnosis. In its current form in DSM–IV, classification of SD stigmatizes patients, is overtly dualistic, overlaps with depression and anxiety in many shared symptoms, is unreliable, lacks a defined threshold, and has unclear medico–legal status. Mayou et al. (2005) gave the example of IBS as a disorder that could be diagnosed as an undifferentiated Axis I SD as well as an Axis III general medical condition. Clearly, this is an untenable position. More broadly, McWhinney, Epstein, and Freeman (1997) criticized the label *somatization* as a product of Western medicine's dualistic perspective. In many other cultures, the idea that emotions can be embodied physically is overtly accepted, and a biopsychosocial model is implicitly accepted.

Associations Among Depression, Anxiety, and Somatization

The World Health Organization has documented that depression, anxiety, and somatic complaints are more common among women than men. These conditions are related to risk factors such as gender-based roles, stressors, and negative life experiences. The World Health Organization report (2007) described gender-specific risk factors such as gender-based violence, socioeconomic disadvantage, low or subordinate social status, and constant care of others. These risk factors constitute a psychological burden that have the potential to be expressed in depression, anxiety, or somatization symptoms.

R. C. Smith et al. (2005) set out to determine the prevalence of *DSM–IV* somatoform and nonsomatoform disorders in patients with MUS in a community-based health maintenance organization. Patients with MUS were those picked from a chart review of 1,646 high utilizers; trained raters assessed documented (severe MUS) and undocumented (mild MUS) nonorganic disease. Patients who met the criterion for a high proportion of undocumented and documented nonorganic symptoms were recruited into the study. Two hundred six patients with MUS averaged 13.6 hospital visits in the year preceding the study, 79.1% of them were women, and the average age was 47.7 years. Patients with full or abridged *DSM–IV* somatoform diagnoses were labeled "DSM somatoform-positive," whereas those without such diagnoses were labeled "DSM somatoform-negative." R. C. Smith et al. found that 60.2% had a nonsomatoform *DSM–IV* diagnosis, primarily anxiety or depression. Only 4.4% had any full *DSM–IV* somatoform diagnosis, and only 18.9% had abridged SD. Thus, depression and anxiety characterized MUS patients better than the somatoform disorders. Correlates of *DSM* somatoform-negative status were female gender and less severe psychiatric and physical dysfunction. These data suggest that multiple unexplained symptoms are not the same as SD, are more closely related to depression and anxiety, and are more common in women.

MOOD AND ANXIETY DISORDERS IN MEDICALLY UNEXPLAINED ILLNESSES

The majority of patients with depression and anxiety who go to primary care physicians do not present with psychological symptoms but rather with somatic symptoms such as fatigue, pain, headache, gastrointestinal complaints, and disturbed sleep (Kroenke, 2001). Patients with MUIs in both primary care and medical specialty samples have significantly higher rates of depression and anxiety than do comparable patients with clearly defined medical diseases (Katon, Sullivan, & Walker, 2001; Wessely, Nimnuan, & Sharpe, 1999). In a comprehensive meta-analysis, Henningsen, Zimmerman, and Sattel (2003) examined the relationship between MUIs (FMS, CFS, IBS, and nonulcer dyspepsia) and anxiety and depression. They reviewed 244 studies and concluded that depression and anxiety are a common feature of these MUIs. The association with depression and anxiety is higher than in healthy controls or in patients with similar symptoms explained by a medical diagnosis. Compared with patients with IBS, patients with FMS were significantly less anxious and patients with CFS were significantly more depressed.

Depression, Anxiety, and Gender

It is well established that anxiety and depression have a higher prevalence among women than among men and that these conditions are also strongly related to symptom reporting (Wool & Barsky, 1994). One might reasonably ask whether the higher rate of MUIs in women can be explained by their higher rates of depression and anxiety. The data do not support this parsimonious explanation, however. Haug, Mykletun, and Dahl (2004) examined the association between anxiety, depression, and somatic symptoms in a large population-based study of all inhabitants in a Norwegian county who were 20 years old or older. The association between anxiety and depression and number of functional somatic symptoms was found to be strong, and it was as strong among men as among women, although women consistently reported more symptoms.

Likewise, Kroenke and Spitzer (1998) assessed whether gender disparities in symptom reporting were attributable to psychiatric comorbidity in the PRIME-MD 1000 study. Although physically unexplained symptoms were more frequent among women, and depressive and anxiety disorders were the strongest correlate of symptom reporting, gender had an independent effect that persisted even after adjusting for psychiatric comorbidity. Thus, women's tendency to report more unexplained symptoms is not solely explained by women's higher rates of depression and anxiety.

Women with unipolar depression outnumber men 2:1. The gender difference in depression is robust, with a female preponderance in prevalence, incidence, and morbidity risk for major depression, dysthymia, atypical depression, and seasonal affective disorder (Piccinelli & Wilkinson, 2000). A consistent factor that differentiates female and male depression is the preponderance of somatic symptoms in female depression. Women are much more likely than men to report depression with appetite loss, sleep disturbances, and fatigue, but they are not more likely than men to report depression without these symptoms (i.e., "pure depression"; Silverstein, 2002). In a study of 201 opposite-sex twin pairs in which both twins fulfilled *DSM–III–R* criteria for major depression, the female twins reported significantly more fatigue, hypersomnia, and psychomotor retardation than their male twins (Khan, Gardner, Prescott, & Kendler, 2002). In an international study of 14 countries, females in all of the centers were twice as likely to report more somatic symptoms than men (Maier et al., 1999). Thus, it is well established that higher levels of somatic symptoms do characterize depression among women.

In a review of gender differences in depression, several social factors were found to contribute to the higher incidence of women among depressed individuals. These factors included adverse events in childhood, depression and anxiety disorders in childhood and adolescence, crises involving children and housing, reproductive problems, and poor coping skills (Piccinelli & Wilkinson, 2000). Girls are more likely than boys to be victims of sexual abuse in childhood, which may contribute to their greater risk for depression and anxiety disorders (Weiss, Longhurst, & Mazure, 1999).

Women are more likely to use a ruminative response style, dwelling on negative events and focusing on their symptoms and the possible causes and consequences of their symptoms. People who ruminate show longer lasting depressions than people who take action to distract themselves from their symptoms (Nolen-Hoeksema, Larson, & Grayson, 1999). Ruminative responses prolong depression because they allow the depressed mood to negatively bias thinking and interfere with coping behavior. This rumination may extend to health problems. In a series of studies, Silverstein and colleagues (Silverstein & Blumenthal, 1997; Silverstein, Caceres, Perdue & Cimarolli, 1995; Silverstein & Lynch, 1998) found that anxious, somatic depression (but not pure depression) in adolescent girls was associated with distress over the achievement and occupational limits experienced by their mothers.

Klonoff, Landrine, and Campbell (2000) found that in a sample of 255 university students, women scored higher on anxiety, depression, and somatization symptoms than men. Critically, women with low exposure to sexist stress did not differ from men on these symptoms, whereas women with frequent exposure to sexist stress accounted for the gender difference in symptoms. These findings were not explained by ethnicity, marital status, education or income differences, or reporting bias. Klonoff et al. hypothesized that an accumulation of stress contributes to women's symptoms of depression, anxiety, and somatization. Because women experience gender-specific stressors that men do not (e.g., discrimination, battering, and sexual harassment), women exhibit more symptoms because they experience more stress. Gender-related stress, as well as rumination about that stress, appears to be related to depression, anxiety, and somatization.

Gender, Depression, and Pain

Gender may moderate the relationship between distress and pain. Findings in this area have been inconsistent; some studies have found that depression among women is associated with greater pain-related disability and that anxiety is related to greater pain severity in men, whereas other studies find no gender differences (Keogh, McCracken, & Eccleston, 2006). Keogh et al. (2006) examined whether gender moderated the relationship between anxiety and depression and pain and pain-related disability in 260 patients enrolled in a British pain management center. When depression was high, women reported greater disability than men, whereas men took more medications than women. Social gender roles may be operating here, with women having a stronger belief in the link between depression and pain than men, thus rendering women more vulnerable to disability. We know that health care practitioners are more likely to prescribe antidepressants and antianxiety drugs for women than men, even for similar symptoms (Hohmann, 1989). Women are also more likely to make psychologizing attributions for symptoms, whereas men are more likely to make normalizing attributions (Nykvist, Kjellberg, & Bildt, 2002).

Depression and Anxiety in Medical Illness

Medical patients generally report higher rates of depression and anxiety than matched healthy controls. Some of this may be attributable to confounding of symptoms. There is ample evidence that somatic symptoms can artificially elevate depression levels in a variety of medical populations (Frank et al., 1992; Nyenhuis et al., 1995; Plumb & Holland, 1977; A. Williams & Richardson, 1993). Yet the core elements of depression, such as negative self-evaluations, depressed affect, and suicidal ideation, are lower in many medical populations than those seen in clinical depression. The high rates of depression and anxiety in MUIs may also be partially explained by confounding of symptoms on self-report and interview surveys. Symptoms such as fatigue, pain, difficulty concentrating, difficulty sleeping, loss of appetite, and excessive health worry can be part of a psychiatric assessment of depression or anxiety but are also common in medical illness. In a study that specifically examined depressive symptoms in CFS, S. K. Johnson, DeLuca, and Natelson (1996b) found that although individuals with CFS may meet criteria for depressive disorder or score in the depressed range on a self-report inventory, they had significantly higher somatic and significantly lower self-reproach scores than a clinical depressed comparison group. It may be more than a confounding of symptoms and closer to a common pathophysiology, however. In a review of mood disorders in medical illness, Evans et al. (2005) posited that a growing body of evidence indicates that biological mechanisms underlie a bidirectional relationship between depression and many medical conditions.

Simple explanations seem to elude us yet again. Clearly the high rates of depression and anxiety in individuals with MUIs are not just a reporting artifact of confounding symptoms and may be more than a reaction to disability wrought by illness. Lifetime history of depression and anxiety is higher among individuals with MUIs than among those with comparable medical diseases. Individuals with similar symptoms caused by medical disease have higher psychiatric morbidity than healthy people, but they have consistently lower levels of psychiatric distress than their counterparts with MUIs.

Rief, Martin, Klaiberg, and Brahler (2005) surveyed a representative German sample of 2,507 people and identified those with panic disorder, somatic syndrome, and depression on the Scale for the Assessment of Illness

Behavior (Rief, Ihle, & Pilger, 2003). Those with panic disorder showed the highest scores for illness behavior and health care use. Depression was associated with illness consequences (e.g., "'Illnesses influence the way I act toward family and friends") and illness expression (e.g., "Everyone can see when I am suffering"). People with somatic syndromes had the highest scores on medication and treatment (i.e., relied on and had confidence in pharmacological treatment) and scanning the body for symptoms. This study illustrates the connection between mood and anxiety disorders and greater illness expression and health care utilization—the intimate connection that often exists between psychiatric morbidity and multiple somatic symptoms. The presentation of multiple somatic symptoms also can mean an individual meets criteria for several MUIs concurrently, which leads to the issue of overlap among the MUIs.

The tendency for substantial overlap among the various MUIs reinforces the view that these disorders involve somatization. Numerous investigators have noted this overlap—that is, individuals with one of these conditions are more likely to have another of these conditions (Aaron & Buchwald, 2001, 2003; Barsky & Borus, 1999; Buchwald & Garrity, 1994; Clauw, 1994, 2001; Clauw & Chrousos, 1997; Deary, 1999; Hudson & Pope, 1989; Manu, 2004; Peres, 2003; Wessely et al., 1999; Whitehead, Palsson, & Jones, 2002; Yunus, 2001, 2002). Specifically, the tendency to report a history of any one unexplained symptom is associated with a tendency to report many others (Deary, 1999). Additionally, those who seek care for MUIs are more likely to have overlapping conditions than those identified within population-based studies.

CONCLUSION

There are numerous reasons why women have more MUIs. It is well established that women generally report more symptoms than men. Women appear to somatize more than men. Women have higher rates of depression and anxiety, which increase symptom reporting. This chapter has shown that somatization, depression, and anxiety commonly co-occur in MUIs. It appears, however, that psychiatric disorder is neither necessary nor sufficient to explain MUIs. Although the higher prevalence of somatization, depression, and anxiety in women undoubtedly contributes to their greater prevalence of MUIs, it is just one piece of the biopsychosocial puzzle. Further pieces of the puzzle are discussed in chapters 3 and 4.

3

PSYCHOSOCIAL AND COGNITIVE FACTORS IN MEDICALLY UNEXPLAINED ILLNESS

The biopsychosocial model of illness is premised on the well-established fact that psychosocial, contextual, and cognitive factors play a major role in the experience of symptoms. A number of psychological factors may contribute to gender differences in medically unexplained illnesses (MUIs). Some of the factors examined in this chapter are lowered thresholds for symptom perception and reporting, health care utilization, and the effects of gender roles and expectations on illness behavior. Compared with men, women may accumulate more stressful experiences such as abuse, have differing beliefs and attributions for symptoms, and use different coping styles.

There are many potential psychosocial explanations for the higher prevalence of MUI in women. The sick role is generally more accepted in women because gender role stereotypes promote the notion that women are more delicate and weaker than men. Evidence suggests that women who have strong feminine gender role identification have more MUIs (Ali, Richardson, & Toner, 1998; Toner, 1995; Toner & Akman, 2000). Illness behavior, emotional expression, and attributional style can be affected by gender roles. Women experience more childhood abuse and other stressors, which are associated with higher numbers of unexplained symptoms. Higher rates of child-hood abuse can lead to hypervigilance regarding physical symptoms and the perception of symptoms as threatening. Additionally, unexplained symptoms may be a way to seek care through the medical system.

ILLNESS BEHAVIOR

Mechanic (1972) introduced the term *illness behavior* to describe the observation that people with the same illness display a spectrum of illness behaviors. Illness behavior encompasses characteristics such as health care use, taking medications, work disability, avoiding activity, expression of symp-toms to significant others, and doctor shopping. Pilowski (1969) coined the term *abnormal illness behavior* to describe behaviors such as having a hypo-chondriacal attitude and multiple somatic complaints, engaging in inappro-priate treatment seeking, and displaying disability disproportional to physi-cal findings. Illness behavior is only moderately associated with illness severity. Compared with men, women engage in more illness behavior, spend more days in bed, restrict more of their activities because of illness, and use more prescription drugs (Kandrick, Grant, & Segall, 1991).

The concept of illness behavior is clearly relevant for the MUIs, wherein disability levels appear in excess of organic pathology. A similar concept, the *sick role*, refers to adopting behaviors such as staying in bed, restricting activi-ties, and taking medications on their own initiative rather than having them prescribed by medical professionals. Playing the sick role is generally permit-ted in those diagnosed with medical conditions, but Western society does not easily give people permission to be ill in the absence of recognized dis-ease (Nettleton, 2006).

Learned Illness Behavior

Excessive illness behavior may have its origins in childhood learning experiences. Children may imitate illness behavior modeled by parents. Al-ternately, adults with excessive illness behaviors may have had stressful ex-periences as children, such as early separation or loss of a parent or illness-specific stressors like hospitalization. Secondary gains may also be operating in some contexts. Whitehead, Winget, Fedoravicius, Wooley, and Blackwell (1982) found that patients with irritable bowel syndrome (IBS) reported that their parents were more likely to give them special attention, foods, or treats when they were sick compared with healthy controls or patients with peptic ulcers.

Levy et al. (2004) interviewed 208 mothers with IBS and their 296 children and 241 healthy mothers (controls) and their 335 children. Factors assessed were stress, mothers' and children's psychological symptoms, children's perceived competence, and pain coping style. Children of women with IBS reported more frequent stomachaches and nongastrointestinal symptoms, made more physician visits for gastrointestinal symptoms, had more nongastrointestinal clinic visits, and missed more school than control children. Children whose mothers made solicitous responses to illness complaints independently reported more severe stomachaches, and they also had more school absences for stomachaches, but solicitous behavior did not significantly impact nongastrointestinal symptom reporting, clinic visits, or school absences.

To rule out the possibility that children were imitating their parents' illness behavior, Crane and Martin (2004) looked at mothers of infants younger than 18 months. They compared mothers taking medication for functional gastrointestinal symptoms (mostly IBS) with mothers with stomach ulcers, who completed questionnaires when their children were 6 and 18 months old. The infants of mothers with IBS were taken to the doctor for a significantly greater number of symptoms than were children whose mothers had ulcers. The mothers did not differ on psychiatric distress variables. This finding provides evidence for potential reinforcement of illness behavior in childhood experiences, which may increase vulnerability to MUIs in adulthood. Studies of these childhood experiences indicate that children of parents with IBS were more likely than children with non-IBS parents to report secondary gain and to have more symptom reports, health care use, and disability, suggesting an intergenerational transmission of illness behavior.

Symptom Reporting

It is well established that women report more symptoms than men across various age spans (Borglin, Jakobsson, Edberg, & Hallberg, 2005; Haug, Mykletun, & Dahl, 2004; Kroenke & Spitzer, 1998; Tibblin, Bengstsson, Furunes, & Lapidus, 1990; Verbrugge, 1985, 1989). In a review paper on gender and symptom reporting, Gijsbers van Wijk and Kolk (1997) concluded that researchers using health surveys and symptom and physician reports found that adult women reported more frequent or more intense symptoms, particularly when symptoms were measured in retrospect. It is interesting to note that most of this review was concerned with reports from healthy, community-residing individuals. Conversely, when actual disease was present, men tended to report more symptoms than women.

Researchers conducting large population-based studies found that women reported more symptoms. In a Norwegian study of both men and women that included 50,377 women, Haug et al. (2004) reported an average of 3.8 symptoms in women compared with 2.9 in men. The most common symptoms reported were tiredness, gastrointestinal symptoms, headache, back pain, and pain in arms and shoulders. Tibblin et al. (1990) studied 30 symptoms and their prevalence in different age cohorts in men and women from a

Swedish population based study. They found that most symptoms, particularly depression and tension, were more common among women, and this difference was more pronounced in younger age groups. Higher levels of symptom reporting do not completely diminish with age, however; in a study of community-dwelling elderly individuals aged 75 to 99 years, women had a significantly lower health-related quality of life than men and a significantly higher degree of self-reported health complaints (Borglin et al., 2005).

These studies also make clear that the core symptoms of many MUIs, such as fatigue, pain, gastrointestinal complaints, and headaches, are present in very high base rates in the general population (Kroenke, 2001). The gender difference in symptoms is not due to women's more complex reproductive system, gynecological disorders, or menstrual events. In the U.S. Epidemiological Catchment Area study, 20 out of 22 nonmenstrually related symptoms were more common in women; only chest pain and difficulty walking were more common in men (Kroenke & Price, 1993).

Kroenke and Spitzer (1998) also found that increased symptom reporting in women was a generic phenomenon and not restricted to particular types of symptoms. They assessed gender differences in symptoms and investigated whether these differences were attributable to psychiatric comorbidity. They analyzed data from the PRIME-MD 1000 study (1,000 patients from four primary case sites evaluated with the Primary Care Evaluation of Mental Disorders interview; Spitzer et al., 1994) examining the reporting of 13 common physical symptoms. This study controlled for a lower threshold for seeking care than is often found in women, because all the individuals in the PRIME-MD study were seeking health care. After adjusting for depressive and anxiety disorders as well as age, race, education, and medical comorbidity, all symptoms except one (sexual problems) were reported more commonly by women, with statistically significant differences for 10 of 13 symptoms. Medically unexplained symptoms were also more frequent in women. Gender was the most important demographic factor associated with symptom reporting, followed by lower education and younger age. Total symptom count was similar to that found by Haug et al. (2004), with women on average reporting 1.47 more symptoms than men.

Symptom Perception

Under most circumstances, women report more symptoms than men. What are some possible explanations for this phenomenon? Hibbard and Pope (1983) showed that women were more likely to perceive symptoms than men, that women place a higher value on health, and that women have a higher preventive orientation than men do. Their study population included 1,648 adults between the ages of 18 and 59. Medical record data covering 7 years of outpatient services were linked with survey data on the respondents. The findings showed that although women were more likely to perceive symptoms than men, there was no apparent sex difference in a tendency to adopt the sick role when ill. Gender role factors such as level and type of role responsibility and concern with health were related to female but not male symptom reports. Illness orientation variables were related to rates of medical utilization for both genders. However, it was primarily the greater perception of symptoms and an interest and concern with health in women that contributed to sex differences in medical utilization rates.

Several gender factors may influence symptom perception and symptom reporting. Women may have lower thresholds for many sensations. There is evidence that women have lower perceptual thresholds and sensitivity (Dalton, Doolittle, & Breslin, 2002; Else-Quest, Shibley Hyde, Hill Goldsmith, & Van Hulle, 2006). Wool and Barsky (1994) have argued that women are more sensitive to sensations.

Pennebaker (1994) summarized a series of laboratory and field studies noting consistent gender differences in how individuals perceive and react to symptoms. His studies have found that women are particularly sensitive to situational and environmental cues, whereas men are more sensitive to internal physiological cues. In controlled laboratory studies, men are more accurate at detecting heart rate, stomach activity, blood pressure, and blood glucose levels. In field studies or in the home, there are no gender differences in accuracy. Pennebaker speculated that women's symptom-reporting patterns reflect a context that is stressful or potentially toxic, whereas men are more oblivious to setting and focus on physiological cues.

Personality tendencies that increase symptom reporting may be more common in women. Subjectively reported symptoms have been shown to be systematically biased by neuroticism, which is strongly correlated with health complaints but not actual health status (P. T. Costa & McCrae, 1987). The personality trait of neuroticism is associated with a tendency to experience emotional distress, including anxiety, anger, sadness, and other emotions with negative valence (P. T. Costa & McCrae, 1992). In a healthy student population, Neitzert, Davis, and Kennedy (1997) found that depression and neuroticism levels were significantly associated with higher symptom reporting and that symptom reporting was higher in women.

P. T. Costa, Terracciano, and McCrae (2001) analyzed Revised NEO Personality Inventory (P. T. Costa & McCrae, 1992) data from 26 cultures (N = 23,031) and found that adult women reported themselves to be higher in neuroticism. However, in a large meta-analysis, Else-Quest et al. (2006) studied children up to age 13 years and found few gender differences in negative affectivity, aside from slightly higher levels of fearfulness in girls. It is possible that small childhood differences in negative emotions are later magnified by gender stereotypes. Neuroticism, anxiety, and negative affect appear to be associated with a cognitive style of heightened vigilance toward body sensations (Pennebaker, 1994). It appears that stereotypes and gender expectations allow women to more readily express negative emotions, which may contribute to higher symptom reporting.

A study using the Tridimensional Personality Questionnaire (Cloninger, 1987) found increased scores on harm avoidance and lower scores on reward dependence (constructs similar to neuroticism) in individuals with chronic fatigue syndrome (CFS) and multiple sclerosis relative to healthy controls (Christodoulou et al., 1998). Generally, studies reveal trends toward higher neuroticism among persons with CFS (Buckley et al. 1999; Cristodoulou et al., 1998; S. K. Johnson, DeLuca, & Natelson, 1996c), although not as high as is seen in clinically depressed persons.

Health Care Seeking

Physicians have reported that female patients disproportionately present to medical practices with vague and medically unexplained symptoms (Gijsbers van Wijk & Kolk, 1997). Celentano, Linet, and Stewart (1990) found in a random sample of 10,167 Washington County, Maryland, residents that women were more attentive to headache symptoms and were more likely to use medical care for relief of symptoms than men. Depression and health beliefs may directly influence health care seeking, whereas factors such as life stress, poor coping skills, and catastrophizing about symptoms are more likely to contribute to exacerbation and chronicity of symptoms (Naliboff, Heitkemper, Chang, & Mayer, 2000).

L. K. Smith, Pope, and Botha (2005) performed a qualitative synthesis of international research on cancer patients' experiences of help seeking and what accounted for delays in help seeking. They looked for shared concepts and themes in research published between 1985 and 2004 and found that gender influenced help seeking. Themes that emerged were that men viewed help seeking as unmasculine, did not want to appear neurotic, and associated consultation with weakness. Men believed that women found help seeking easier because they have more contact with health services for themselves and families. When women delayed help seeking, it was because of competing priorities of work and family over their own needs.

Verbrugge (1985) found that women generally are more apt to label their symptoms as physical illness and to adopt the sick role. She cited a number of reasons for this: Men may tolerate more physical discomfort, have fewer concerns about their personal health, and feel it is not "masculine" to adopt the sick role. Conversely, women may be more likely to adopt the sick role for a variety of reasons ranging from poor coping responses to stress, a history of physical or sexual abuse, more learned helplessness, and dependency to more trust in authority compared with men (Verbrugge, 1985, 1989).

Physicians usually cannot formulate coherent causal explanations for the symptoms of MUIs that are meaningful to their patients. This contributes to illness uncertainty (Mischel, 1999). Illness uncertainty is especially salient in MUIs because they are characterized by problems with diagnosis, unknown etiology, unpredictable symptoms and outcomes, and largely ineffective treatments. Illness uncertainty is a strong predictor of psychological distress and difficulty in social relationships (L. M. Johnson, Zautra, & Davis, 2006; Reich, Olmsted, & van Puymbroeck, 2006).

Not surprisingly, the medical encounters of women with MUIs are often difficult and frustrating for physician and patient alike (R. M. Epstein et al., 2006; Malterud, 2000; Stone et al., 2002). Women with fibromyalgia (FMS) and CFS report being judged as suffering from an imagined illness or are given a psychiatric label (Asbring & Narvanen, 2002; Zavestoski et al., 2004). Werner, Isaksen, and Malterud (2004) describe the themes from a qualitative interview study of women with chronic pain. These women were cognizant of the gendered views of women with MUIs as "whiners and complainers," and they were vigilant about avoiding this taboo. Their narratives, paradoxically, recognized other women's chronic pain complaints as attention seeking, avoidant, or psychological, but they emphasized their own strength and credibility in suffering with chronic pain symptoms.

DISEASE CONVICTION BELIEFS

Do those with MUIs become any more obsessed with illness and illness careers than people diagnosed with organic diseases who become excessively involved with their illness? Data show higher rates of disability in individuals with MUIs compared with patients with organic disorders. For example, Assefi, Coy, Uslan, Smith, and Buchwald (2003) surveyed 630 patients evaluated at the University of Washington Chronic Fatigue Clinic regarding the functional consequences of their fatiguing illness. They measured self-reported disability in patients with CFS, FMS, and *chronic fatigue* (fatigue that is of at least 6 months' duration but that does not meet all the symptom criteria of CFS), compared with a chronically fatiguing but unrelated medical condition. Among the groups, the FMS group was the least likely to be employed. Likewise, the FMS and CFS groups more frequently reported loss of material possessions, valued activities, jobs, and support by friends and family as a result of their illness than those with medical conditions.

Zavestoski et al. (2004) noted that MUI prevalence is increasing as media coverage spreads awareness of these conditions. Diagnostic disputes can arise among physicians, scientists, and sufferers over the struggle for legitimacy of MUIs and how this influences the clinical interaction. Hadler (1996) raised concerns over this struggle for legitimacy in FMS with the notion that if patients must expend effort to prove they are sick, they are never going to get well. Patient activism is largely motivated by the challenge of legitimating symptoms and receiving a medical diagnosis (Nettleton, 2006; Zavestoski et al., 2004).

Dumit (2006) monitored the content of Internet chat rooms among people with CFS, multiple chemical sensitivities (MCS), and FMS. He noted that many posts reflected the dilemma of "proving" the legitimacy of these illnesses to doctors. Such research provides evidence that MUIs require tremendous amounts of work to achieve diagnosis and acknowledgement. Patients recognize that psychiatric diagnosis carries a stigma and delegitimizes their claim to the sick role. A medical diagnosis achieves social recognition that validates sick role behaviors. The biomedical model that asserts "biological primacy" is widely accepted by people with MUIs (J. A. Hamilton, 1994). These beliefs can lead to excessive doctor shopping in search of a legitimate diagnosis.

To use a specific MUI as an example, a tendency to minimize psychological risk and maximize somatic risk has been found in IBS. Crane and Martin (2004) used a questionnaire to assess worry about deep vein thrombosis and perceived future risk of developing the condition in individuals with IBS and controls following a media scare concerning this condition. Individuals with IBS reported higher perceived lifetime risk of deep vein thrombosis than did healthy controls or individuals with asthma. This study showed that a perception of enhanced vulnerability to illness is not specific to cognitions about IBS but may spread to unrelated health issues.

Doctor shopping may arise out of strong disease conviction. Alternatively, it may be related to somatization and dissociative tendencies. Individuals with MUIs may be out of touch with the connection between emotions and bodily symptoms. Dissociation may work as a coping response to blunt the horror of abuse. People with MUIs may be searching for an authority figure to validate the suffering they are experiencing.

Aceves-Avila, Ferrari, and Ramos-Remus (2004) have described FMS, CFS, MCS, Gulf War syndrome, and other conditions as "culture driven disorders" and have contended that the physiological abnormalities found are insufficient to explain the level of illness behavior. Because symptoms are disregarded in Western societies if they cannot be interpreted as disease, it is the drive to establish the legitimacy of symptoms that shapes symptom reports. Aceves-Avila et al. observed that MUIs share a number of factors: a focus on the legitimacy of these disorders as diseases; similar symptomatology; and a focus on causative external agents such as injury, environmental exposure, or infection. A diagnosis that implies a psychological problem is more offensive to MUI patients because it does not provide social sanction of the sick role (J. Stone et al., 2002). Looper and Kirmayer (2004) directly examined the stigma experienced by MUI patients matched to patients with comparable medical conditions with clear etiology. Thus, CFS was compared with multiple sclerosis, FMS was compared with rheumatoid arthritis, and IBS was compared with inflammatory bowel disease (IBD). Only the CFS group was found to have a significantly higher level of perceived stigma compared with its matched control group, although the overall group of MUI reported a higher level of perceived stigma.

An example of striving toward greater legitimization is the active movement to change the name of CFS. The label "chronic fatigue syndrome" is viewed by advocates as connoting a vague, subjective condition thought to carry a negative stigma with medical professionals and the general public, which hinders access to medical care and social services (Jason, Holbert, Torres-Harding, Taylor, et al., 2004). The name itself may influence the type of medical care a person is offered. Medical trainees were presented with identical patient case studies labeled with the diagnoses CFS, myalgic encephalomyelitis (the name used in the United Kingdom), or Florence Nightingale disease (so named because Nightingale is rumored to have had a CFS-like illness). Trainees who received cases labeled CFS were less likely to attribute the illness to medical causes and more likely to prescribe psychotherapy and psychotropic medications (Jason, Holbert, Torres-Harding, & Taylor, 2004).

Somatic Attribution

Feminist critiques of medical practice have pointed out that illnesses that disproportionately affect women are more likely to be seen as psychiatric or sociocultural in origin because medical power is dominated by "male-centered" thinking (Findley & Miller, 1994; J. A. Hamilton, 1994). Gijsbers van Wijk and Kolk (1997) have suggested that medicalization of the female body may explain women's greater tendency to attribute physical symptoms to physical illness as opposed to normalizing symptoms.

The flip side of overmedicalization is the finding that physicians are more likely to attribute health problems to psychological causes in women than in men. Chrisler and O'Hea (2000) have suggested that women with autoimmune disorders often go through a long diagnostic process because the vague symptoms of immune disorders are thought to be emotionally caused.

Individuals generally emphasize one of three types of attributions for the cause of common symptoms. *Somatic* attributions maintain that the symptoms are caused from a physical problem, *psychological* attributions stress psychological processes causing symptoms, and *normalizing* attributions emphasize a transient, nonthreatening physiological or environmental process (Robbins & Kirmayer, 1991). Somatic attributions and the concomitant tendency to minimize psychological contributions to their illness are common in MUIs. Many people with MUIs have strong disease convictions, are well-defended psychologically (S. K. Johnson et al., 1999; Nettleton, 2006), and prefer biomedical explanations (Binder & Campbell, 2004).

Robbins and Kirmayer (1991) reported that patients with unexplained symptoms tend to make disease-related attributions for everyday somatic sensations. Kolk, Hanewald, Schagen, and Gijsbers van Wijk (2002) found that individuals who paid selective attention to bodily sensations had a distinct preference for disease-related attributions for somatic symptoms. Furthermore, individuals with MUIs and strong organic illness attributions tend to have higher health care use (Kolk et al., 2004).

It is interesting to note that although some studies have found that people with MUIs prefer somatic attributions, women in the general population are much more likely than men to consider psychological and multifactorial explanations for their symptoms. Nykvist et al. (2002) obtained data from 678 persons after surveying a randomly selected Swedish community sample regarding causal explanations for symptoms they had experienced. Results showed that women rated a higher number of causes as important compared with men. Men were significantly more likely to rate no cause as important or a physical work situation as important, whereas women were significantly more likely to cite illness, psychological causes, high demands and responsibility, and strained work situations as important. Women were also more likely to have chronic symptoms than men. Kessler, Lloyd, Lewis, and Gray (1999) also found that men were more likely to make normalizing attributions for symptoms, explaining them as being due to environmental irritants or overexertion and thus playing down the symptoms' significance. These studies suggest that women possess more of an implicit biopsychosocial explanatory model for somatic symptoms than men do.

Women's ratings of self-assessed health are based on a wider range of health-related and non-health-related factors. In a 5-year follow-up study of 830 community-dwelling elderly people, Benyami, Leventhal, and Leventhal (2000) found that high levels of negative affect were related to lower self-assessed health in both men and women and to higher mortality in men but to lower risk of mortality in women. Presumably, this was because in men high negative affect was linked to serious disease, whereas in women a variety of negative life events could increase negative affect. Furthermore, men's self-assessed health was related to serious disease, whereas women's self-assessed health was associated with mild and serious disease.

M. Martin and Crane (2003) examined attributions in 28 university students who fulfilled diagnostic criteria for IBS, comparing those who sought treatment for symptoms with those who had not. The two groups did not differ in terms of depression and anxiety. Treatment seekers were more likely than non–treatment seekers to make somatic attributions across 21 common symptoms. Treatment seekers made more somatic attributions for gastrointestinal symptoms and for nonspecific symptoms characteristic of depression and anxiety, even when symptoms were placed in a context that indicated the presence of a psychological stressor. Treatment seekers also perceived themselves to be significantly less resistant to illness and to have a more negative health outlook than non–treatment seekers. These findings suggest that premorbid illness attitudes and attributional style influence the decision to seek treatment. In a second study, M. Martin and Crane (2003) examined attributions in a community sample with persistent IBS. In this group, a variety of nonspecific symptoms became incorporated into the cognitive representation of IBS. This tendency to view all symptoms as a part of IBS may increase the perception of IBS as a pervasive, unmanageable illness and contribute to chronicity of illness.

In individuals with MUIs, somatic attributions and disease conviction appear to be paramount. These beliefs contribute to high rates of medical utilization in attempts at establishing legitimacy and easing suffering. The drive for legitimacy is fueled by patients' awareness that the medical establishment perceives MUIs to be women's illnesses and thus implicitly less serious than organic conditions, a perception that MUI patients resist.

Childhood Maltreatment and Unexplained Symptoms

According to the National Clearinghouse for Child Abuse and Neglect, girls are three times more likely to be victims of sexual abuse than boys (Snyder, 2000). It is possible that females may be more willing than males to disclose histories of sexual abuse and to participate in consequent studies, but this is unlikely to account entirely for the difference. Exposure to childhood sexual abuse has many detrimental psychological, behavioral, cognitive, and physiological consequences for both sexes. Some of the psychological problems exhibited by victims of child sexual abuse include depression, anxiety, reduced self-esteem, sleep disturbances, personality disorders, and cognitive dysfunction. Victims of child sexual abuse may also have behavioral problems such as substance abuse, conduct problems, externalizing disorders, or sexualized conduct (Arias, 2004).

The psychological consequences of child sexual abuse are relatively well-known, and now emerging research has shown that a multitude of physiological problems are associated with this as well, such as somatic complaints, gastrointestinal problems, fatigue, headaches, migraines, and pain disorders (Nelson, 2002). Among the MUIs, FMS and IBS in particular have been associated with high rates of reported child sexual abuse. A large epidemiologic study showed that as the number of abuse and neglect experiences increased, so did the number of unexplained symptoms. Walker, Gelfand, et al. (1999) surveyed 1,225 randomly selected women from the membership of a large health maintenance organization in Seattle, Washington. Women with and without histories of childhood maltreatment experiences were compared. A history of childhood maltreatment was associated with perceived poorer overall health, greater functional disability, increased numbers of distressing physical symptoms, and a greater number of health risk behaviors. Women with multiple types of maltreatment showed the greatest health decrements for both self-reported symptoms and physician-coded diagnoses.

A preponderance of studies indicates that exposure to adverse childhood experiences increases sensitivity to somatic complaints. This hypersensitivity may predispose individuals with this exposure to use the health care system more often than individuals without it. Individuals who have experienced childhood adversity are more likely to report a health problem (Sachs-Ericsson, Blazer, Plant, & Arnow, 2005). Women who have experienced sexual assault have more lifetime health care contacts (Ullman & Brecklin, 2003), significantly higher primary care and outpatient costs, and more frequent emergency department visits than women without such a history (Walker, Unutzer, et al., 1999).

Individuals who report childhood adversity are more likely to report medically unexplainable symptoms such as abdominal pain, headaches, fatigue, limb or back pain, or noncardiac chest pain (Fiddler, Jackson, Kapur, Wells, & Creed, 2004). In a study of 219 women military veterans, Stein et al. (2004) found that the 44% who reported a sexual assault history were more likely to report headache, abdominal pain, muscle pain, chest pain, face or jaw pain, overwhelming fatigue, shortness of breath, insomnia, and numbness. Again, significantly higher health anxiety and health care utilization were also reported. Emotional abuse and neglect were also correlated with higher reports of doctor visits (Spertus, Yehuda, Wong, Halligan, & Seremetis, 2003). Walker, Keegan, Gardner, Sullivan, Bernstein, and Katon (1997) have pointed out that abuse may be linked to multiple unexplained symptoms because for many women this may be the most acceptable strategy, although oblique, for trying to secure treatment for traumatic experiences.

Although medically unexplained symptoms in victims of child sexual abuse are widely interpreted as somatization, underlying physical problems may actually be the cause of the symptoms (Nelson, 2002). Adults with a history of child sexual abuse have more surgeries, are hospitalized more often, and have more visits to general practitioners than do those without a history of abuse (Finestone et al., 2000).

Both an individual's perception of a traumatic event and a determination of available resources are important in determining that individual's emotional reaction and connection to potential pain pathways. Negative emotional states, such as depression and anxiety, have been linked to pain sensitivity and general overestimation of painful experiences (Keefe, Lumley, Anderson, Lynch, & Carson, 2001). Understanding the perception of an event is particularly important to note when discussing high rates of child sexual abuse in individuals with MUIs. Studies cited here relied almost exclusively on retrospective reports of abuse. In an important study, Raphael, Spatz Widom, and Lange (2001) conducted a prospective study on documented child sexual and physical abuse and neglect and unexplained pain complaints. They followed up 908 children with court-substantiated cases of child abuse or neglect who were matched to 667 nonabused children. They were able to locate and interview 76% of the original sample 20 years later. One surprising finding was that the odds of reporting one or more unexplained pain symptoms were not associated with any childhood victimization experience. Raphael et al. argued that their findings contradicted the widespread belief that unexplained pain is psychogenic; they maintained that the Freudian view of expressing past trauma through current symptoms is too simplistic. Certainly, this study suggests adopting a cautious approach to associations between child sexual abuse and unexplained symptoms.

Linton (2002) conducted a more limited prospective survey study of the Swedish general population and found that women with self-reported sexual and physical abuse were at increased risk for pain 1 year later. However, there was no increased risk for worse pain or poorer function for women who reported back pain at baseline. Linton studied only women because an earlier study had indicated that abuse was not a strong risk factor for men to report back pain, whereas it was a powerful risk factor for women. Linton interpreted this finding as indicating that abuse may affect reporting or occurrence of new pain episodes but not worsening of an initial pain problem.

Although child sexual abuse is implicated in MUIs, there is no specific diagnosis or symptom cluster unique to this history. The extent to which a history of childhood abuse influences adult health may be molded by the dynamics of families characterized by sexual abuse or by inherent physiological vulnerabilities. It is postulated that family dysfunction and insecure attachment precedes the onset of sexual abuse (Lackner, Gudleski, & Blanchard, 2004). It is also notable that a review of long-term effects of child sexual abuse concluded that up to one third of children who are sexually abused remain free of symptoms (Finkelhor, 1990). These children are more likely to have been abused for shorter periods of time without force or penetration by a nonfather figure and to have received support from their family. This confirms that it is the context of attachment relationships before and after the abuse and the severity of abuse that determines the effects of abuse.

In a series of studies, Pennebaker (1994) found that undisclosed traumas in particular result in elevated symptom reports. He speculated that this could be due to altered stress response resulting from trauma; using symptom reporting as a distraction to avoid thinking about trauma; or trauma thought suppression, wherein a person experiences emotion but because the trauma is suppressed he or she labels the emotion as a physical symptom. Secondary gain of avoiding work or eliciting attention may also be operative in high levels of symptom reports in someone with a trauma history (Pennebaker, 1994). Failure to recover positive affect after traumatic life events seems to characterize the MUI; this has been shown specifically in FMS (Zautra et al., 2005; Zautra, Johnson, & Davis, 2005).

GENDER AND COPING STYLES: CATASTROPHIZING

The cognitive coping style people adopt can influence the perception of symptoms. There is some evidence for gender differences in coping styles, with women generally using more emotion-focused strategies and men engaging in more problem-solving strategies, although in specific types of stressful situations these differences are less evident (Sigmon, Stanton, & Snyder, 1995). Rollnik et al. (2003) examined gender differences in coping with tension headaches. Female episodic tension headache sufferers scored significantly higher than males on the subscales that measured distracting and encouraging oneself. Among chronic headache sufferers, women scored lower on active coping, were more depressed, and reported their pain as more intense than the men with chronic headache.

Catastrophizing is a particularly dysfunctional coping response. Catastrophizing entails worrying about symptoms and their negative impact on a patient's activities and future and ruminating over worst case scenarios. Persons who catastrophize have difficulty shifting their attention away from painful stimuli and tend to magnify the threat value of pain stimuli (Peters, Vlaeyen, & van Drunen, 2000; M. Sullivan et al., 2001). Catastrophizing is positively correlated with neuroticism, negative affectivity, and emotional vulnerability.

M. J. L. Sullivan, Bishop, and Pivik (1995) developed a Pain Catastrophizing Scale consisting of subscales of rumination, helplessness, and magnification. Women report significantly higher total scores on this scale, accounted for by women's higher scores on rumination and helplessness. This is consistent with findings that women are more likely to use ruminative and expressive styles when under stress (Nolen-Hoeksema et al., 1999).

M. J. L. Sullivan, Tripp, and Santor (2000) hypothesized that catastrophizing may be a critical mediator in explaining gender differences in pain experience. Perhaps women report more intense and disabling pain because they are more likely to catastrophize. They examined the role of catastrophizing on an experimental pain procedure. During immersion of the forearm in ice water for 1 minute, men reported significantly less pain and displayed pain behavior for a shorter duration than women. Men also reported lower scores on the Pain Catastrophizing Scale; for women the Helplessness subscale was the most predictive of pain duration, whereas the Rumination subscale was more critical for men's pain duration. When catastrophizing was statistically controlled, gender no longer contributed to pain intensity and duration. M. J. L. Sullivan et al. suggested that although catastrophizing has typically been viewed as a maladaptive response, it may play an important communicative function. By expressing distress, women may be able to recruit the caregivers and support that they need, which suggests that it is an adaptive coping response. The problem with this interpretation is that catastrophizing is universally reported to be associated with poorer outcomes, so communicating distress does not appear to lead to improved functioning.

According to Crombez, Van Damme, and Eccleston (2005), attentional hypervigilance to pain has been found to be automatic and unintentional in experimental tasks. This does not mean that it is uncontrollable; Crombez et al. noted that participants can switch attention back to tasks and complete them. Individuals who catastrophize, however, have difficulty performing distracting tasks and experience less analgesia from distraction. Crombez et al. proposed that amplification of pain is due to repeated failure to distract oneself from pain. Thus, pain may evoke a more intense and defensive fear response in those who are hypervigilant.

I. Jensen, Nygren, Gamberale, Goldie, and Westerholm (1994) compared men and women with long-term intractable musculoskeletal pain in a large rehabilitation sample. They found that women, particularly those in unskilled occupations, were more likely to use dysfunctional coping strategies such as catastrophizing. McGeary, Mayer, Gatchel, Anagnostis, and Proctor (2003) examined gender differences in 1,827 consecutively treated patients with chronically disabling spinal disorder undergoing a tertiary functional restoration program. Patients were assessed before the start of the program, on completion of the program, and 1 year later. Male patients showed lower disability and depression scores than women and had higher levels of physical functioning before and after treatment. The authors suggested that men came into the program with less fear avoidance–induced inhibition of physical activity. Women showed higher levels of depression, pain, and disability self-report and a higher rate of searching out new health care providers. In rehabilitation samples, women showed differences in pain perception, pain report, and coping skills.

Gender Role Expectations

Gender role expectations endorse a stoic, brave role for boys in messages such as "big boys don't cry," whereas greater expressiveness is sanctioned for girls and women. Girls and women are more likely to be reinforced for emotional expressiveness than boys and men (Helgeson, 2005; Plant, Shibley Hyde, Keltner, & Devine, 2000). It is generally more socially acceptable for women to report subjective symptoms and seek medical care than men. To some extent, complaining of symptoms and admitting illness violates gender role norms for boys and men (Helgeson, 2005).

Higher levels of catastrophizing, helplessness, fear of pain, and avoidance in women is consistent with gender role behavior. Men may demonstrate more tolerance for pain because it fits into the masculine gender role to be stoic and to "tough it out." Similarly, the finding that men get back to work sooner after pain episodes is consistent with the primacy of the breadwinner role for many men. Lower self-efficacy in women can contribute to lower pain threshold and tolerance and to experiencing pain as more unpleasant and intense.

Some investigators have highlighted modern social strains on women, particularly multiple roles, that cause women to unconsciously seek relief in the sick role (Ware & Kleinman, 1992). The theory is that women who cannot successfully integrate a fulfilling career and a rich family life may escape into MUIs (Richman, Jason, Taylor, & Jahn, 2000). Hadler (2003) also argued that FMS is a way of medicalizing the burdens of life with a socially acceptable reason for coping failures. Although popular in the media, there seems to be little scientific evidence to support this view.

Stress, Gender, and Medically Unexplained Illnesses

Documenting gender differences is useful, but one must also attempt to explain them. Yoder and Kahn (2003) have noted that consideration of the social context when gender differences are found is often overlooked. Gender should be regarded as a marker or a moderator, not a cause of differences in the health of women and men (Barnett, 1997). Women's health is broadly influenced by social realities, reproductive life events, and the demands of multiple roles. In terms of the social context of MUI, chapter 1 in this volume illustrates the idea that symptoms could change according to the zeitgeist of the times. One leitmotif of our times is that of the overstressed woman, the woman who has to balance everything—marriage, children, and career—and make it all work. Perhaps these social role demands and expectations increase vulnerability to MUI.

Verbrugge (1989) summarized the view that too little or too much social involvement causes distress for women. The female nurturant role can place continual burdens on women's lives. Davis, Matthews, and Twamley (1999) performed a meta-analysis to determine whether there were gender differences in stressful life events. They found that women reported greater exposure to stressful events and that there was an even stronger gender difference in terms of appraisal of stressful life events. This self-reported intensity appeared to be partially due to female gender role expectations of emotional expressiveness. Women were also more likely to report interpersonal stressors than males, consistent with the gender role of communality. Women's tendency to report more psychological symptoms, however, was not an important predictor of differences in stress exposure and appraisal.

In their Swedish population-based study, Tibblin et al. (1990) found that the biggest gender differences were in the symptoms of depression and tension, which were more prevalent in women. Tibblin et al. explained these differences as being due to women's situation of "double work"—being responsible for their job, their home, and bringing up the children. Repetti (1998) echoed the theme that overwork, family pressures, and hassles can be understood as role-related stressors that impact women's health. Lundberg (2005) noted that Scandinavian countries have seen a dramatic increase in absenteeism among women caused by what are often described as stress-related health problems. The pace of modernity and continuous adjustment to changes and ever-increasing demands may disrupt allostatic processes. An investigation into this widely accepted idea, however, found that people living in simpler, nonindustrial settings actually reported significantly more musculoskeletal complaints, fatigue, mood changes, and gastrointestinal complaints than a representative Norwegian sample (Eriksen, Hellesnes, Staff, & Ursin, 2004). These findings suggest that MUIs are not specific to the stress of modern industrialized societies; concerns about modernity may be the key issue, because worries about modern hazards such as toxins, pesticides, and pollution are associated with more reporting of subjective health concerns (S. K. Johnson & Blanchard, 2006; Petrie et al., 2005). Thus, it is the perception of threat that is critical in linking stress to ill health.

Unruh (1996) hypothesized that women may attend to pain sooner than men because the painful condition may result in more interference with gender-related social roles. Because women have such pervasive duties, pain needs to be attended to quickly, whereas for men pain is important only if it interferes with occupational responsibilities. Becker (2005) contended that the view of the overstressed woman with its subsequent health consequences places too much emphasis on the individual and that it is persistent structural gender inequalities that are the important culprits in women's health.

CONCLUSION

A number of psychosocial and cognitive factors may contribute to the higher prevalence of MUIs in women compared with men. This chapter has presented evidence for robust differences in symptom reporting that may be influenced by higher rates of depression and anxiety, negative affect, more frequent and more intense stressful life events, lower thresholds for seeking health care, higher likelihood of catastrophizing, and lower thresholds for pain.

All of the above may be associated with gender role expectations wherein it is more permissible within the feminine gender role to have a low threshold for pain, report illness symptoms, and be more expressive and dependent. Women's tendency to encounter more social stressors and childhood traumas also appears to contribute to a vulnerability to MUIs, which could be a result of physiological alterations subsequent to traumas. Stress-related symptoms could also represent an avenue through which to get help.

4

BIOLOGY OF MEDICALLY UNEXPLAINED ILLNESS

This chapter examines the evidence for gender differences in physiology that may help illuminate the higher incidence of medically unexplained illnesses (MUIs) among women than among men. There is evidence that physiological factors such as hormonal influences on pain, lower thresholds for pain, immune and hypothalamic–pituitary–adrenal (HPA) axis reactivity, and central nervous system hypersensitivity differ between men and women. Specific physiological factors that have been investigated for each MUI are examined, but the general issues relevant to the biology of MUI and gender are discussed as well.

GENETIC EXPLANATIONS

MUIs may have genetic components. There is a coaggregation within families of many of these disorders, such as fibromyalgia (FMS), chronic fatigue syndrome (CFS), and migraine. This genetic vulnerability may then be triggered by emotional stress, physical trauma, or infections (Clauw & Crofford, 2003). Several population-based twin studies have examined whether MUI symptoms (somatic distress) are distinct from anxiety and depression. Hickie, Kirk, and Martin (1999) found that 44% of the genetic variance in chronic fatigue was not shared by anxiety and depression. Gillespie, Zhu, Heath, Hickie, and Martin (2000) found that 33% of genetic variance in somatic distress was due to specific gene action unrelated to depression or phobic anxiety, and 74% of environmental influence on somatic distress was unrelated to depression or anxiety. Collectively, these studies have concluded that fatigue is etiologically distinct from anxiety and depression. Conversely, Roy-Byrne et al. (2002) studied a sample of 100 female twin pairs and found a strong association between fatigue and psychological distress without evidence of genetic covariation. Relatives of patients with FMS, particularly female relatives, have a higher prevalence of FMS and more tender points than the general population (Buskila & Neumann, 2005). Evidence for a genetic contribution to FMS and CFS has been explored and is discussed in chapters 6 and 7, respectively. Genetics and familial transmission may play a role in MUIs, but the specific mechanism is still unclear.

PHYSIOLOGY OF SOMATIZATION

Chapter 2 reviewed the evidence that MUIs involve somatizing tendencies. Although one of the hallmarks of somatization is that objective findings do not explain symptoms and levels of disability, several studies have found physiological abnormalities in somatoform disorders (SDs).

Hakala et al. (2002) found that 10 women with chronic SD and no other Axis I diagnosis had significantly lower cerebral metabolism compared with 17 healthy female volunteers. In a study of regional brain glucose metabolism, 10 women with SD or undifferentiated SD were compared with 12 healthy women. Low caudate and low putamen glucose metabolism, as well as low novelty seeking and high harm-avoidance temperament, were significantly associated with severe somatization (Hakala, Vahlberg, Niemi, & Karlsson, 2006).

Winfried Rief and her colleagues have performed a number of studies investigating the physiology of SDs. In a replication and extension of Rief, Shaw, and Fichter (1998), Rief and Auer (2001) found that people with SD showed less physiological habituation in a mental challenge task. In controls, heart rate decelerated when the experimental procedure changed from task to break and reaccelerated when the task began again. Participants with SD, however, did not show heart rate deceleration, and they stayed aroused during break periods. The authors stated that these results confirmed a cognitive–psychobiological model of somatization.

Rief, Pilger, Ihle, Bosmans, Egyed, and Maes (2001) examined the inflammatory response system in patients with SD compared with patients with major depression. They found T-cell activation (increased CD8), monocytic activation (IL-1RA), and a lowered anti-inflammatory capacity of the serum (lower CC16) in depression, whereas in SD there was monocytic activation and lowered T-lymphocytic activity (lowered CD8 and IL-6). These results suggest different immune alterations in SD compared with depression. In a study examining serotonergic and noradrenergic monoamino acids in 150 participants from four groups (SD, depression, depression and SD, and healthy controls), tryptophan, serotonin, and monoamines were decreased in patients with SD (Rief et al., 2004). This research is preliminary, and more study is needed to establish whether there are any consistently replicated physiological patterns in individuals with SD that may illuminate the pathophysiology of MUI.

Stress Physiology

Stress is implicated in the etiology of MUIs, whether through stressful life events, poor coping responses, dysfunctional stress regulation, or an interplay between these factors. In both sexes, the sympathetic nervous system–adrenal–medullary (SAM) and the HPA axis are the primary physiological systems involved in responding to stressful stimuli. The stress response consists of the sympathetic nervous system producing epinephrine and norepinephrine and the HPA axis producing glucocortocoids. Corticotropin-releasing hormone (CRH) is synthesized in hypothalamic neurons. When CRH acts on the anterior pituitary, endocrine cells secrete adrenocorticotropic hormone (ACTH; Silverthorn, 2001). ACTH stimulates the adrenal cortex of the adrenal glands. A group of stress hormones called *corticosteroids*, including cortisol, is then released from the adrenal cortex into the body's circulatory system. Components within the HPA axis have the ability to positively or negatively regulate other components within the system. For example, when cortisol is secreted from the adrenal cortex, it negatively regulates its own secretion by sending hormonal signals to the hypothalamus and anterior pituitary. This halts the synthesis of CRH and ACTH, respectively, which in turn decreases the amount of cortisol (Comer, 2005; see Figure 4.1). Although the HPA axis is self-regulating, chronic hyperarousal may cause permanent changes in the release of hormones.

It was not until Marianne Frankenhaeuser's work in the 1980s that the stress hormone responses of women began to be systematically studied and were found to be different from those of men. Laboratory stressors resulted in greater epinephrine response in men than women (Frankenhaeuser, Lundberg, & Forsman, 1980), and mothers taking their children for check-ups had higher norepinephrine levels than fathers (Lundberg, de Chateau, Winberg, & Frankenhaeuser, 1981). Krantz, Forsman, and Lundberg (2004) compared different physiological stress responses (systolic and diastolic blood pressure, heart rate, urinary epinephrine and norepinephrine, salivary cortisol) as well as trapezius muscle activity during mental and physical stress in women and

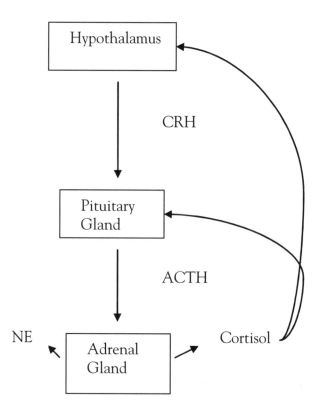

Figure 4.1. Hypothalamic–pituitary–adrenal (HPA) axis. CRH = corticotropin-releasing hormone; ACTH = adrenocorticotropic hormone; NE = norepinephrine.

men. They found significantly increased activity on all measures except cortisol and a significant association between sympathetic arousal and muscle activity, which helps explain the high prevalence of musculoskeletal disorders in mentally stressful but physically light work tasks. Men had higher blood pressure and a more pronounced increase in epinephrine output than women, whereas women had higher heart rate. It was concluded that sympathetic activity is more sensitive to moderately intense stress exposure than cortisol activity and that men respond to performance stress with more epinephrine output than women.

Other Swedish studies have found that although men and women respond similarly to stress at work, gender differences appear at the end of the working day, with men relaxing and women's physiological stress levels remaining high at home (Lundberg & Frankenhaeuser, 1999). The conclusion drawn from these studies was that gender roles and psychological factors were more important than biological factors in explaining gender differences in epinephrine response (Lundberg, 2005).

S. E. Taylor et al. (2000) have proposed an alternate biobehavioral stress response in women that they labeled *tend and befriend*. They posited that it would have been evolutionarily adaptive for women to develop social networks to protect themselves and offspring when the "fight or flight" response would endanger their young. Thus, women may exhibit relatively increased parasympathetic responses as opposed to sympathetic ones during stress. Taylor et al. proposed that the tend and befriend response is mediated primarily by the lactational hormone oxytocin and endogenous opioids whose effects are moderated by estrogens. They marshal a prodigious amount of animal research in support of this claim. This cumulative downregulation of the stress response may contribute to women's consistently greater longevity relative to men. Only a limited amount of data for humans addresses the validity of this theory. Ennis, Kelly, and Lambert (2001) collected cortisol before and after an examination in college students. The men in the challenge appraisal group demonstrated a significant increase in cortisol production from baseline to pretest with the increased anxiety level compared with the threat appraisal group. Women had a significant decrease in cortisol excretion in the challenge appraisal group and no difference in the level of anxiety between the challenge and threat groups. The authors interpreted these findings as consistent with the tend-and-befriend framework. It remains to be seen whether this gender difference in stress response has any bearing on the prevalence of MUIs or is more relevant to an evolutionary understanding of healthy women's stress responses.

Hypothalamic–Pituitary–Adrenal Axis and Medically Unexplained Illnesses

Alterations or malfunctions with components of the HPA axis have been implicated in a number of conditions. Fries, Hesse, Hellhammer, and Hellhammer (2005) reported that 20% to 25% of patients with "stress-related" disorders such as CFS, chronic pelvic pain, FMS, inflammatory bowel syndrome (IBS), posttraumatic stress disorder (PTSD), low back pain, burnout, and atypical depression show evidence of hypocortisolism. Rief and Barsky (2005) described the "overadjustment" of the HPA axis that can occur in "somatoform-associated disorders" (p. 996). The HPA axis may change from an initial hypercortisolism when a stressor becomes chronic. After prolonged periods of stress, whether from infection, work pressures, or interpersonal stress, an individual may begin to report fatigue, widespread pain, and stress sensitivity that signal a hypocortisolemic state. Different patient subgroups within one "stress-related" disorder can also be characterized by different patterns of hypocortisolism, such as decreased free cortisol, cortisol resistance, and reduced biosynthesis of CRF, ACTH, or cortisol (Fries et al., 2005).

Early life stressors may result in acute and chronic changes in the activity and regulation of the brain's biological stress response system that creates a vulnerability or increased sensitivity to stressors in adulthood (Bremner, 2005; Diseth, 2005; Weber & Reynolds, 2004). There is substantial evidence that early childhood trauma influences stress reactivity, behavioral sensitization, brain function, and pain processing. Brain areas that are particularly affected by emotion are the prefrontal cortex, amygdala, thalamus, hypothalamus, hippocampus, and anterior cingulate cortex (ACC; Bremner et al., 1997; Bremner, Vermetten, et al., 2003; Bremner, Vythilingam, Vermetten, Southwick, McGlashan, Nazeer, et al., 2003; Bremner, Vythilingam, Vermetten, Southwick, McGlashan, Staib, et al., 2003; Carrion et al., 2001; De Bellis et al., 1999; Vermetten & Bremner, 2002).

Girls are more likely than boys to be victims of sexual abuse in childhood and subsequently are at greater risk for depression and anxiety disorders (Weiss et al., 1999). Adverse events in childhood, particularly sexual abuse, may activate the HPA axis and result in a perpetuating negative feedback loop; this hypercortisolism can contribute to symptoms such as fatigue and depression (Kiecolt-Glaser, McGuire, Robles, & Glaser, 2002). PTSD is an example wherein differences in cortisol levels may be associated with duration of the stressor and symptoms. Putnam and Trickett (1997) conducted longitudinal studies of sexually abused girls and found that the girls had an increased cortisol level around the time of the stressor, and those who developed PTSD symptoms later had a decreased level of cortisol. Women are more likely to develop PTSD than men; approximately 8% of men and 20% of women who have been traumatized develop PTSD (Schnurr, Friedman, & Bernardy, 2002). Rape victims are more likely to develop PTSD than accident and natural disaster victims (Brewin, 2005). Leserman, Li, Drossman, and Hu (1998) found that symptoms consistent with PTSD were common among women with functional gastrointestinal disorders, particularly those who had abuse histories.

Studies on the effects of chronic stress report converging evidence for decreased cortisol secretion in a variety of MUIs (A. J. Cleare, 2003; Heim, Ehlert, & Hellhammer, 2000; Jerjes et al., 2006). Early childhood sexual abuse and trauma can result in hypercortisolism in some cases; in others it appears to result in hypocortisolism (Heim et al., 2000). Thus, early abuse can initiate a trajectory toward depression, anxiety, and a hyperactive HPA axis (Bhagwagar, Hafizi, & Cowen, 2005; Burke, Davis, Otte, & Mohr, 2005) or PTSD, FMS, CFS, or other fatigue and pain disorders characterized by a hypoactive HPA axis. The HPA axis is clearly relevant in the MUIs, although further research is needed to determine whether the HPA axis elucidates etiological and treatment issues.

McEwen and Lasley (2003) proposed a concept they called *allostatic load*, meaning that recurrent stress responses and prolonged activation of cardiovascular and neuroendocrine systems lead to wear and tear on the body and increase the risk for a variety of health problems. Mellner, Krantz, and Lundberg (2005) investigated whether the construct of allostatic load could be used to explain high levels of medically unexplained symptoms. They studied 222 healthy Swedish women who were part of a longitudinal health initiative; all of the women were 43 years old. They were assessed with a multisystem summary index of allostatic load and were examined on physiological indicators including blood pressure, heart rate, blood lipids, and stress hormones as well as self-reported symptoms. Women with a high symptom load were found to have significantly higher levels of cortisol and higher heart rate than those with low symptom load, whereas women with low symptom load had significantly higher levels of epinephrine on a work-free day. No differences were found in norepinephrine or in the summary measure of allostatic load. Although the differences between high- and low-symptom groups were not consistent over all physiological stress indicators, there were signals of dysregulation in stress-related biomarkers.

Several studies have found that CFS was associated with a high level of allostatic load. The allostatic load components that best discriminated CFS patients from controls were waist:hip ratio and aldosterone and urinary cortisol levels (Maloney et al., 2006). Among CFS patients, a high allostatic load was significantly associated with worse bodily pain, poorer physical functioning, and greater symptom frequency and intensity (Goertzel, Pennachin, de Souza Coelho, Maloney, et al., 2006). At least in the case of CFS, allostatic load appears to be a potentially fruitful avenue for research.

Stress, Immune System, and Endocrine Interactions

The immune system is closely integrated with the nervous and endocrine systems, and social factors influence the immune system through these systems. Psychological stress can downregulate the immune system by affecting the interplay between the HPA axis, autonomic nervous system, and endocrine and immune systems (Glaser & Kiecolt-Glaser, 1998; Kiecolt-Glaser, Bane, Glaser, & Malarkey, 2003). A large body of literature associates perceived stress with vulnerability to illness and slower recovery from illness (Kiecolt-Glaser et al., 2002; Kiecolt-Glaser, Page, Marucha, MacCallum, & Glaser, 1998). Segerstrom and Miller (2004) examined the relationship between stress and the immune system in a meta-analysis that included more than 300 empirical studies. They found that chronic stressors were associated with suppression of immunity and that those who were more vulnerable because of age and disease were more likely to experience immune changes during stress. There is evidence that women differ from men in terms of stress experiences, appraisals of stress, and stress physiology.

Serotonin regulates the circadian fluctuations of the HPA axis and the release of CRH from the hypothalamus (Silverthorn, 2001). There is evidence for low brain serotonin levels or function in a number of MUIs, particularly FMS and CFS. Nishizawa et al. (1997) were able to measure serotonin synthesis in living brains of 8 male and 7 female healthy participants using positron emission tomography (PET). They found that the mean rate of serotonin synthesis was 52% higher in the male individuals and noted that this is one of the largest gender brain differences not related to hormone binding sites. They went on to speculate that the lower rate of synthesis in the women's brains may mean that women are not as efficient at maintaining adequate stores of serotonin. They proposed that in stressful situations, serotonin would decline more in female than in male individuals, making them more vulnerable to depression. Gender linkages between serotonin synthesis and its interactions with HPA axis function could prove an important avenue for future MUI research.

Autoimmunity and Gender

It has been suggested that several MUIs, particularly CFS, involve alteration in immune function. It is well established that women are about 2.7 times more likely than men to acquire an autoimmune disease (Jacobson, Gange, Rose, & Graham, 1997; Walsh & Rau, 2000). Women have enhanced immune systems compared with men, which increases women's resistance to many types of infection but also makes them more susceptible to autoimmune diseases (Cannon & St. Pierre, 1997). Sinaii, Cleary, Ballweg, Nieman, and Stratton (2002) surveyed 3,680 women with physician-diagnosed endometriosis. Compared with published rates in the general population, women with endometriosis had higher rates of diagnosed CFS, FMS, hypothyroidism, autoimmune diseases, allergies, and asthma. The clustering of pain and fatigue syndromes with autoimmune and atopic disorders suggests a common interactive pathophysiology involving autoimmune inflammatory processes.

Markers of inflammatory response have shown gender differences. For example, the plasma activity level of phospholipase A2, a key enzyme involved in chronic inflammatory diseases, is significantly higher in Caucasian and Asian Indian women than their male counterparts (Kuslys, Vishwanath, Frey, & Frey, 1996). Conversely, interleukin-1-receptor-II, which is important in reducing the inflammatory response, is present in higher concentration in white blood cells from men than from women (Daun, Ball, & Cannon, 2000). These biological factors indicating greater susceptibility to autoimmune processes and increased inflammatory responses in women may play a role in CFS, FMS, and IBS pathophysiology. Researchers should investigate these connections.

SENSITIZATION AND MEDICALLY UNEXPLAINED ILLNESSES

There is evidence that women have lower odor thresholds and sensitivity (Dalton, Doolittle, & Breslin, 2002), which may have implications for multiple chemical sensitivity (MCS). Women also have lower thresholds for pressure touch (Komiyama & De Laat, 2005) and pain (Chesterton, Barlas,

Foster, Baxter, & Wright, 2002), which has implications for IBS, FMS, and CFS. In a large meta-analysis of gender differences in children's temperament, Else-Quest et al. (2006) found small to moderate gender differences in perceptual sensitivity. Girls were better at perceiving low-intensity environmental stimuli than boys, which may translate into greater female awareness of subtle environmental changes. Women may have an innately greater sensitivity to bodily sensations (Wool & Barsky, 1994).

Lee, Mayer, Schmulson, Chang, and Naliboff (2001) surveyed 714 consecutively screened IBS patients to explore gender differences in reported symptoms. Women reported more symptoms that involved increased sensitivity to food, medications, taste, and smell. Lee et al. concluded that these differences in sensitivity may represent altered sensory processes, autonomic responses, or cognitive hypervigilance. These differences in autonomic and sensory processes may parallel male and female differences in the general stress response.

Sensitization describes the phenomenon that the same signals can lead to more and more amplified perceptions. Sensitization includes biological sensitization, such as visceral hyperalgesia, and psychological sensitization, when hypervigilance to a subjective symptom leads to amplification of the symptom (Wilhelmsen, 2005). Psychobiological sensitization mechanisms may be operating in MUIs, wherein chronic stress contributes to increased sensitization of the central nervous system, autonomic nervous system, and the HPA axis.

Eriksen and Ursin (2004) have maintained that subjective health complaints become intolerable conditions through a process of sensitization. Sensitization occurs at the central and peripheral levels of the nervous system and then at a higher level through cognitive bias. Similarly, Rief and Barsky (2005) described a "filter model" for explaining subjective health complaints. They described MUIs as disorders that involve altered perceptions, which may amplify sensory input resulting from increased arousal, distress, chronic HPA stimulation, deconditioning, and sensitization. This amplification reduces filtering capacity, as does vigilance, anxiety, depression, and lack of distraction, and this leads to a lower threshold for perception of symptoms.

Individuals with MUIs may have more labile or reactive physiological systems that make them more prone to experience a number of physical symptoms in response to stressful events or negative emotional experiences (Kirmayer, Robbins, & Paris, 1994). It is even possible that a trait like neuroticism is associated with increased symptom reporting through a physiological tendency to experience higher levels of symptoms.

Sex Differences in Pain

Female gender and increasing age are the primary determinants of decreased pain tolerance and pain threshold. Most of the MUIs involve pain experiences; IBS and FMS are defined by pain. Gender differences in behavioral responses to pain are clear and well-investigated. Women report more health care utilization and disability in response to pain (Unruh, 1996). Additionally, studies have shown that somatosensory perception and pain sensitivity are influenced by sex hormones (Aloisi, 2003).

Pain Perception

Most experimental paradigms show that women have lower pain thresholds and tolerance and rate pain as more intense and more unpleasant than do their male counterparts (Jensen, Rasmussen, Pederson, Lous, & Oleson, 1992; Weisenberg, Tepper, & Schwarzwald, 1995). Tactile detection, pressure pain detection thresholds, and pressure pain tolerance threshold have been found to be significantly lower in healthy women, using a variety of paradigms and testing at various body sites (Chesterton et al., 2002; Komiyama & De Laat, 2005). Women show greater perceptual sensitization and "wind-up," which is a temporal summation of pain, indicating that women's central nociceptive processing is upregulated compared with that of men (Sarlani & Greenspan, 2002). Sarlani and Greenspan (2005) also found that women's central processing of nociceptive input may be more easily upregulated into pathological hyperexcitability, possibly accounting for the predominance of pain syndromes among women.

Although sex differences in experimental pain perception are well documented, a minority of studies have found no differences. The consistency and magnitude of sex differences vary across pain induction techniques; for example, the smallest differences appear to be in thermal pain stimuli (Riley, Robinson, Wise, Myers, & Fillingam, 1998).

Menstrual cycle changes in pain perception are an important area for examining the role of gonadal hormones on pain sensitivity. The menstrual cycle has been reported to alter pain perception, although patterns differ somewhat among studies. It has been reported that estrogens may influence somatic sensory processes. Women generally have less pain sensitivity during the phases that are associated with higher estrogen levels (Johns & Littlejohn, 1999) and are more sensitive to pain during periods of low estrogen. De Leeuw, Albuquerque, Anderson, and Carlson (2006) found that ACC activation was greater during the low estrogen phase of the menstrual cycle in healthy women.

Riley, Robinson, Wise, and Price (1999) reviewed 16 studies of experimentally induced pain across menstrual cycle phases in healthy women. Meta-analyses found that for pressure stimulation, cold pressor pain, thermal heat stimulation, and ischemic muscle pain, higher thresholds and tolerance for pain were found in the follicular (high estrogen) phase. The authors proposed that menstrual cycle effects on human pain perception are large enough that it should be controlled for in pain studies.

Although biological factors play a role in gender differences in pain experiences, a number of studies have found that psychosocial factors also influence pain perception and report. Wise, Price, Myers, Heft, and Robinson (2002) investigated the accuracy of the Gender Role Expectations of Pain (GREP; Robinson et al., 2001) in measuring pain. The GREP consists of 12 visual analog scales that assess a participant's personal attribution of his or her pain sensitivity, pain endurance, and willingness to report pain relative to a typical man and woman (Robinson et al., 2001). Wise et al. found that GREP scores were significant predictors of threshold, tolerance, and pain unpleasantness, although they did not account for all of the variance. Biological sex remained a significant predictor of pain tolerance after controlling for GREP scores. Wise et al. concluded that both psychosocial factors and biological sex differences are viable explanations for gender differences in pain reports. Similarly, Jackson, Iezzi, Gunderson, Nagasaka, and Fritch (2002) found that men's greater physical self-efficacy and task-specific self-efficacy mediated their higher tolerance and lower reports of pain intensity on a cold pressor test. Anxiety and pain appear to be strongly associated in men. Jones and Zachariae (2004) found no effect of gender on a cold pressor pain procedure, but they did find that low-anxious men tolerated the cold pressor significantly longer than high-anxious men. There was no effect of anxiety on pain response in women. Keogh and Herdenfeldt (2002) manipulated sensory-focused and emotion-focused coping instructions and found that men exhibited lower pain responses when using sensory-focused coping compared with women, whereas emotional focusing increased the affective pain experiences in women.

Pain reports in women may be augmented by a catastrophizing coping style. Altered peripheral or central processing mechanisms are correlated with pain catastrophizing in women with FMS (Geisser et al., 2003). Evidence presented in chapter 3 of this volume indicates that women are more prone to catastrophizing.

Brain and Pain

The ACC plays an important role in pain processing and affective–motivational experiences and affects the impact of pain-related distress on cognitive function through its role in attention. We have seen in the discussion of sensitization that some individuals may be more prone to hypervigilance than others, allocating attention to symptoms and pain and finding it harder to distract themselves. Cognitive efficiency and memory can be affected by chronic stress, which repeatedly activates both the HPA axis and ACC areas. The vigilant anticipation of pain and symptoms, especially in individuals with high trait neuroticism, disrupts attention and cognitive efficiency (Hart, Wade, & Martelli, 2003). This could explain some of the cognitive complaints reported by individuals with MUIs.

CONCLUSION

MUI symptoms can be due to biobehavioral changes that occur with life experiences that modify central brain areas, neuroendocrine, and HPA axis functioning. These include changes in beliefs (catastrophizing), behavioral changes (vigilance to symptoms, amplification, reduced activity, deconditioning), conditioned responses, and sensitization processes. Physiological vulnerabilities can exist in various body systems as a result of genetics, physical insult (viral, accident, toxic exposure, infection), or chronic stressors. Additionally, behavioral and cognitive factors may keep physiological systems from recovering adequately after a physical insult or psychosocial stressor.

II

COMMON MEDICALLY UNEXPLAINED ILLNESSES

Chapters 5 through 8 present comprehensive research findings on the most common medically unexplained illnesses (MUIs): irritable bowel syndrome (IBS), fibromyalgia (FMS), chronic fatigue syndrome (CFS), and multiple chemical sensitivity (MCS). Clauw and Crofford (2003) divided MUIs into "systemic" conditions such as FMS and CFS; "regional" syndromes such as IBS, temporomandibular disorders, migraine, and tension headaches; and "exposure" syndromes such as MCS, Gulf War syndrome, and sick building syndrome. MUIs have been termed *chronic multisymptom illnesses* because population-based studies using factor analysis to identify key symptoms have found that multifocal pain, fatigue, memory difficulties, and mood disturbance are coaggregated (Clauw, 2001; Gray, Reed, Kaiser, Smith, & Gastanaga, 2002; McLean & Clauw, 2004).

It is notable that there is more comorbidity among the MUIs in women than in men (Aaron & Buchwald, 2001; Buchwald & Garrity, 1994; Tseng & Natelson, 2004; Yunus, 2001). For example, overlap between IBS and FMS is 40% in women and only 14% in men (Yunus, Inanici, Aldag, & Mangold, 2000). Overlap between CFS and FMS is 36% in women and 12% in men (Buchwald, Pearlman, Kith, & Schmaling, 1994). Tseng and Natelson (2004) found that 65.5% of women with CFS also met criteria for FMS or MCS, whereas 38.6% of men with CFS had FMS or MCS comorbidly. This is consistent with women reporting more symptoms in various systems (Creed & Barsky, 2004; Yunus, 2001).

Wessely, Nimnuan, and Sharpe (1999) have argued that there are many similarities in 12 common functional somatic syndromes, and the distinctions are just an artifact of medical specialization. They noted that there is substantial overlap among definitions: eight syndromes contained "bloating," "abdominal distension," or "headache"; six contained "fatigue"; and six contained "abdominal pain" as core symptoms. Furthermore, a number of nonsymptom characteristics are shared among these 12 syndromes (discussed below).

Aaron and Buchwald (2001) reviewed studies that assessed overlap among MUIs. They found that in referral clinic populations, up to 70% of patients with FMS met criteria for CFS and that 35% to 70% of patients with CFS have FMS. Studies also have shown that 32% to 80% of patients with FMS and 58% to 92% with CFS also have IBS. In 53% to 67% of people with CFS, illness worsens with exposure to various chemicals, and 30% of patients diagnosed with MCS meet criteria for CFS. In people with FMS, 55% have symptoms consistent with MCS. The large percentages of people who meet criteria for more than one MUI signal that many people with MUIs have a broad array of symptoms in many body systems.

A Dutch study followed 182 primary care patients diagnosed with functional somatic symptoms from 1998 through 2002 and compared them with matched control patients (olde Hartman, Lucassen, van de Lisdonk, Bor, & van Weel, 2004). Compared with controls, the functional symptom patients had a greater diversity of symptoms, higher prescription drug use, higher rates of referrals, and higher psychiatric morbidity. The authors argued that patients with chronic functional symptoms do not cluster into distinct syndromes and should not be classified into medical subspecialty syndromes (olde Hartman et al., 2004). Collectively, these studies suggest a common mechanism in many MUI conditions.

EXPLAINING COMORBIDITY

Several factors may account for the high rates of comorbidity among the MUIs. Wessely et al. (1999) noted that the following nonsymptom characteristics are shared among 12 MUI syndromes: female predominance, increased rate of depression and anxiety, altered central nervous system functioning, history of childhood maltreatment and abuse, and difficulties in doctor–patient relationships.

Hudson and colleagues (Gruber, Hudson, & Pope, 1996; Hudson, Goldenberg, Pope, Keck, & Schlesinger, 1992; Hudson & Pope, 1989) and Yunus (2001, 2002) cited overlapping features and a common neuroendocrine mechanism between migraines, CFS, temperomandibular disorders,

MCS, and FMS. These MUIs involve central sensitivity, a hypersensitivity to various sensory stimuli, and responsiveness to low doses of antidepressants. Clauw (1994) has added that these MUIs share strong female predominance, are usually worsened by stress, and improve with aerobic exercise and antidepressants. In both FMS and IBS, women have more symptoms than men, but their severity of pain is not different from that of men (Yunus, 2001).

Although common psychiatric vulnerabilities are seen in MUIs, statistically controlling for traits such as somatization and depression does not explain all of the overlap among MUIs (Whitehead, Palsson, & Jones, 2002). A related vulnerability would be childhood maltreatment and abuse; a number of studies have found significantly more unexplained symptoms in women with a history of abuse compared with women with no such history (Walker, Keegan, Gardner, Sullivan, Bernstein, & Katon, 1999).

Overlapping symptoms and a sheer multitude of symptoms also contribute to overlap among MUIs. Core symptoms such as pain and fatigue rarely occur alone. As Claudius states in *Hamlet*, "When troubles come, they come not single spies but in battalions" (act IV, scene 5), and nothing could be more apt for the symptom of fatigue. Fatigue is a good example of a vague, subjective symptom more commonly reported in women that co-occurs with numerous other symptoms such as pain, weakness, headaches, sleep problems, cognitive problems, and depression (Hartz, Kuhn, & Levine, 1998; Manu et al., 1989; Nisenbaum, Reyes, Mawle, & Reeves, 1998).

MEDICALLY UNEXPLAINED ILLNESSES AS DISTINCT DISORDERS

Although many investigators have argued that MUIs are really one disorder with variations in the predominant symptom, in this volume the research findings collected on each disorder are presented separately. Whitehead et al. (2002) found that individuals with IBS were twice as likely as comparison groups to be diagnosed with FMS, CFS, chronic pelvic pain, and temporomandibular joint disorder. They acknowledged the features shared by these disorders: They disproportionately affect women; are stress-related; and involve sleep difficulties, fatigue, anxiety, and depression. Nonetheless, Whitehead et al. did not believe that the case for a common etiology is convincing, because the pathophysiology of each disorder is different. Whitehead et al. marshaled the evidence for overlap in IBS, CFS, FMS, temporomandibular joint disorder, and chronic pelvic pain and concluded that they have independent etiologic mechanisms, yet their extensive overlap suggests common factors. Whitehead et al. suggested that the common factors could be stress reactivity and selective attention and amplification of somatic sensations. Hyperalgesia may account for the vague, overlapping symptoms; discomfort; and pain common to MUIs. Mayer, Fass, and Fullerton (1998) proposed that symptoms are vague in MUIs because visceral afferents converge with somatic afferents on the same dorsal horn neurons in the spinal cord, and this overlapping of pathways results in nonspecific symptoms. Individual vulnerabilities in the digestive system may increase the likelihood of IBS, whereas vulnerabilities in immune functioning may predispose some people to CFS.

Robbins, Kirmayer, and Hemami (1997) used latent variable models of functional somatic symptoms for a sample of 686 family medicine patients. Symptom items were selected to approximate diagnoses of FMS, CFS, and IBS. Confirmatory factor analysis showed that hypothesized latent variables of somatic depression, somatic anxiety, FMS-like, CFS-like, and IBS-like illness offered tentative confirmation of functional somatic syndromes as discrete entities. Still, there was moderately high overlap among patients who endorsed the five distinct clusters of symptoms. These findings are similar to those of Ciccone and Natelson (2003), who found some support for a distinct syndrome yet with considerable overlap. They examined people with CFS only and compared them with those with CFS and FMS, with CFS and MCS, and with all three disorders. There were few differences in physical functioning except that people with FMS had higher tender point counts and higher pain levels. Ciccone and Natelson found that those with only CFS had fewer psychiatric diagnoses. Each overlapping syndrome was associated with a corresponding increment in major depression; for example, 85% of those with all three syndromes (i.e., CFS, FMS, and MCS) had at least one psychiatric disorder, whereas only 44% of those with CFS alone had some psychiatric disorder. This is consistent with Kroenke's work (Kroenke, 2001; Kroenke et al., 1994), which showed that the number of unexplained symptoms was positively associated with psychiatric disorder; the more unexplained symptoms, the higher the percentage of psychiatric disorders.

Linder, Dinser, Wagner, Krueger, and Hoffman (2002) used artificial neural networks, a computer-based model, rather than conventional methods to generate classification criteria for CFS compared with other fatiguing illnesses, systemic lupus erythematosus, and FMS. Ninety-nine case patients with CFS, 41 with systemic lupus erythematosus, and 58 with FMS were recruited from an outpatient population. Clinical symptoms were documented with help of a predefined questionnaire. Classification criteria developed by artificial neural networks were found to have a sensitivity of 95% and a specificity of 85% in accurately identifying CFS, which was a higher ratio than any of the other methods. The CFS symptoms that had the highest accuracy ratios were "acute onset of symptoms" and "sore throat."

R. R. Taylor, Jason, and Schoeny (2001) found diagnostic distinctions between CFS, FMS, somatic depression, somatic anxiety, and IBS by using a confirmatory factor analysis of self-reported symptoms. Jason and colleagues (Jason et al., 1997; Jason, Taylor, Song, Kennedy, & Johnson, 1999) insisted that the MUIs be viewed as distinct disorders, because the core features of the syndromes do not overlap.

Whitehead et al. (2002) proposed a "dual etiology" hypothesis to explain the heterogeneity of symptoms of people with IBS. In some patients, symptoms are primarily physiological, whereas others have a stronger psychological basis for their symptoms. People with IBS with comorbid MUIs and excessive numbers of symptoms have somatization tendencies and predominantly psychological etiology, whereas those without comorbid conditions and few excess symptoms are more likely to have a physiologic etiology for IBS.

A similar approach has been attempted with CFS by Natelson's research group. CFS groups were stratified according to psychiatric status and mode of onset of symptoms. The results of the stratification studies suggest at least two subgroups of CFS patients: one subgroup with a gradual onset of symptoms, concurrent psychiatric disturbance, and relatively mild cognitive impairment; and another subgroup with sudden onset, lack of psychiatric disturbance, and more serious cognitive deficits (S. K. Johnson, DeLuca, & Natelson, 1999). In a factor analytic study, Hickie et al. (1995) also found two "distinct clinical subgroups" within CFS: one small subgroup with clinical characteristics suggestive of somatoform disorder, and a larger subgroup with a symptom profile consistent with what the authors called "acquired neurasthenia" (p. 109). The "acquired neurasthenia" group would roughly correspond to S. K. Johnson et al.'s (1999) sudden onset, nonpsychiatric, cognitively impaired subgroup.

Moss-Morris and Spence (2006) performed a prospective study to determine whether they could distinguish precipitating factors for IBS and CFS. They followed 592 general practice patients with an acute episode of *Campylobacter* gastroenteritis and 243 patients with an acute episode of infectious mononucleosis at 3- and 6-month time points. Patients had no prior history of IBS or CFS and were assessed for distress at baseline using the Hospital Anxiety and Depression Scale (Zigmond & Snaith, 1983). The nature of the infections did predict onset of MUI; the odds for developing IBS were significantly greater after *Campylobacter* infection, whereas the odds for developing chronic fatigue or CFS were significantly greater after mononucleosis infection. Female gender was a significant risk factor for both IBS and chronic fatigue or CFS. However, the presence of baseline depression or anxiety was the most important predictor of chronic fatigue or CFS at 3 and 6 months; for IBS it was the type of infection, with anxiety playing a smaller role. At 6 months, only 7 of the 118 identified cases met criteria for both CFS and IBS, indicating minimal overlap. Moss-Morris and Spence argued that their data suggest distinctions between postinfectious IBS and CFS, at least in primary care patients.

Biopsychosocial models recognize the frequent inapplicability of simple either–or models. The taxing of a weak and vulnerable system (induced by infection, stress physiology imbalance, anterior cingulate and amygdalar dysregulation, and sleep neurohormone dysregulation) can produce significant impairment in attention focusing and other cognitive processes and exacerbation of underlying psychological vulnerabilities such as depression, chronic stress, anxiety, and history of abuse. Deary (1999) commented that neither lumping all MUIs together nor splitting them into distinct syndromes would provide a satisfactory descriptive taxonomy of MUIs. Understanding the valid arguments on both sides (MUI as a single syndrome, MUIs as distinct syndromes), the chapters that follow examine what is known about these perplexing disorders. Even though these disorders are presented in separate chapters, we must remain ever mindful of the extensive overlap among them.

5

IRRITABLE BOWEL
SYNDROME

Irritable bowel syndrome (IBS) is a complex, multidetermined syndrome involving altered gut reactivity, altered pain perception, and brain–gut dysregulation that is modulated by psychosocial and biological factors (Bose & Farthing, 2001; Mayer, 1999, 2000; Naliboff, Chang, Munakata, & Mayer, 2000; Palsson & Drossman, 2005). The symptomatology of IBS is a combination of abdominal pain or discomfort, rectal distension, and altered bowel habit (either altered stool frequency, such as diarrhea or constipation, or altered stool form). Symptoms commonly associated with IBS include abdominal bloating, passage of mucus with a bowel movement, sensation of incomplete evacuation after having a bowel movement, and abdominal pain or discomfort. Four subgroups of IBS are described according to their most predominant symptom: constipation predominant, diarrhea predominant, having an alternating pattern of constipation and diarrhea, or abdominal pain (Horwitz & Fisher, 2001; Talley, Zinsmeister, & Melton, 1995). No pathologic pattern of gut motility can be identified specifically with IBS, in contrast with other functional or organic disorders of the gut (McKee & Quigley, 1993).

DIAGNOSIS

Three diagnostic sets of criteria have been commonly used for research and diagnosing IBS: the Manning criteria, Rome I criteria, and Rome II criteria. The Manning criteria were developed in 1978 and required pain relieved by defecation, pain followed by change in frequency or form of stool, abdominal distension, mucus in stool, and a feeling of incomplete evacuation (Talley et al., 1990). A diagnosis using the Rome criteria requires the presence of two or more of these symptoms in addition to abdominal pain. IBS can currently be diagnosed using the Rome II criteria (Thompson et al., 2000). See Exhibit 5.1. The Rome I and Rome II criteria were developed using a consensus approach adopted by a panel of international experts and are generally found to be both sensitive and specific for the diagnosis of IBS (Vanner et al., 1999). This consensus has allowed a standardization of entry criteria into clinical studies and more expeditious diagnosis (Talley & Spiller, 2002). Recently, Rome III criteria have been developed emphasizing subtyping according to bowel habit (Longstreth et al., 2006). Four subtypes have been proposed: IBS with constipation, IBS with diarrhea, mixed IBS, and unsubtyped IBS.

In studies of people who are clinically diagnosed with IBS according to Manning or Rome criteria, a higher percentage of women compared with men fulfill Manning and Rome criteria. R. C. Smith et al. (1991) found that the Manning criteria were of no diagnostic value in men. Thus, it appears that the Manning and Rome I criteria are more sensitive and reliable in women than men. Thompson (1997) found no gender differences in the three pain symptoms; however, mucus, incomplete evacuation, and abdominal distension and bloating were less common in men. Thompson suggested that women may remember these more subtle symptoms better than men, and in fact other studies have indicated that women are more likely than men to remember symptoms. Gender differences have not been examined using the newer Rome II criteria, so it remains to be seen if this problem of differential sensitivity and reliability persists. The studies discussed below used Manning or Rome criteria unless otherwise indicated.

Medical professionals have moved away from the concept of "diagnosis of exclusion" toward a so-called "positive approach" to diagnosis. The positive approach sets a partnering tone for the physician–patient relationship. Thus, patients who fit the epidemiologic profile for IBS and have IBS-like symptoms that meet the Rome II diagnostic criteria for IBS are considered to have IBS, unless so-called "alarm factors" are present. The symptoms of IBS can also occur in many other structural disorders of the gastrointestinal tract. Physicians using the framework provided by the Rome II diagnostic criteria must rapidly exclude the possibility of other disorders and determine whether alarm factors exist and require evaluation (Olden, 2002). Hammer, Eslick, Howell, Altiparmak, and Talley (2004) found that older age, rectal bleeding,

EXHIBIT 5.1
Diagnostic Criteria for Irritable Bowel Syndrome
(IBS; Revised Rome Criteria)

At least 12 weeks or more, which need not be consecutive, in the preceding 12 months of abdominal discomfort or pain that has two of three features:
- relieved with defecation, *and/or*
- onset associated with a change in frequency of stool, *and/or*
- onset associated with a change in form (appearance) of stool.

Symptoms that cumulatively support the diagnosis of IBS are as follows:
- abnormal stool frequency (for research purposes, *abnormal* may be defined as more than three bowel movements per day or fewer than three bowel movements per week),
- abnormal stool form (lumpy and hard or loose and watery stool),
- abnormal stool passage (straining, urgency, or feeling of incomplete evacuation),
- passage of mucus, and
- bloating or feeling of abdominal distension.

Note. From *Rome II: The Functional Gastrointestinal Disorders* (p. 360), by D. A. Drossman, E. Corazziari, N. J. Talley, W. G. Thompson, and W. E Whitehead (Eds.), 2000, McLean, VA: Degnon Associates. Copyright 2000 by Degnon Associates. Adapted with permission.

and unexplained weight loss are alarm features that separate IBS from organic gastrointestinal disease.

ETIOLOGY

Etiologic mechanisms for IBS include visceral hypersensitivity, autonomic dysfunction, postinfectious IBS, and psychosocial factors. The pathophysiology of IBS remains incompletely understood. Much research attention has focused on altered gut motility as a cause of IBS symptoms (McKee & Quigley, 1993). However, this approach is limited because although altered motility of the colon and small bowel can be demonstrated in IBS, there is a poor correlation between IBS symptoms and the presence of alterations in motility (Whitehead et al., 1992). Likewise, drugs that alter gastrointestinal motility alone do not provide any significant relief of IBS symptoms (Noor et al., 1998; Page & Dirnberger, 1981). It appears that altered motility in IBS is currently seen as one of many factors associated with the disorder rather than a cause of the disorder itself.

Several triggering events have been associated with the onset of IBS. Such triggers include pelvic surgery, use of antibiotics, psychological trauma, and acute gastroenteritis (Gwee et al., 1999). Yet, in many individuals who develop IBS there do not appear to be any discernable triggers. Gwee et al. (1999) prospectively studied 94 consecutive patients hospitalized for gastroenteritis who had completed standardized psychometric and life events scales for the previous 12 months. Twenty-two patients were subsequently diagnosed with IBS. Anxiety, neuroticism, and somatization were higher in those who developed IBS, and stepwise regression showed that disruptive life events and higher hypochrondriasis scores predicted IBS independent of the other psychological measures. Three months after the gastroenteritis hospitalization, both IBS-positive and IBS-negative patients showed rectal hypersensitivity, hyperreactivity, and rapid colonic transport compared with healthy controls. Only the IBS-positive patients showed higher chronic inflammatory response 3 months after infection. Gwee et al. speculated that a gastroenteritis attack might sensitize the bowel and that psychological factors bring out the perception of these changes as symptoms.

Zar, Kumar, and Benson (2001) reviewed the evidence for food hypersensitivity in the etiology of IBS. Seven studies of dietary exclusion followed by food challenge found response rates from 15 to 67%, and the best response was in those with diarrhea predominant IBS. This suggests that diet may be implicated in a significant subgroup of IBS. Like the other medically unexplained illnesses (MUIs) discussed in this volume, the etiology of IBS is multidetermined through interactions of physiological, psychosocial, and behavioral factors (Drossman, 1998). Drossman (1998) proposed that early life factors (genetics and environmental exposures) influence the later interaction of psychosocial and physiological functioning with the central nervous system—enteric nervous system axis, which affects clinical expression and outcomes such as physician visits, functional status, and quality of life.

PREVALENCE

A number of studies using standardized diagnostic criteria have been performed to help determine the true prevalence of IBS. IBS is estimated to affect between 10% and 20% of the population (Horwitz & Fisher, 2001; Talley, Zinsmeister, & Melton, 1995). Its incidence varies by age; it is higher in individuals in the 2nd to 5th decades of life and declines considerably thereafter. In individuals younger than 50 years of age, IBS affects between 15% and 20% of the population, and in individuals older than 50 years of age, prevalence is approximately 10% to 12% (Longstreth & Wolde-Tsadik, 1993).

IBS accounts for about 12% of patients seen in primary care practice, although most IBS sufferers do not seek medical treatment. Studies have indicated that IBS is the largest diagnostic group seen in gastrointestinal practices; an estimated 50% of patient visits to gastroenterologists were related to IBS symptoms (Mitchell & Drossman, 1987; M. W. Russo, Gaynes, & Drossman, 1999).

An estimated 70% of persons with IBS symptoms do not seek medical attention (Drossman, Sandler, McKee, & Lovitz, 1982; Thompson & Heaton, 1980). Patients with IBS, when compared with individuals with IBS symptoms who do not seek medical treatment, have more nongastrointestinal complaints and consult physicians more for these symptoms (Levy et al., 2001; Sandler, Drossman, Nathan, & McKee, 1984; Sperber et al., 2000). Consulters have been found to be much higher on measures of psychological dysfunction (depression and anxiety) than nonconsulters. Whitehead, Bosmajian, Zonderman, Costa, and Schuster (1988) found that women who met restrictive criteria for IBS but had not consulted a physician had no more symptoms of psychological distress than asymptomatic controls. Conversely, medical clinic patients with both IBS and lactose malabsorption had significantly more psychological symptoms than asymptomatic controls or nonconsulters with the same diagnoses. Similarly, Drossman et al. (1988) studied 72 IBS patients, 82 persons with IBS who had not sought medical treatment, and 84 controls. When controlling for symptoms of pain and diarrhea, they found that IBS consulters had a higher proportion of abnormal personality patterns, greater illness behaviors, and fewer positive life events than IBS nonconsulters and controls. The IBS nonconsulters had higher coping capabilities, viewed IBS as less disruptive, and exhibited less denial than consulting patients. Collectively, these studies indicate that psychological factors influence who consults a doctor for IBS symptoms and who does not.

Much research in IBS is based on samples from specialty referral centers, so Thompson, Heaton, Smyth, and Smyth (2000) examined the prevalence in general practice prospectively in all patients of British clinics in six locations. Of 255 patients with gastrointestinal complaints, 30% had IBS and 14% had other functional disorders. Compared with the 100 patients found to have "organic" disease, those with IBS were more often women, had a greater number of unexplained symptoms, and were more likely to fear that they had cancer.

An increasing number of transcultural and transracial population studies have documented a fairly constant prevalence for IBS across national boundaries and ethnic and racial lines. No particular country or geographic area stands out as having a higher or lower prevalence of IBS, although individuals who live in countries with universal health care are more likely to consult a physician for IBS symptoms (Talley, Boyce, & Jones, 1997).

OVERLAP WITH OTHER MEDICALLY UNEXPLAINED ILLNESSES

Abdominal pain or discomfort is the distinctive symptom for the diagnosis of IBS. This combination of altered bowel habits with abdominal pain or discomfort is thought to separate IBS from other functional bowel disorders, such as functional dyspepsia, functional constipation, or functional diarrhea. However, IBS and functional dyspepsia overlap to a large extent. Because the symptoms of both conditions involve a lower threshold for reporting pain from intraluminal distension, Whitehead (1999) suggested that they may have a common pathophysiologic basis. Lembo et al. (1999) reported that out of 443 new referrals to a tertiary functional gastrointestintal disorders center who met criteria for IBS, 35% also had functional dyspepsia.

Interstitial cystitis is a chronic syndrome characterized by bladder and pelvic pain, with urinary problems but with no distinctive tissue pathology. It is 9 times more likely to occur in women than in men (Alagiri, Chottiner, Ratner, Slade, & Hanno, 1997). In a survey of 2,405 individuals with interstitial cystitis, the most commonly co-occurring disorders were allergies (45%) and IBS (38%), followed by fibromyalgia (FMS), sensitive skin, vulvodynia, migraine headaches, and endometriosis (Alagiri et al., 1997). Ninety seven percent of those responding to the survey were women.

Naliboff, Heitkemper, et al. (2000) reported that dyspareria (painful intercourse) is a specific problem for women with IBS and that 43% report some sexual dysfunction, most often decreased libido. The authors speculated that this may be due to an altered central stress response (increased secretion of corticotropin-releasing hormone), similar to what is found in chronic fatigue syndrome (CFS) and FMS. Walker, Gelfand, Gelfand, Green, and Katon (1996) evaluated a sequential sample of 60 women with IBS and 26 women with inflammatory bowel disease in an urban gastroenterology clinic. Chronic pelvic pain was reported in significantly more of the IBS (35%) than the inflammatory bowel disease group (14%). Compared with women with IBS alone, those with both IBS and chronic pelvic pain were significantly more likely to have a lifetime history of dysthymic disorder, current and lifetime panic disorder, somatization disorder (SD), childhood sexual abuse, and hysterectomy. The mean number of somatization symptoms was the best predictor of comorbid IBS and chronic pelvic pain compared with either inflammatory bowel disease or IBS alone. These findings indicate that high rates of psychopathology associated with IBS and chronic pelvic pain independently are even higher in women with both syndromes. It is possible that women with IBS report more dysmenorrhea, interstitial cystitis, and pelvic pain because of heightened visceral hypersensitivity.

In addition to functional disorders that affect the gastrointestinal system and pelvic area, a number of conditions, such as fibromyalgia, CFS, and certain psychiatric disorders, have been found more often in IBS patients than in non-IBS controls (Barsky & Borus, 1999; Manu, 2004). Whitehead, Palsson, and Jones (2002) found that individuals with IBS were twice as likely as comparison groups to be diagnosed with nongastrointestinal somatic disorders, most commonly FMS, CFS, chronic pelvic pain, and temporomandibular joint disorder. These four conditions share certain features: They disproportionately affect women; are stress related; and are associated with fatigue, sleep difficulties, anxiety, and depression. These disorders overlap not only with IBS but also with each other (as is discussed extensively in the introduction to Part II, this volume).

Vandvik, Wilhemsen, Ihlebaek, and Farup (2004) did not investigate the comorbidity of IBS with specific MUIs; rather, they investigated the correlation of IBS with level of subjective health complaints. They conducted a prospective study of 208 consecutive patients with IBS (Rome II) in nine general medical practices. They assessed comorbid symptoms, psychosocial factors, and quality of life. Subjective health complaint data were collected from 1,240 adults (controls). Health care seeking was assessed after 6 to 9 months. Patients with IBS reported comorbid symptoms significantly more frequently than controls. Patients with high somatic comorbidity reported higher levels of mood disorder, health anxiety, neuroticism, adverse life events, reduced quality of life, and increased health care seeking when compared with those with low and intermediate somatic comorbidity. These findings indicate that people with IBS and numerous additional symptoms tend to have more psychopathology and poorer functioning.

Perkins, Keville, Schmidt, and Chalder (2005) investigated the connection between eating disorders and IBS. Similarities between the two conditions include strong female predominance; high prevalence of childhood sexual abuse; and characteristics of perfectionism, negative self-evaluations, and self-blame (Ali et al., 2000; Toner, 1994). Perkins et al. found that two thirds of individuals with a current or past eating disorder fulfilled criteria for IBS. They also found an association between the severity of attitudinal eating disorder symptoms, such as weight and shape concerns, and IBS. The authors suggested this may be due to a common underlying factor of hypervigilance to internal sensations and excessive self-focused attention.

ECONOMIC IMPACT

The economic impact of IBS on U.S. society is impressive and disturbing. More easily quantified direct costs of medical care (i.e., medications, hospitalizations, and emergency room and office visits) have estimated in excess of $8 billion (Talley et al., 1995). Indirect costs, which encompass the cost of absence from work, school, and other productive activities, have been estimated to be about $20 billion a year (R. Martin, Barron, & Zacker, 2001). Not captured in these estimates are the costs associated with unnecessary *cholecystectomy* (gall bladder removal; Kennedy & Jones, 2000) and hysterectomy (Walker et al., 1996), two types of operations that patients with IBS frequently undergo. A study of HMO attendees with physician-diagnosed IBS reported that patients with IBS are 3 times as likely to undergo cholecystectomies and twice as likely to undergo appendectomies, hysterectomies, and back surgery, compared with HMO patients without IBS (Longstreth & Yao, 2004). The staggering cost of care for IBS patients, estimated to be in the 10s of billions of dollars, does not even include the significant negative impact on quality of life that is induced by IBS. It is difficult to measure the intangible costs in human suffering, isolation, and social restrictions because of IBS-related symptoms.

Levy, Whitehead, Von Korff, and Feld (2000) studied 631 children of parents with IBS (cases) and 646 matched children (controls) in the database of a large HMO to explore the intergenerational transmission of gastrointestinal illness behavior. Adult patterns of health care use for IBS predicted child visits; case children had significantly more ambulatory care visits for all causes as well as more visits for gastrointestinal symptoms. These patterns were associated with increased health care costs.

DISABILITY AND QUALITY OF LIFE

As with other MUIs, IBS is not associated with excess mortality. A number of large retrospective studies have shown that patients diagnosed with IBS do not go on to develop inflammatory bowel disease, colorectal or other gastrointestinal cancers, or other life-threatening disorders in excess of non-IBS controls. Overall life expectancy for individuals with IBS is as good as (or somewhat better than) that of the population at large. However, IBS is associated with significant levels of disability and impaired quality of life (Hahn, Yan, & Strassels, 1999). Patients with IBS have been shown to have rates of absenteeism from work that are almost 3 times that of non-IBS controls. Likewise, studies have shown that absence from school and work; difficulty in activities of daily living; and the need to modify one's work setting, work fewer hours, or give up one's occupation because of IBS are common consequences. In this respect, patients with IBS differ significantly from patients with many other chronic medical illnesses, and they differ dramatically from controls.

In addition to income and productivity losses associated with IBS, a number of studies have shown, as might be expected, that the health-related quality of life of patients with IBS is significantly lower than that of population-based controls. However, these studies also showed that compared with individuals with rheumatoid arthritis, asthma, diabetes, and gastroesophageal reflux disease, IBS patients showed significantly lower levels of quality of life as measured by the SF-36 Health Survey (El-Serag, Olden, & Bjorkman, 2002; Gralnek, Hays, Kilbourne, Naliboff, & Mayer, 2000). Using the SF-36, Gralnek et al. (2000) compared the health-related quality of life of IBS patients (N = 877) with previously reported SF-36 data for the general U.S. population and for patients with gastroesophageal reflux disease, diabetes mellitus, depression, and dialysis-dependent end-stage renal disease. On all SF-36 scales, IBS patients had significantly worse health-related quality of life than the general population. Compared with patients with gastroesophageal reflux disease, IBS patients scored significantly lower on all scales except physical functioning. Similarly, IBS patients had significantly worse health-related quality of life on selected SF-36 scales than patients with diabetes mellitus and end-stage renal disease. IBS patients did

health SF-36 scale scores than patients with
) studied 104 consecutive patients referred
nts met Rome II diagnostic criteria as deter-
nterologist; the number of overall unhealthy
ated that of patients with cancer and ex-
s, diabetes, heart disease, stroke, or morbid
he dramatic impact that IBS has on quality

GENDER AND IRRITABLE BOWEL SYNDROME

IBS is more prevalent in women. Among individuals with IBS who do not seek care, the number of women is double the number of men (Drossman, Camilleri, Mayer, & Whitehead, 2002). Among individuals who seek care for IBS, the female:male ratio jumps to 4:1 (Mitchell & Drossman, 1987; Toner & Akman, 2000). Gender disparity in IBS may, in part, reflect the general tendency of women to seek medical care for symptoms. However, it is reasonable to assume that most patients with IBS who are seen in clinical practice are women. One community sample of women in England found a prevalence of IBS of almost 23% (Kennedy & Jones, 2000). One often cited study found that in an Indian clinic sample, men outnumbered women (Jain, Gupta, Jajoo, & Sidhwa, 1991), but more international studies are needed to determine whether there is a consistent cross-cultural difference in gender ratios.

Women generally have slower gut transit times than men. E. J. Bennett et al. (2000) used imaging techniques to track the transit time of food through the gastrointestinal track. Their main finding was that for the 110 outpatients with functional gastrointestinal disorders, those with the most widespread delay of gut transit were more likely to be female and older and to have a low level of hypochondriasis, more severe gastric stasis, and high levels of depression and anger control. Those with normal transit were more likely to be male and have high levels of hypochondriasis. E. J. Bennett et al. made the point that gut motor function changes in terms of the function of the whole individual; consequently, depression and controlled anger affect objectively measured gut stasis.

Men and women differ in terms of symptom expression in IBS; men report more diarrhea and women report more bloating, pain, and constipation. Mayer, Berman, Chang, and Naliboff (2004) reviewed sex-based differences in gastrointestinal pain and concluded that there is a common core of IBS symptoms across sexes but that women seem to report a larger number of symptoms. Simren, Abrahamsson, Svedlund, and Bjornsson (2001) examined the impact of gender and bowel patterns on quality of life in IBS patients seen in referral centers versus primary care settings. They found lower quality of life in women and in referral center patients, but they did not find differences in bowel patterns.

Several studies have investigated menstruation and IBS symptomatology. Whitehead, Cheskin, et al. (1990) compared women with and without IBS and found that although 34% of controls reported exacerbations of gas, diarrhea, or constipation during menstruation, the women with IBS were significantly more likely to experience these problems. Self-reports of bowel symptoms during menstruation were not associated with psychological traits or with menses-related changes in affect. Houghton, Lea, Jackson, and Whorwell (2002) compared rectal responses to balloon distension during Days 1 to 4 (menses), 8 to 10 (follicular phase), 18 to 20 (luteal phase), and 24 to 28 (premenstrual phase) of the menstrual cycle in 29 women with IBS. Their data confirmed that IBS symptomatology and rectal sensitivity are exacerbated during menses in women with IBS compared with healthy women. However, anxiety and depression remained unaltered throughout the menstrual cycle.

Although there is extensive literature on gender differences in somatic pain perception (discussed in some detail in chaps. 3 and 4, this volume), there are few studies of gender differences in visceral pain perception. It is a much more common experience for women to experience pain or discomfort in the pelvic region related to menstrual or reproductive system events. Women may be more vigilant regarding sensory input from the pelvic viscera. Lee, Mayer, Schmulson, Chang, and Naliboff (2001) surveyed 714 consecutively screened IBS patients to explore gender differences in reported symptoms. They found that men and women were similar in terms of illness severity, abdominal pain, psychological symptoms, and illness impact. However, women reported more bloating, constipation, nausea, alterations of taste and smell, morning stiffness, and greater food and medication sensitivity. They concluded that these differences in sensitivity may represent altered sensory processes, autonomic responses, and cognitive hypervigilance.

Chang and Heitkemper (2003) concluded in a review of IBS that no differences have been found in healthy controls in perception of visceral stimuli. In contrast, research has found that women with IBS show enhanced colorectal perception compared with men with IBS, particularly after a visceral stressor.

S. Berman et al. (2000) performed positron emission tomography scans on men and women with IBS who were undergoing moderately aversive rectal pressure. They found that despite similar ratings of stimulus intensity and discomfort, men displayed stronger regional activation of anterior cingulate, prefrontal cortex, thalamus, and cerebellum. Rectal pressure activated the insula bilaterally in men but not in women. The insula receives extensive visceral input and also plays a role in autonomic responding and emotional processing. The authors speculated that the gender differences may be due to greater variability of insula activation in women because of hormonal fluctuation or differences in the processing of emotional content; further investigation is required to address these issues.

Naliboff et al. (2001) performed a positron emission tomography study with 26 female and 24 male nonconstipated patients undergoing a visceral stimulus (moderate rectal inflation) and a psychological stimulus (anticipation of noxious visceral distension). Although there was overlap, this imaging study showed differences between men and women in both conditions. Men with IBS showed greater activation of cognitive areas (dorsolateral prefrontal cortex) and central autonomic areas (insula, periaqueductal gray) and inhibition of limbic regions (amygdala, infragenual cingulated) during the stressors, whereas women showed greater activation of autonomic regions (ventromedial prefrontal cortex, infragenual cingulate, amygdala).

Noting that the female predominance in IBS may be partially due to hormonal influences, Houghton, Jackson, Whorwell, and Morris (2000) investigated whether testosterone mediated some protection from IBS by comparing 50 male patients with IBS with 25 control men. There was a significantly lower level of luteinizing hormone in men with IBS relative to controls, which corroborates the dysfunction of the hypothalamic–pituitary axis found in other studies. Although findings for testosterone were equivocal, luteinizing hormone may play a role in IBS by stimulating hormones detrimental in women (estrogen, progesterone) and protective in men (testosterone).

Although there is more research on gender differences in IBS than on any other MUI, it is clear that there are many unanswered questions. The female preponderance, male and female physiological and behavioral responses to stress, the role of hormones in pathophysiology of IBS, and male and female mechanisms of bowel symptoms are still not understood (Chang & Heitkemper, 2003).

GENDER ROLE AND IRRITABLE BOWEL SYNDROME

Several investigators have examined the association of typical feminine gender role characteristics and illness behavior in IBS. Clinical observation had revealed that IBS patients appear to exhibit certain stereotypically feminine traits such as nurturing, putting others' needs first, suppressing anger, being servile, and seeking approval from others (Ali et al., 1998; Toner, 1995; Toner & Akman, 2000). These gender role behaviors were found to be associated with strong disease conviction in a study by Ali et al. (1998), who examined 34 women and 16 men with IBS on the Communal Femininity subscale of the Personal Attributes Questionnaire (Spence, Helmreich, & Stapp, 1974) and found significant positive correlations between disease conviction and general hypochondriasis. The relationship between stereotypically feminine subordination and the conviction that physical disease accounts for IBS symptoms was significant for male as well as female participants. Thus, it may be, as Toner and Akman (2000) have suggested, that women and men with IBS are more similar than different. The feminine gender role (rather than female sex) is influential in affecting illness attributions. Toner and Akman proposed that the connection between feminine gender role and disease conviction could come from focusing on others' needs, which leads to neglect of self, and that this lack of self-nurturance exacerbates stress. The distressing symptoms of IBS cannot be ignored, but IBS patients who go to specialists tend to selectively attend to physiological symptoms and are less likely to acknowledge stress than are individuals with IBS who do not see gastrointestinal specialists (Toner, 1994). Strong disease convictions also contribute to high levels of doctor shopping to confirm somatic attributions.

Dancey, Hutton-Young, Moye, and Devins (2002) studied psychosocial burdens in 63 women and 54 men with IBS. They found that with increased illness intrusiveness, quality of life declined more rapidly among men compared with women. This could be because men have different coping skills and are more distressed by lifestyle disruptions and restrictions on personal freedom than women. Dancey et al. (2002) also suggested that the belief that IBS is mostly a woman's disorder may make the lifestyle disruptions more acceptable to women than men.

Ali et al. (2000) investigated whether emotional abuse was associated with IBS over and above the association of physical and sexual abuse with IBS. Their study investigated the presence of emotional abuse, self-blame, and self-silencing in a sample of 25 women with IBS compared with 25 women with inflammatory bowel disease. They found that the IBS group reported significantly higher levels of emotional abuse, self-blame, and self-silencing than the inflammatory bowel disease group. It is interesting that depressive symptoms did not correlate significantly with emotional abuse, self-blame, or self-silencing in either sample. Ali et al. speculated that women who experience emotional abuse may be more likely to develop response patterns of self-blame and self-silencing. These response patterns may increase stress, which has been shown to be an important exacerbating factor in IBS.

Blanchard, Keefer, Galovski, Taylor, and Turner (2001) sought to determine where there was a gender difference in psychological distress in IBS. They used dimensional measures, the Beck Depression Inventory, the State–Trait Anxiety Inventory, and the Minnesota Multiphasic Personality Inventory (MMPI) as well as categorical *Diagnostic and Statistical Manual of Mental Disorders* (3rd ed., rev. [DSM–III–R]; American Psychiatric Association, 1987) diagnoses. The women (n = 238) were significantly more depressed and trait anxious than the men (n = 83), but they did not differ on state anxiety. Women scored significantly higher on the Depression and Hysteria scales of the MMPI, whereas men scored significantly higher on the Mania scale. There were no significant gender differences on any *DSM–III–R* Axis I disorder; a total of 66% had at least one Axis I disorder. The most frequently occurring disorders were Generalized Anxiety Disorder, Social Phobia, Dysthymia, and

Panic Disorder with Agoraphobia. Because there were no differences in diagnosable psychiatric disorders, and the differences on dimensional measures were small, Blanchard et al. argued that their data do not support the idea that the higher prevalence of IBS among women is explained by more neurosis than men that drives health care seeking.

PATHOPHYSIOLOGY

IBS involves both diffuse smooth muscle dysmotility and lower visceral pain thresholds. Because there is no correlation between motility and pain perception, these symptoms are thought to be mediated through two separate mechanisms (Clauw, 1994). The finding that IBS patients experience pain and bloating at lower levels of balloon inflation in the rectum and lower bowel than do controls has been replicated in numerous studies, and the concept of "visceral" hypersensitivity has been postulated (Mertz, Naliboff, Munakata, Niazi, & Mayer, 1995).

In an important study, Whitehead, Holtkotter, et al. (1990) discovered that after balloon distention in the rectum, individuals suffering from IBS were more sensitive to distention than were individuals from a variety of comparison groups. Tolerance for stepwise distention of a balloon in the sigmoid colon was compared with tolerance for holding one hand in ice water in 16 IBS patients, 10 patients with functional bowel disorder who did not meet criteria for IBS, 25 lactose malabsorbers, and 18 asymptomatic controls. IBS patients had significantly lower tolerance for balloon distention but not ice water, and balloon tolerance was not correlated with neuroticism or other measured psychological traits. Whitehead, Holtkotter, et al. proposed a peripheral–visceral mechanism such as altered receptor sensitivity as the cause of distention pain in IBS patients.

However, not all IBS study participants showed hypersensitivity; it was found most reliably when using ascending stimuli wherein individuals anticipate greater discomfort as the magnitude of stimuli increase predictably. Because hypersensitivity is less likely to be found when rectal pressures are unpredictable, Naliboff, Chang, et al. (2000) have surmised that there is strong evidence for hypervigilance for visceral sensations influenced by fear and anticipation, whereas hypersensitivity caused by true sensory alterations is less consistently found. Generally, noxious sigmoid colon stimulation causes hypersensitivity in patients with IBS but not in controls.

These findings indicate that under certain conditions individuals with IBS have a unique local rectal response to visceral stimulation. Neuroimaging studies have also shown that a visceral stimulus (e.g., rectal distention) is processed in the brain differently than in non-IBS controls. Neuroimaging studies have shown that compared with controls, IBS patients have differential responses in the anterior cingulate cortex (ACC) and other areas of the brain when stimulated with rectal or sigmoid colon distention (Mertz et al., 1995, 2000; Silverman et al., 1997). The ACC is a cerebral cortical area that is rich in opiate receptors and is thought to be a major component of cognitive circuits relating to perception as well as descending spinal pathways involving pain. Silverman et al. (1997) found that in healthy individuals, perception of pain during actual or simulated delivery of painful stimuli was significantly associated with activity of the ACC, whereas no ACC response to perception of nonpainful stimuli was observed. However, in patients with IBS, the ACC did not respond to the same stimuli, whereas significant activation of the left prefrontal cortex was seen. Thus, the perception of acute rectal pain is associated with activation of the ACC in healthy individuals, and patients with IBS show an aberrant brain activation pattern both during noxious rectal distention and during the anticipation of rectal pain.

Mayer et al. (2005) found that certain areas of the ACC were activated in IBS. They compared men with ulcerative colitis, IBS patients, and controls using regional cerebral blood flow (analyzed in positron emission tomography scans) during actual and anticipated (but undelivered) rectal distensions. No differences in anterior insula or dorsal ACC were found. However, IBS patients showed greater activation of the limbic and paralimbic brain areas (amygdale, hypothalamus, ventral/rostral ACC, dorsolateral prefrontal cortex), indicating increased activation of pain pathways in IBS.

The enteric nervous system acts directly on effector systems such as smooth muscles, endocrine cells, and blood vessels, facilitating serotonin-mediated secretion and motility. However, the parasympathetic and sympathetic nervous systems have a pivotal role in gastrointestinal function through autonomic integrative processes that facilitate the brain–gut interaction (Gershon, 1999). The discovery of altered processing of neural sensation in IBS patients has led to the search for the specific neurotransmitters involved in this abnormal signal transmission. Serotonin has provoked the greatest research attention because it influences motility, visceral perception, and secretion in the gut. The pervasive role of serotonin in normal and pathological gastrointestinal conditions is apparent in its pattern of distribution: 95% of serotonin in the body is in the gastrointestinal tract, and approximately 5% is localized in the brain (Gershon, 1999; Talley, 1992).

Modulation of serotonin action in the gut could influence IBS and other functional bowel symptoms. The subtypes of serotonin contained in the gut consist mainly of $5\text{-}HT_3$ and $5\text{-}HT_4$, thus, drugs have been developed that are designed specifically to act on these serotonin subtypes. Cholecystokinin antagonists to block cholecystokinin and neurokinin are also being investigated for their potential to influence IBS symptoms (D'Amato, Labum, & Whorwell, 1999).

Collectively, these data suggest the possibility of a "brain–gut axis," where peripheral symptoms are processed in the end organ (i.e. the colon), and then neural signals are carried via visceral afferents to the spinal cord and then to the brain, where they are subject to additional processing that can influence descending pathways (Mertz, 2002; Talley, 1992). This bidirectional pathway is modulated by a number of neurotransmitters; cholecystokinin, enkephalins, serotonin, and corticotropin-releasing factor. Visceral signals from the gut ascend to the midbrain, thalamus, limbic system, and somatosensory cortex. The somatosensory cortex registers the location and intensity of pain, whereas the limbic system (ACC, insula, medial thalamus) mediates the affective and motivational aspects of pain. The limbic system can activate the descending endorphin analgesic system to the dorsal horn of the spinal cord and up or down regulate incoming visceral signals (Halpert & Drossman, 2005). Uncovering differential activation of the brain–gut axis in IBS relative to various comparison groups appears to indicate that pain is experienced more intensely in IBS.

Mayer et al. (2004) summarized the perceptual findings in IBS as follows:

1. IBS is associated with hypersensitivity in the upper gastrointestinal tract and the colon.
2. IBS is associated with heightened perception of normal intestinal contractions.
3. IBS (unlike FMS) is not associated with a generalized hypersensitivity to noxious somatic stimulation (I. J. Cook, van Eeden, & Collins, 1987; Whitehead, Holtkotter, et al., 1990).
4. Perception of colonic distensions can be modified by attention, anxiety, and relaxation.

Because IBS is associated with an exaggerated response to stress, Sagami et al. (2004) investigated whether a corticotropin-releasing hormone (CRH) receptor antagonist would reduce IBS symptoms. They administered the CRH antagonist intravenously to 10 diarrhea-predominant IBS patients and 10 healthy controls. The CRH antagonist successfully suppressed motility induced by rectal electrical stimulation, abdominal pain, and anxiety in IBS patients but not in controls. The authors concluded that the CRH pathway must be involved in the mechanism of increased colonic motility to stimuli in IBS.

PSYCHOLOGICAL DISORDERS

A number of studies have documented high rates of Axis I disorders in people with IBS. Studies using the Diagnostic Interview Schedule (Robins, Cottler, & Keating, 1991) and standardized criteria for IBS (Manning, Rome I, or Rome II criteria) have found lifetime rates of psychiatric disorders at 90% or higher in patients with IBS (Lydiard, Fossey, Marsh, & Ballenger, 1993; Walker et al., 1990; Woodman et al., 1998). In these samples, about 80% of the patients in the IBS group were women. The most common psychiatric diagnosis in these studies was major depression, followed by anxiety disorders. Woodman et al. (1998) found a high percentage of substance use disorders (35%). It is important to note that it is past history of Axis I disorders that is so high rather than current psychiatric disorder. Active psychiatric disorder has been found in only about 25% of participants. After summarizing findings regarding depression, anxiety, and somatization in IBS, Manu (2004) concluded that the severity of somatization phenomena predicts the burden of psychopathology and psychological distress in IBS.

The high rates of psychiatric disorders in IBS have been based largely on patients who present to referral centers for care. In a general community cohort, Talley, Howell, and Poulton (2001) investigated the rate of psychiatric disorders in 26-year-old adults ($N = 890$) in New Zealand. Prevalence of IBS was assessed, with 12.7% meeting the Manning and 4.3% meeting the Rome II criteria. Although prevalence rates were somewhat higher in women, this difference was not significant. It is important to note that diagnosis of IBS was not associated with a Diagnostic Interview Schedule DSM–III–R (American Psychiatric Association, 1987) psychiatric diagnosis. They did not separate out consulters from nonconsulters for IBS symptoms in this study. Although some studies have found people with gastrointestinal symptoms in general to be more neurotic and anxious, it is likely that psychological distress increases consulting behavior (Drossman et al., 1988; Whitehead et al., 1988).

In a study of 709 college students, Hazlett-Stevens, Craske, Mayer, Chang, and Naliboff (2003) found that 11% met Rome II criteria for IBS. As in the Talley et al. (2001) study, women predominated, but gender differences were not significant. It is possible that increasing female predominance in IBS develops later in the life course. In this group, Hazlett-Stevens et al. found a significant association between IBS and anxiety-related measures of worry, neuroticism, anxiety sensitivity, and generalized anxiety disorder. There was a particularly strong association between IBS and anxiety about visceral sensations. Hazlett-Stevens et al. speculated that a vicious cycle may develop, with fears about gastrointestinal sensations leading to increased vigilance toward these sensations and the visceral sensations increasing as a result of anxiety and vigilance, leading to greater fear and avoidance of gastrointestinal sensations and situations associated with them.

A. R. Miller et al. (2001) explored psychiatric symptoms and illness behavior in IBS in relation to SD. A total of 50 outpatients with IBS or ulcerative colitis were evaluated with the Diagnostic Interview Schedule and Illness Behavior Questionnaire in a university-based office setting. Although no ulcerative colitis patients were diagnosed with SD, 42% of IBS patients met criteria for SD. IBS patients with SD, but not those without SD, reported more psychiatric symptoms and abnormal illness behaviors than did ulcerative colitis patients. Thus, comorbidity with SD accounted for the association of psychiatric symptoms with IBS.

Emmanuel, Mason, and Kamm (2001) examined the relationship between psychological factors and gut innervation in women with functional gut disorders. Women with constipation had greater levels of anxiety, depression, and somatization and felt "less feminine" compared with healthy controls. The more impaired the score on psychological testing, the lower the mucosal blood flow reading, suggesting a link between psychological state and gut function.

Whitehead et al. (2002) found that among IBS patients with other comorbid MUIs, psychiatric disorders were higher than in those with just IBS. This fits in with the patterns of somatizing and doctor shopping that separate consulters from nonconsulters. Thus, those who meet criteria for IBS and other MUIs are more likely to be vigilant about symptoms, be distressed by symptoms, and seek treatment for symptoms. It is the consulters who present the impact on the health care system and are most likely to need psychological treatment. Hersbach, Henrich, and von Rad (1999) summarized the difference between nonconsulters and consulters by saying that nonconsulters with IBS tend not to differ from controls (healthy individuals or individuals with organic disorders); conversely, consulters with IBS have more psychopathology, more fear of "serious illness," more health complaints, and are more affected by stress than nonconsulters.

Whitehead et al. (2003) performed a large, comprehensive study designed to overcome the methodological pitfalls of previous examinations of psychiatric prevalence in IBS, such as small sample, inappropriate controls, and tertiary care settings. They matched 3,153 patients with IBS to 571 patients with inflammatory bowel disease and to 3,153 individuals without gastrointestinal diagnosis and examined the psychiatric diagnoses in the electronic records of a large HMO. The presence of at least one psychiatric diagnosis was found for 51.2% of IBS patients, 21.4% of inflammatory bowel disease patients, and 29.1% of controls. The most prevalent diagnoses were depression, stress reaction, and anxiety. In summary, in IBS clinic and treatment trial samples that used standardized psychological assessment through interview, about half of the patients met criteria for psychiatric disorder.

ILLNESS BEHAVIOR

Dancey et al. (2002) examined illness intrusiveness in IBS and found that the burden in IBS was similar to that seen in more serious disorders such as rheumatoid arthritis, bipolar disorder, and end stage renal disease. Crane and Martin (2004) found that individuals with IBS have a perception of increased susceptibility to unrelated health threats (deep vein thrombosis, arthritis, bowel cancer) but not to nonhealth risks. This perception may increase illness behaviors and partly explain the overlap with other MUIs.

Koloski, Boyce, and Talley (2005) examined the correlates of health care seeking in IBS and functional dyspepsia in an Australian population-based survey. They found that there were no differences between consulters and nonconsulters in social learning of abnormal illness behaviors such as encouragement, reinforcement of the sick role, and modeling of illness behavior. The only important factor predicting IBS or functional dyspepsia status was disease conviction, which operated independently of age, gender, psychiatric diagnoses, and symptom severity. Other studies of determinants of health care consulting have found symptom severity and fears of serious illness to be the most important predictors. Similarly, M. Martin and Crane (2003) found that attributional style was key to consulting versus nonconsulting for IBS symptoms among university students. Treatment seekers were more likely to make somatic attributions for gastrointestinal symptoms as well as physiological symptoms usually characteristic of depression and anxiety than nonconsulters.

To summarize the differences between those who consult for IBS symptoms and those who do not, IBS consulters display increased illness behavior, greater psychological distress, more fears of serious illness, and more overlap with other MUIs. They are also more likely to be women.

CHILDHOOD SEXUAL ABUSE

A number of studies have documented the high prevalence of reported childhood sexual abuse in individuals with IBS (Blanchard et al., 2004; Drossman et al., 1990; Walker et al., 1990; Walker, Katon, Roy-Byrne, Jemelka, & Russo, 1993). Drossman, Talley, Leserman, Olden, and Barreiro (1995) found that generally about one third of women with IBS report a history of sexual abuse. Drossman et al. (1990) conducted a survey of consecutive women patients seen in a gastroenterology practice over a 2-month period. Compared with patients with organic disease, patients with functional bowel disorders (including IBS, dyspepsia, chronic pelvic pain, and constipation) reported significantly more experiences of sexual exposure, threatened sex, incest, rape, and physical abuse.

In a controlled study using a structured psychiatric interview (abridged DIS), Walker et al. (1993) examined sexual victimization in 28 IBS patients compared with 19 inflammatory bowel disease patients. The IBS group had significantly higher rates of lifetime history of severe sexual victimization (with *severe* defined as any form of penetration). All of the individuals with IBS who had experienced sexual victimization were women. Compared with IBS patients with no sexual trauma, those with severe trauma had more medically unexplained symptoms, anxiety symptoms, and psychiatric diagnoses.

Drossman, Li, Leserman, Toomey, and Hu (1996) evaluated 239 female outpatients at gastroenterology clinics in North Carolina and found that on interview, 60% reported a history of physical or sexual abuse. There was no difference in prevalence of abuse between those with functional as opposed to structural disease. Regardless of diagnosis, those with self-reported abuse reported more pain and more disability than those not reporting abuse. Talley and Boyce (1996) argued that the Drossman et al. study was subject to selection bias. They also asked whether self-reported abuse identifies people who are "positive reporters" and who are more predisposed to distress. Additionally, there is a need to define abuse more clearly; the Drossman et al. study encompassed a wide range of experiences; however, it appears that the context of the abuse is critical—that is, whether it is a single episode or repeated episodes, how severe the abuse is, and whether there is emotional support for the victim.

Talley, Boyce, and Jones (1998) performed a population-based survey of 730 individuals and found that 12% met Rome II criteria, with significantly more women meeting the criteria than men. They explored the association between IBS, abuse, and psychological disturbance. Almost half of the respondents reported some abuse history, and abuse was associated with IBS. However, after they controlled for neuroticism and psychological morbidity, there was no significant link between childhood abuse and IBS.

Selected symptoms associated with abuse were examined by Leserman, Li, Drossman, and Hu (1998) in 239 women from a gastroenterology clinic with a variety of organic and functional gastrointestinal disorders. Leserman et al. found that women with sexual and physical abuse histories were much more likely to report panic; depression; skin rashes; and musculoskeletal, genito–urinary, and respiratory symptoms. As in other studies, a dose–response effect was observed, with a more severe abuse history associated with more symptoms, greater health care use, and worse functional disability.

Reilly, Baker, Rhodes, and Salmon (1999) examined the association of sexual and physical abuse in patients presenting with IBS and nonepileptic attack disorder and compared them with organic (Crohn's disease and epilepsy, respectively) control groups. Although presenting with very different symptom profiles, the IBS and nonepileptic attack disorder groups recalled more sexual and physical abuse, both as children and adults, than their controls. The IBS and nonepileptic attack disorder groups were also very similar in terms of higher anxiety and depression, stronger disease conviction, somatization symptoms, and poorer social function than their respective comparison groups.

A model for the relationship between early abuse and gastrointestinal disorders was developed by Scarinci, McDonald-Hale, Bradley, and Richter (1994) using sensory decision theory tasks. Early traumatic stress can lead an individual to develop hypervigilance, which results in low response bias and low pain thresholds. Hypervigilance may predispose patients to experience symptoms as more salient; the past trauma may make physical symptoms more threatening. Scarinci et al. demonstrated, among patients with gastroesophageal reflux disease, noncardiac chest pain, and IBS, that abused patients had significantly lower pain thresholds to finger pressure stimulation; lower cognitive standards for judging stimuli as noxious; higher levels of functional disability; and a greater number of psychological disorders, daily hassles, and other pain syndromes than their nonabused counterparts. In terms of treatment implications, patients with an abuse history more frequently blamed themselves for their pain and were more likely to use maladaptive pain strategies. Self-blame is common in abuse victims, and this tendency, combined with multiple painful symptoms, appears to engender catastrophic coping responses, hopelessness, disability, and doctor shopping to achieve ever-elusive relief. Medicinal treatment, however, is unlikely to relieve their symptoms. Drossman et al. (2000) found that among 239 women referred for gastrointestinal disorders, catastrophizing, low perceived ability to decrease symptoms, and a history of abuse significantly predicted poor outcome over a 1-year follow-up period. These findings are consistent with the Scarinci et al. model.

Numerous studies have documented that individuals with IBS who have an abuse history have worse outcomes than those without such a history. Creed, Guthrie, et al. (2005) assessed 257 patients with severe IBS and found that 12.1% reported a history of rape and 11% reported forced touching. Those who reported abuse were more impaired on pain and physical function scales of the SF-36. They found that the association between abuse history and impaired functioning was mediated by somatization tendencies. The good news was that those with an abuse history also got the most out of therapy. In a 15-month trial of psychotherapy and paroxetine, Creed et al. (2003) found the greatest beneficial response in those with abuse history, particularly those with a reported history of rape.

Several studies have found that women with IBS and no history of abuse have lower pain thresholds than women with a history of abuse (Ringel et al., 2004; Whitehead, Crowell, Davidoff, Palsson, & Schuster, 1997). Whitehead et al. (1997) suggested that lower pain thresholds are due to perceptual response bias. Thus, modifying the psychological processes that affect pain perception may be more effective than drug therapies. These studies indicate that the greater pain reporting and poorer health status in IBS patients with abuse history are not related to increased rectal pain sensitivity.

Guthrie et al. (2003) performed a cluster analysis to differentiate subgroups in 107 treatment-resistant individuals with IBS. They investigated the relationship between symptoms, psychological variables, and rectal sensitivity and produced three clinically meaningful subgroups. The three groups were not different in terms of age, sex, type of IBS, or symptom severity as measured by daily diary. Group I was called "distressed high utilizers" because they had low rectal distension discomfort thresholds, highest prevalence of a history of childhood sexual abuse, higher doctor consultations, more psychiatric diagnoses, more interpersonal problems, and higher unemployment. Group II, "distressed low utilizers," also had low distension thresholds and high prevalence of psychiatric disorders but a lower prevalence of childhood sexual abuse, less disability, and less consulting behavior. Group III, "tolerant low utilizers," consisted of patients with high distension thresholds; they were constipation predominant, had lower levels of psychological and interpersonal problems, and low consultation rates. This study illustrates the complex interaction between past trauma, distress, pain thresholds, functioning, and help seeking.

The prior studies demonstrate that a significant percentage of people with IBS are likely to report a history of sexual and physical abuse and that they tend to have worse health outcomes than those without reports of such abuse. Salmon, Skaife, and Rhodes (2003) attempted to implicate dissociation as a mechanism that could link abuse history to IBS. Specifically, they examined the role of dissociation in explaining the relationship between abuse and somatization, and then they looked at whether somatization could, in turn, explain the relationship of abuse and dissociation to IBS. They compared 67 outpatients with IBS with 61 patients with Crohn's disease or ulcerative colitis. They developed a regression model that found increased dissociation was associated with abuse and could account statistically for the link between childhood sexual abuse and somatization. This study also found that individuals with IBS recalled more sexual abuse as adults, more physical abuse as children, and more psychological abuse as adults than those in the organic disease group. Only childhood sexual abuse and adult psychological abuse were uniquely associated with IBS (Salmon et al., 2003).

When discussing high rates of childhood sexual abuse in IBS patients, studies have almost exclusively relied on retrospective reports of such a history. Raphael, Spatz Widom, and Lange (2001) conducted a prospective study on documented childhood sexual and physical abuse and neglect and unexplained pain complaints. Surprisingly, they found that reporting one or more unexplained pain symptoms was not associated with any childhood victimization experience. Their findings indicate that explaining MUIs as expressions of past trauma through current symptoms is too simplistic. Lackner, Gudleski, and Blanchard (2004) also contended that investigators need to move "beyond abuse," because an emphasis on severe stressors may overlook the importance of less extreme parenting variables in influencing somatic complaints. Lackner et al. investigated whether negative parenting behaviors may be more strongly associated with IBS symptoms than abuse-specific factors in 81 consecutively evaluated IBS patients (70 women, 11 men). They found that although both abuse and a negative, rejecting parenting style were correlated, only parenting style correlated with somatization. They argued that their findings were consistent with stress physiology and abuse research, which has found that family social climate is a stronger predictor of adult health issues than abuse-specific variables. Although the abuse is certainly related to IBS, the extent to which it influences adult health may be molded by day-to-day parental nurturance. As discussed in great detail in chapters 3 and 4, this volume, there is substantial evidence that early caregiving influences stress reactivity, brain function, and pain processing.

CONCLUSION

Although various physiologic and psychological mechanisms are implicated in IBS, no one mechanism explains the majority of patients with IBS (Whitehead et al., 2002). The biopsychosocial model applied to IBS has been explicated by Drossman (1998, 1999), who maintained that (a) many factors contribute to symptom development, (b) no one factor is necessary to develop IBS, and (c) factors interact in different combinations. Thus, in some patients, higher levels of stress predict who develops IBS after a bout of gastroenteritis, whereas patients with a low sensory threshold are more susceptible to gastrointestinal pain in IBS (Whitehead et al., 2002). Whitehead et al. (2002) also suggested that people with IBS with comorbid MUIs have somatization tendencies and predominantly psychological etiology, whereas those without comorbid conditions and few excess symptoms are more likely to have a physiologic etiology for IBS. The female predominance in IBS is likely due to a number of biopsychosocial factors. Women's higher levels of somatic reporting, higher rates of a history of childhood sexual abuse, different brain–gut axis, and sensitivity could all be important contributors.

6

FIBROMYALGIA

Fibromyalgia syndrome (FMS) is a common rheumatic disorder characterized by chronic, widespread pain that does not radiate from a particular region of the body. The term *fibrositis* was used for the same condition before *fibromyalgia* became the accepted label in the 1990s. *Chronic widespread pain* is another rubric seen in the literature, and fibromyalgia is often viewed as existing on a continuum of chronic widespread pain (Gran, 2003); others view FMS as a distinct disorder (Russell, 1999).

DIAGNOSIS

The diagnosis of FMS is based on a history of at least 3 consecutive months of widespread bilateral pain. The pain is in response to stimuli not normally considered painful (*allodynia*), as well as a reduced threshold for reporting pain (*hyperalgesia*; Price & Staud, 2005; Staud, 2005). The pain must be accompanied by excessive tenderness on application of pressure to at least 11 of 18 muscle–tendon sites (tender points) during clinical examination (Wolfe et al., 1990; see Exhibit 6.1 and Figure 6.1). These American College of Rheumatology (ACR) 1990 classification criteria (Wolfe et al., 1990) for the diagnosis of fibromyalgia provide a sensitivity (88%) and speci-

EXHIBIT 6.1
American College of Rheumatology Criteria for Fibromyalgia

1. Widespread muscular and joint pain for over 3 months. Pain is bilateral and appears above and below the waist.
2. Extreme tenderness in 18 specific "tender points." Digital palpation should be performed with an approximate force of 4 kilograms. For a tender point to be considered positive, the subject must state that palpation was "painful."

Patients will be classified as having FMS if both criteria are satisfied.

Note. Data from Wolfe et al. (1990, p. 171).

ficity (81%) in differentiating FMS from other forms of chronic musculoskeletal pain. Sleep disturbance, fatigue, and morning stiffness are common in FMS, but these symptoms do not distinguish the syndrome as reliably as widespread pain and tender points. The ACR criteria have been useful in guiding research, although FMS remains a controversial disorder, with debate surrounding its etiology and treatment.

No definitive physical findings or laboratory or imaging abnormalities exist in FMS. A number of nonpain symptoms commonly occur in FMS, including morning stiffness, nonrestorative sleep, headache, numbness, chilliness, low blood pressure, mood and cognitive problems, fatigue, and bowel problems (Hazlett & Haynes, 1992; Neeck, 2002). These symptoms can be modulated by activity, weather, and stress (Goodnick & Sandoval, 1993). Clauw (1994) noted that the multiple nonrheumatic symptoms associated with FMS can be clustered into cohorts of patients with (a) primary neurologic symptoms (sleep disturbances, paresthesias, cognitive and mood problems); (b) primary smooth muscle dysmotility (bowel and bladder symptoms, migraine); (c) increased skeletal tone (myalgias, temporomandibular disorder, tension headache); and (d) inflammatory symptoms (cystitis, rhinitis, pharyngitis).

One of the distinguishing characteristics of FMS is the presence of tender points. The presence of tender points is associated with psychological distress and a tendency toward increased medical utilization (McBeth, Macfarlane, Benjamin, Morris, & Silman, 1999). A high tender point count is associated with intermediate levels of fatigue; low levels of self-care; and reports of more somatic symptoms, more medical consultations, and psychological symptoms (McBeth et al., 1999). Researchers have also found that individuals with a high tender point count are more likely to have been exposed to childhood adversity, such as abuse or parental loss.

Common assessment measures for individuals with FMS in clinical practice and research paradigms are tender point and dolorimeter evaluation. Tender points are generally assessed by manual palpation of the 18 tender points specified by the ACR (see Figure 6.1). Individuals indicate when they first feel pain (not just pressure), and the sum of positive tender points is reported. Dolorimetry is generally conducted with a pressure algometer, which

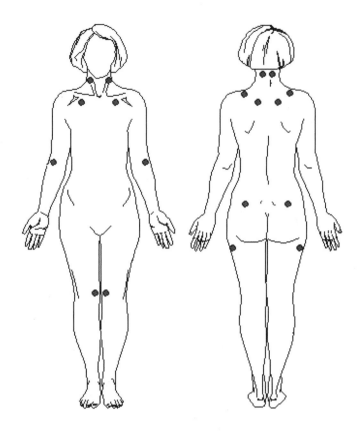

Figure 6.1. Eighteen tender point sites. Digital palpation should be performed with an approximate force of 4 kilograms. A tender point has to be painful at palpation, not just "tender." From *Diagnosing Fibromyalgia Syndrome*, by We Are FMily (2002). Copyright 2002 by Tigi Higgins. Reprinted with permission.

applies pressure uniformly to tender points and control points. Pressure is applied at a rate of 1 kilogram/second, and individuals also indicate when they first feel pain.

The course of FMS varies from individual to individual. Fluctuating, intermittent symptoms characterize the course for some individuals. For many individuals with FMS, however, the syndrome follows a progressive course, with symptoms worsening over time and with few or no periods of remission (Boissevain & McCain, 1991a, 1991b).

PREVALENCE

Fibromyalgia is the most common cause of chronic, widespread muscular pain. Six to 10 million Americans meet the classification criteria for FMS; as many as 10% of women aged 50 to 60 may be affected (Meisler, 2000). In the overall population, it has been estimated that 3.4% of women and 0.5% of men have FMS (Wolfe, Ross, Anderson, & Russell, 1995). Given these numbers, most FMS patient visits are to the primary care physician, whereas specialists provide care for about 20% of Americans with FMS (Goldenberg, 1995). Weir et al. (2006) recently conducted a population-based retrospective cohort study of 62,000 enrollees in a nationwide health insurance claims database. Cases of FMS were identified from 1997 through 2002. Weir et al. found that female preponderance was not as substantial as reported in previous studies, although incidence was 6.9 cases per 1,000 person years for men and 11.3 cases per 1,000 person years for women. Patients with FMS were 2 to 7 times more likely to be diagnosed with one or more of the examined comorbid conditions: chronic fatigue syndrome (CFS), irritable bowel syndrome (IBS), depression, anxiety, headache, systemic lupus erythematosus, and rheumatoid arthritis.

FMS is primarily an illness of middle age. However, adolescents, particularly female teenagers, may present with symptoms of FMS, and initial attempts have been made to classify a disorder called *juvenile primary fibromyalgia syndrome* (Kashikar-Zuch, Graham, Huenefeld, & Powers, 2000). Nevertheless, the median age of onset for fibromyalgia is between the ages 29 and 37, whereas the average age of diagnosis is between the ages of 34 and 54. The gap between these medians indicates that it generally takes several years before an appropriate diagnosis is made (Boissevain & McCain, 1991a). One reason for the delay may be that some patients are mistakenly diagnosed with connective tissue disorders. Additionally, some physicians may be hesitant to assign a diagnosis of FMS because they perceive that the label may precipitate illness behavior or learned helplessness. K. P. White, Nielson, Harth, Ostbye, and Speechley (2002) explored prospectively whether labeling with FMS has adverse effects on outcome. They surveyed southwestern Ontario residents using random digit dialing and identified 100 individuals who met criteria for FMS by screening 3,395 adults. Only 28 had already been diagnosed, all of them women, and 14 of those newly diagnosed were men. White et al. then compared those who had a prior label with the newly labeled at study entry and at 18- and 36-month follow-up points. Although those carrying a preexistent diagnosis at baseline were clinically worse than the undiagnosed, those assigned and informed of their FMS label did not worsen over time. It appears that the label of FMS did not adversely affect clinical course or health care utilization, so fears of learned helplessness may be unfounded.

OVERLAP WITH OTHER MEDICALLY UNEXPLAINED ILLNESSES

Rheumatologists continue to argue over whether FMS is a distinct disorder (Hadler, 2003; Malleson, 2002). No sharp boundaries distinguish FMS from other functional disorders such as CFS, IBS, or muscular headaches

(Aaron & Buchwald, 2001). Although FMS is the only diagnosis that re-quires tender points on examination, many patients with these other condi-tions also feel pain in tender point areas. In many patients who meet the criteria for diagnosis for CFS, the only difference between them and a typical FMS patient is the degree of pain. Seventy percent of patients with FMS meet the criteria of the Centers for Disease Control and Prevention for CFS (Aaron & Buchwald, 2003; Buchwald, Goldenberg, Sullivan, & Komaroff, 1987), and 66% of patients with CFS meet the ACR criteria for FMS (Goldenberg, 1989a). It seems unlikely that these patients have two separate disease processes. Perhaps dividing these two groups of patients on the basis of whether they have prominent pain is as artificial as division on the basis of prominence of any other associated symptoms. In summarizing studies of FMS overlap with other medically unexplained illnesses (MUIs), Aaron and Buchwald (2003) found that the greatest overlap was with CFS (21%–80%), IBS (32%–80%), temporomandibular disorder (75%), headache (10%–80%), multiple chemical sensitivity (33%–55%), interstitial cystitis (13%–21%), and chronic pelvic pain (18%).

Veale, Kavanagh, Fielding, and Fitzgerald, (1991) examined overlap in groups of patients with FMS and IBS compared with healthy and disease control populations. They studied four patient groups (those with FMS, IBS, inflammatory arthritis, and inflammatory bowel disease) and controls. There were 20 people in each group. Seventy percent of the FMS patients had IBS, and 65% of the IBS patients had FMS. In the disease control groups, 12% met FMS criteria and 10% met IBS criteria. Clearly, there is consistently strong evidence that FMS overlaps substantially with CFS, IBS, temporo-mandibular disorders, and headache. When people with FMS also meet cri-teria for other MUIs, they obviously have a number of additional symptoms, but they also have been found to have greater impairment, disability, dis-tress, and economic problems than those with only the FMS diagnosis (Wolfe et al., 1997a). Aaron and Buchwald (2003) hypothesized that the best expla-nation for the overlap is that both a genetic predisposition and environmen-tal triggers alter the balance between hypothalamic–pituitary–adrenal (HPA) axis, autonomic nervous system, and pain processing.

PROGNOSIS

Although FMS is generally viewed as a chronic condition, outcomes for FMS have varied across studies, with some finding significant improve-ment or remission over time and others finding very little improvement. Granges, Zilko, and Littlejohn (1994) assessed the outcome of patients with FMS who were diagnosed and treated with minimal intervention in a com-munity rheumatology practice. Forty-four ambulant patients with FMS, first seen and treated with a simple 2-month pain management program, were reviewed 2 years after diagnosis. Forty-seven percent no longer fulfilled criteria for FMS, and remission was objectively identified in 24.2% of assessed patients. Regular physical exercise, rather than drug or specific physical therapies, correlated highly with low FMS scores, whereas mood and coping strategies at the 2-year review were not related to FMS. Granges et al. concluded that community FMS has a better prognosis than the literature suggests and that simple intervention may be associated with good outcome in a significant number of patients with FMS.

Wolfe et al. (1997a) conducted a longitudinal outcome study by mailed questionnaire administered every 6 months to 538 patients at six rheumatology centers over 7 years. Measures of pain, global severity, fatigue, sleep disturbance, anxiety, depression, and health status were markedly abnormal at study initiation and were essentially unchanged over the study period. Although there was a great deal of variability in scores at one center compared with another, there was very little change from patient to patient from baseline over the 7 years of the survey.

Hamilton, Gallager, Thomas, and White (2005) performed a longitudinal survey of 18,122 patients diagnosed by their general practitioner with FMS, CFS, myalgic encephalitis, or postviral fatigue syndrome from 1988 to 2001 using electronic records from the General Practice Research Database in England. The length of illness was calculated as the interval between the diagnosis and the last recorded fatigue symptom, expressed as days per year. Patients with CFS and myalgic encephalitis combined had a worse prognosis than patients with FMS or postviral fatigue syndrome. There were differences in outcome between the various fatigue labels, with myalgic encephalitis having the worst prognosis and postviral fatigue syndrome the most favorable. Hamilton et al. suggested that the myalgic encephalitis label itself has an adverse effect. (In chap. 7, this volume, the effects of numerous treatment approaches on the prognosis of FMS are examined.)

ETIOLOGY

The etiology of FMS appears to be multifactorial in nature. Genetics, lower pain threshold, neural sensitization, neuroendocrine alterations, hormonal perturbations, sleep abnormalities, and psychosocial factors have all been implicated in FMS. The evidence for these factors is detailed below.

Genetic Contributions

Familial studies have suggested that genetic and familial factors may play a role in the etiology of FMS. Several studies have reported an elevated prevalence among first degree relatives of those diagnosed with FMS, but these studies had small sample sizes and did not use standardized criteria or direct interviews with relatives. Arnold et al. (2004) examined 533 relatives of 78 probands with ACR criteria FMS and 272 relatives of 40 probands with rheumatoid arthritis. They found that FMS aggregated strongly in families (much more so than rheumatoid arthritis), suggesting a possible genetic contribution to the etiology. They used a dolorimeter and found that tender point and myalgic scores were strongly associated with FMS in families, indicating a possible inherited factor in pain sensitivity. The results for familial aggregation were almost entirely attributed to the effect of female relatives. Hudson, Arnold, Keck, Auchenbah, and Pope (2004) further found that fibromyalgia coaggregated with other forms of affective spectrum disorder in families. Several recent genetic studies suggest the possibility of an increased prevalence of specific genotypes of neurotransmitters and their receptors in FMS (R. M. Bennett, 2005). There is evidence that polymorphisms of genes in the serotoninergic and catecholaminergic systems are linked to the pathophysiology of FMS and related conditions and are associated with personality traits. Although the mechanisms of genetic factors in FMS remain unknown, it is likely that several genes are operating together to initiate FMS (Buskila & Neuman, 2005). The burgeoning of genotype research will undoubtedly shed more light on this topic.

Pain Hypersensitivity and Central Sensitivity

Pain research in FMS has demonstrated abnormalities in neurotransmitter and neuroendocrine function, and FMS appears to fit the model of sensitization in central pain mechanisms with peripheral modulation (Eriksen & Ursin, 2004; Goldenberg, 1999; Yunus, 1992). A number of studies have assessed pain sensitivity in FMS through experimental paradigms. The methods generally used to measure altered pain sensitivity involve pain stimuli delivered to various body sites administered in ascending or random series of intensities. Thresholds for reporting pain as well as hypervigilance, responsivity, and aversion for pain sensations have been measured.

Maquet, Croisier, Demoulin, and Creilaard (2004) measured pressure pain sensitivity in FMS by blunt pressure applied to tender point areas. They studied 50 healthy men, 50 healthy women, and 20 women with FMS. Force was applied by a dolorimeter and was increased gradually until the participant asked the researcher to stop. They found that the pressure pain threshold was lower in women than men and even lower in women with FMS in all examined areas.

Because the ascending paradigm used by Maquet et al. (2004) presented stimuli in a predictable pattern, it is possible that participants were biased toward increased sensitivity because of expectation of pain; conversely, bias could decrease reported sensitivity because the predictable ascending pattern could reduce anxiety and instill a greater sense of control than a random stimulus. Petzke, Clauw, Ambrose, Khine, and Gracely (2003) addressed this question by varying stimulus type, using both pressure, heat, and mode of presentation, comparing ascending with random presentation in 43 FMS patients (4 men and 39 women) and 28 healthy controls (2 men and 26 women). Manual tender point counts and dolorimetry can also induce bias, because FMS patients might expect to be tender at the tender points. Therefore, Petzke et al. used a remote hydraulic stimulation device to apply pressure to the thumbnails to eliminate direct examiner–subject interaction. Increases in heat pain sensitivity paralleled those in pressure sensitivity, indicating that central as well as peripheral pain mechanisms are involved. Contrary to expectations, both groups of participants rated pain intensity as higher in the random compared with the ascending paradigms. The results suggest that expectancy, response bias, and hypervigilance may not play an important role in pain sensitivity in FMS, because random paradigms are not as influenced by distress or bias. Ascending methods, such as dolorimeter and tender point count, correlate more with psychological state. The number of positive tender points is even more influenced by distress than dolorimetry, where the subject exerts some control by stating when his or her pain threshold has been reached (Wolfe et al., 1997a).

Peters, Vlaeyen, and van Drunen (2000) similarly found no evidence for hypervigilance in FMS patients compared with healthy controls. Thirty women with FMS did not show a faster reaction time for detecting a weak electrocutaneous stimulus in four body locations when compared with 30 healthy women. Women with FMS did not evidence hypervigilance under single task or dual task conditions where two tasks competed for attention.

The lack of response bias or hypervigilance is contrary to what has been reported in IBS. Naliboff et al. (1997) delivered rectal distension stimuli to IBS patients and controls using an ascending series and a random threshold tracking task and found that discomfort levels were lower for patients in the ascending series, but there was no difference between groups on the random task. Chang et al. (2003) used the same method to examine female patients with IBS alone ($N = 10$) and those with IBS and comorbid FMS ($N = 10$) to somatic pressure stimuli applied to the skin. Although IBS patients had similar pain thresholds during the ascending series as healthy controls, they were found to have higher pain thresholds and lower pain frequency and severity during random stimulus series than IBS and FMS patients and controls. Chang et al. concluded that people with IBS and FMS had somatic hyperalgesia with lower pain thresholds and higher pain frequency and severity than those with IBS alone.

Geisser et al. (2003) examined the perception of contact thermal heat at both noxious and innocuous intensities in 20 women with FMS and 20 healthy women. Women with FMS displayed significantly lower pressure pain thresholds at tender point locations as well as at five control sites. Compared with the controls, women with FMS had significantly lower heat pain thresholds and tolerances when stimulated on the volar surface of the left forearm.

Women with FMS gave consistently higher pain intensity and unpleasantness ratings at both noxious and innocuous temperatures. These findings support the idea that people with FMS display perceptual abnormality to varied stimuli, although other investigators have not found differences in response to electrical or laser stimuli (Peters et al., 2000). Geisser et al.'s results do not support a generalized hypervigilance hypothesis, because self-reported pain scores were not related to pain threshold and tolerance. Geisser et al. also reported that greater pain catastrophizing was associated with decreased pain thresholds and tolerances in the entire sample, although surprisingly, self-report of depressive symptoms was associated with increased thresholds and tolerances. These findings indicate that people with FMS display altered perception of both pressure and thermal stimulation even at innocuous levels, and catastrophic cognitions appear to increase pain perception.

Contrary to Geisser et al. (2003), Petzke, Harris, Williams, Clauw, and Gracely (2005) found lower unpleasantness ratings induced by experimental pressure pain in patients with FMS relative to healthy controls. Ratings were obtained from both ascending and random methods of stimulus presentation. Although the patients with FMS reported greater pain intensity, they reported relative lower unpleasantness compared with healthy controls when stimuli were presented in random fashion. This indicates that FMS patients are less bothered by pain in experimental settings. Perhaps because they are more familiar with pain, their clinical pain becomes a reference point to which they have adapted, and evoked pain is thus less aversive, or they are more adept at modulating pain unpleasantness.

Staud, Robinson, Vierck, and Price (2003) investigated the role of the diffuse noxious inhibitory control system (DNIC) in FMS. The DNIC is part of the central pain modulatory system regulated by the spinal cord and its inputs. Previous studies had reported deficiencies in experimental tests of the DNIC. Lautenbacher and Rollman (1997) reported that FMS patients were unable to induce DNIC in response to painful tonic heat stimulation, whereas healthy individuals could inhibit the painful stimulus. Pain modulation, produced by a concurrent tonic stimulus in healthy persons, was not seen in the FMS group. The patients either had deficient pain modulation or were unable to tolerate a tonic stimulus intense enough to engage a modulatory process. Staud et al. compared the differences between 11 healthy men, 22 healthy women, and 11 women with FMS (to determine whether DNIC was a factor in pain sensitization). They found that it was female gender rather than FMS that was crucial, as both groups of women had less effective central inhibitory mechanisms compared with the men. Individuals with FMS may have deficient pain modulation in the DNIC or may be unable to tolerate a tonic stimulus intense enough to engage a modulatory process.

The experimental paradigms described above seem to indicate that people with FMS have lower thresholds for a variety of pain stimuli, which may be operating through central mechanisms such as the DNIC.

Pain and Emotion

Catastrophizing may augment pain perception through enhanced attention to painful stimuli and heightened emotional responses to pain. Gracely et al. (2004) hypothesized that catastrophizing would be positively associated with activation in pain-processing brain structures. They examined the association between catastrophizing and brain responses to blunt pressure through functional magnetic resonance imaging among 29 individuals with FMS (19 women and 10 men). The results suggest that pain catastrophizing, independent of the influence of depression, was significantly associated with increased activity in brain areas active in anticipation of pain (medial frontal cortex, cerebellum), attention to pain (dorsal anterior cingulate, dorsolateral prefrontal cortex), emotional aspects of pain (claustrum, closely connected to amygdala), and motor control. Results show that catastrophizing influences pain perception through altering attention and anticipation and heightening emotional responses to pain.

It has been hypothesized that widespread pain may affect not only pain threshold but self-monitoring mechanisms as well, particularly in disturbances of central nervous system origin. Karst et al. (2005) investigated whether there was a spectrum of dysfunction in self-monitoring ranging from that seen in 10 patients with acute schizophrenia (4 men, 6 women) to 10 patients with somatoform pain disorder (2 men, 8 women), and 10 patients with FMS (1 man, 9 women) compared with 10 healthy individuals (2 men, 8 women). Karst et al. assessed self-monitoring with a tactile stimulus device that used a plastic pointer to deliver pressure to the palm. Participants either delivered pressure themselves with the opposite hand or pressure was delivered by the experimenter. Controls experienced self-produced stimuli as less intense than identical stimuli produced by the experimenter, whereas the patients with pain disorder, schizophrenia, and FMS gave the same perceptual ratings for both types of stimuli. Karst et al. argued that these results indicate that central pain disorders involve a self-monitoring problem in distinguishing self-produced from externally produced sensations, and disturbances in central tactile processing are not limited to somatosensory processing in the painful areas.

Neuroendocrine System

The findings of greater pain sensitivity in FMS reflect a lower central pain processing threshold. This is likely mediated by imbalances in neurotransmitter and neuropeptides. A wide range of neuroendocrine abnormalities have been documented in FMS (Dessein, Shipton, Stanwix, & Joffe, 2000). Biochemical findings support the hypothesis that there are central changes in pain processing in FMS. Studies have found that FMS patients have higher concentrations of Substance P, a pro-nociceptive peptide, and lower levels of norepinephrine, which mediates pain inhibitory pathways (Clauw & Crofford, 2003). The concentration of Substance P, a peripheral pain neurotransmitter, is several times higher in the cerebrospinal fluid of FMS patients than in pain-free controls, implying a peripheral origin for FMS pain (Russell et al., 1994). Other areas of hypofunction in growth hormone, thyroid, glutamates, and reduced sympathetic nervous system responses have all been reported in FMS (Dessein et al., 2000; Garrison & Breeding, 2003) and point to a central mechanism. Dehydroepiandrosterone sulphate (DHEAS) is a more sensitive marker of HPA axis functioning than glutamate secretion. Low DHEAS levels have been reported in FMS and CFS (Dessein et al., 2000). In women, DHEAS concentrations decrease with age, and the prevalence of FMS increases.

Serotonin deficiencies have been found in FMS with low serum levels of serotonin and its dietary precursor tryptophan (Russell, 1996). Serotonin is important in deep sleep and in central and peripheral pain mechanisms (Chase, Shoulson, & Carter, 1976). Estrogen and progesterone ratios regulate serotonin and norepinephrine levels, and menstrual cycle variations in serotonin levels may modulate tender point sensitivity. Whether serotonin abnormalities are etiologically important in FMS or secondary to the illness process is not yet known.

Gender

Nine out of 10 FMS patients are women (Yunus, 2001). Gran (2003) summarized the prevalence of chronic widespread pain and FMS in general population studies and described FMS as a variant of chronic widespread pain. Both Yunus (2001) and Gran concluded that the most obvious risk factor for chronic widespread pain and FMS is female gender and noted that the factors responsible for the skewed sex distribution remain to be delineated.

Yunus, Inanici, Aldag, and Mangold (2000) studied 536 patients (469 women, 67 men) who had been newly diagnosed with FMS in an outpatient rheumatology clinic. Yunus et al. found that the men experienced significantly less fatigue, IBS, morning fatigue, generalized pain, and fewer tender points than the women. The authors cited the number of tender points as the most powerful discriminator between men and women with FMS. Wolfe et al. (1995) conducted a population based survey of 3,006 randomly selected persons in Wichita, Kansas, and identified 193 persons with chronic widespread pain. These people were given a clinical examination, and 36 of them were found to meet the ACR criteria for FMS. Tender point counts, dolorimetry scores, and clinical and psychological variables were measured. Dolorimetry scores were lower in women than men, and women were almost 10 times more likely to have 11 tender points than men. Women were also more likely to have generalized pain, sleep disturbance, fatigue, and IBS than men. Yunus (2001, 2002) summarized the concordant findings of these two studies; women had greater or more frequent fatigue, morning fatigue, generalized pain, anxiety, IBS, and number of tender points. Features that were similar between men and women were pain intensity, functional disability, and global severity.

Buskila, Neuman, Alhoashle, and Abu-Shakra (2000) examined 40 men with FMS matched by age and educational level with 40 women. All participants were asked about the presence and severity of FMS symptoms; a count of 18 tender points was conducted by thumb palpation, and tenderness thresholds were measured by dolorimetry. Men with FMS reported more severe symptoms than women, decreased physical function, and lower quality of life. Women had lower tender point thresholds than men; however, their mean tender point counts were similar. Buskila et al. concluded that although FMS is uncommon in men, its manifestations in their study population were worse than in women.

In an examination of 40 men compared with 160 women with FMS, Yunus, Celiker, and Aldag (2004) evaluated anxiety, stress, and depression using validated psychological instruments. Both men and women scored much higher than normative values on the psychological variables measured, with no significant differences between them. This was similar to findings of Buskila et al. (2000), who also found no differences between men and women with FMS on measures of anxiety and depression.

Clauw and Crofford (2003) believed that the tender point requirement is what has caused FMS to become an almost exclusively female disorder. Tender points are also tightly associated with high levels of distress, because as pressure is applied, distressed individuals "bail out" so as not to experience even slight pain. Clauw and Crofford argued that dropping the tender point requirement in the criteria would result in a disorder with more equal gender distribution and lower levels of distress. However, one also could argue that dropping the tender point requirement would make FMS akin to CFS, which is also much more common in women.

Hormones are always candidate factors for explaining sex differences in the prevalence of MUI. Associations between hormonal levels and pain reports are inconsistent in healthy women. Hapidou and Rollman (1998) tested 90 healthy students in the four different phases of the menstrual cycle. They found that normally cycling women had more tender points during the follicular phase compared with the luteal phase, whereas those who used oral contraceptives showed no cyclical differences. For all participants, pain thresholds measured by pressure dolorimetry remained stable throughout menstrual cycles. Self-reports of pain and mood on a visual analog scale revealed no phase differences. These findings suggest that tender point counts are more sensitive to global pain than dolorimetry. Johns and Littlejohn (1999) also found that dolorimetry thresholds were not affected by menstrual phases in healthy women.

Macfarlane, Blinkhorn, Worthington, Davies, and Macfarlane (2002) performed a population postal survey of 1,178 women living in the northwest of England. The questionnaires contained the symptoms of the ACR criteria for FMS, menstrual history, premenstrual symptoms, oral contraceptive use, and hormone replacement therapy. Macfarlane et al. found that pain was not related to any of the hormonal or menopausal factors examined in premenopausal, perimenopausal, or postmenopausal women. They speculated that more fruitful explanations for gender differences in FMS prevalence may be that women have a lower threshold for reporting pain symptoms, which in turn may be due to differences in pain processing, coping, and psychosocial factors.

Despite these findings, several other studies appear to indicate that some individuals with FMS do report greater pain and other symptoms in the premenopausal and perimenstrual phases of the cycle. Anderberg, Marteinsdottir, Hallman, and Backstrom (1998) examined pain, stress, anxiety, and other symptoms through prospective daily ratings in healthy women compared with women with FMS and women with FMS and premenstrual dysphoric disorder. Anderberg et al. found that the healthy controls had increased fatigue, headache, and anxiety during the luteal and premenstrual phases compared with the ovulatory and follicular phases. In women with FMS and with both FMS and premenstrual dysphoric disorder, there was a significantly more pronounced difference in fatigue, depression, anxiety, stress, and pain symptoms during luteal and perimenstrual phases compared with the ovulatory and follicular phases. In another study, Anderberg, Marteinsdottir, Hallman, Ekselius, and Backstrom (1999) compared premenopausal and postmenopausal women with FMS and postmenopausal healthy controls. There were no differences between the patient groups on pain measures, threshold, or physical symptoms, but the postmenopausal FMS patients reported greater psychological distress than healthy controls. Anderberg et al. (1998, 1999) have also reported changes in the levels of neuropeptide Y and nociceptin in FMS patients compared with healthy controls. These neuropeptides that regulate pain and stress were found to vary across the menstrual phase in FMS patients (Anderberg, Lui, Berglund, & Nyberg, 1998, 1999). Anderberg (2000) concluded that women with FMS have greater sensitivity in brain areas that regulate pain, affect, and stress and that these are to some extent influenced by female sex hormones.

Alonso, Loevinger, Muller, and Coe (2004) examined the influence of the menstrual cycle on pain and emotion in FMS ($n = 57$) compared with rheumatoid arthritis patients ($n = 20$) and healthy women ($n = 48$). The participants assessed menstrual status and pain symptoms through daily logs for the week before their appointment and tender point and dolorimeter evaluation once during the luteal and once during the follicular phase. The women with FMS experienced more pain, more menstrual symptoms, and more negative affect than comparison women. All women reported less positive affect during the luteal phase, although this was more marked in the women with FMS and rheumatoid arthritis. Collectively, these findings indicate that female hormones influence pain and psychological symptoms in FMS patients, whereas a similar but more subtle effect can be found in healthy women.

Ostensen, Rugelsjoen, and Wigers (1997) performed a retrospective analysis based on personal interviews on the influence of pregnancy, abortion, menstruation, use of oral contraceptives, and breastfeeding on FMS symptomatology. Twenty-six women with an established diagnosis of FMS and a total of 40 pregnancies were included in the study. With the exception of 1 patient, all women described worsening FMS symptoms during pregnancy, particularly the last trimester. A change of FMS symptoms within 6 months after delivery was reported for 37 of the 40 pregnancies; 4 improved and 33 worsened, resulting in a prolonged sick leave for 14 patients. An increase in depression and anxiety was a prominent problem in the postpartum period. FMS had no adverse effect on the outcome of pregnancy or the health of the infant. In the majority of patients, hormonal changes connected with abortion, use of hormonal contraceptives, and breast-feeding did not modulate symptom severity. A premenstrual worsening of symptoms was recorded by 72% of the patients. Pregnancy and the postpartum period appeared to exert a negative effect on FMS symptoms by increased functional impairment and disability.

Women with FMS often have pelvic symptoms, including pelvic pain, dysmenorrhea, and painful sexual intercourse. A study of Turkish women investigated sexual function in FMS and evaluated whether concurrent major depression has an additional negative effect on sexual function. One hundred women were enrolled in the study, including 40 with FMS only, 27 with FMS plus depression, and 33 healthy volunteers as a control group. This study demonstrated that women with FMS had sexual dysfunction compared with healthy controls but that coexistent depression had no additional negative effect on sexual function (Tikiz et al., 2005). In a telephone survey of 442 women with FMS compared with 205 women without FMS, women with FMS were significantly more likely to have had reproductive system or sleep disorder diagnoses, including PMS, dysmenorrhea, breast cysts, bladder cystitis, sleep apnea, restless leg syndrome, and abnormal leg movements during sleep. Women with FMS were less than half as active as control women, had sleep pattern difficulties, more negative changes in sexual function, and lower alcohol use than controls (Shaver, Wilbur, Robinson, Wang, & Buntin, 2006). Although nearly two thirds of the women in their survey had been diagnosed with depression, Shaver et al. (2006) found that the physical impacts of FMS were more severe than mental health impacts according to the SF-12 (derived from the SF-36). They recommended that sexual function should be assessed in FMS. The interference with sexual function and motivation in FMS is likely due to a complex combination of dysphoria and the low threshold for touch pressure to become painful.

It is not obvious why women are more susceptible to FMS than men. The gender and pain issues discussed in chapters 4 and 5 of this volume are certainly contributors. Factors such as reduced pain thresholds, greater sensitivity to pain (which may be mediated by sex hormones), gender role sanctions allowing expression of pain, psychosocial vulnerabilities in stress, and trauma experiences may all play a role. FMS seems to involve alterations in pain processing mediated by central processes that can be influenced by a range of psychosocial factors.

Stress

FMS is widely viewed as a stress-related disorder, and disturbances of the HPA axis and sympathetic nervous system axes may explain some of the symptoms. The neuroendocrine abnormalities found in FMS are strongly influenced by the body's biological stress system. A number of studies have found that the HPA axis and sympathetic nervous system processes are disrupted in FMS and that these stress axes interact with pain processing at many levels. Basal hypocortisolism, overactivity of corticotropin-releasing hormone (CRH), and an altered response to stressful challenge are the primary findings (Parker, Wessely, & Cleare, 2001).

Several studies have found increased levels of adrenocorticotropic hormone (ACTH) in response to CRH injections in FMS, which resembles that seen in depression (Neeck, 2002). CRH is the principal regulator of ACTH release and coordinator of the stress response. CRH can suppress gonadal function by inhibiting luteinizing hormone-releasing hormone from the hypothalamus.

Torpy et al. (2000) examined whether CRH hypoactivity was pathogenic in FMS. The researchers administered interleukin-6, a strong stimulator of the HPA axis via activation of hypothalamic CRH, to female FMS patients and their age-matched controls. They found that ACTH release was delayed in FMS patients, which is consistent with a defect in hypothalamic CRH neuronal function. Basal norepinephrine levels were higher as well in FMS patients, which suggests abnormal regulation of the sympathetic nervous system that may be caused by a chronically deficient level of hypothalamic CRH. The results found by Torpy et al. demonstrate the mediating effects of CRH on the stress system at the hypothalamic and brain stem levels and may contribute to the primary symptoms of FMS. These alterations of the stress system, along with central sensitization, may be factors in the amplification of pain perception (Kashikar-Zuch, Graham, Huenefeld, & Powers, 2000). This hypoactivity is associated with underactivity of the stress system. Clauw (1994) surmised that FMS patients have an impaired ability to respond to stressors, consistent with an exhaustion of the autonomic nervous system.

As has been shown in CFS (see chap. 11, this volume), findings of hypocortisolism are not consistent. In a naturalistic study, Cately, Kaell,

Kirschbaum, and Stone (2000) asked 21 FMS patients, 18 rheumatoid arthritis patients, and 22 healthy controls to complete a diary (assessing psychosocial- and lifestyle-related variables) or provide a saliva sample (for cortisol assessment) during normal daily activities when they received a signal with a preprogrammed wristwatch alarm. Participants were signaled to provide six diary reports and six saliva samples over 2 days. Reports of sleep quality and sleep duration were also made on awakening. FMS and rheumatoid arthritis patients had higher average cortisol levels than controls; however, there were no differences between the groups in diurnal cycles of cortisol or reactivity to psychological stress. The patient groups actually reported less stress than the controls. Furthermore, statistically accounting for psychosocial- and lifestyle-related differences between the groups did not change the cortisol findings. The elevations in cortisol in this study were also not related to ongoing daily stress. Because some studies have reported lower cortisol in FMS, whereas this study reported elevated cortisol, one can only conclude that there is evidence of HPA axis disturbance in FMS but that it is not very specific.

Gur, Cevik, Sarac, Colpan, and Em (2004) attempted to determine whether depression, fatigue, and sleep disturbance affected follicle-stimulating hormone, luteinizing hormone, estradiol, progesterone, prolactin, and cortisol concentrations. Thus, this is the only study that has examined the hypothalamic–pituitary–gonadal and the HPA axes in the same patient. Sixty-three women with FMS were compared with 38 matched healthy controls, all of whom were less than 35 years old. Depression was assessed by the Beck Depression Inventory (BDI), and patients with high and low BDI scores were compared. Additionally, patients were divided according to sleep disturbance and fatigue and were compared both with healthy controls and within the group. No significant differences in follicle-stimulating hormone, luteinizing hormone, estradiol, prolactin, and progesterone levels were found between patients with FMS and controls, but cortisol levels were significantly lower in patients than in controls. In particular, cortisol levels in patients with high BDI scores, fatigue, and sleep disturbance were significantly lower than in controls. Correlation between cortisol levels and the number of tender points in all patients was significant. Despite low cortisol concentrations in young women with FMS, there was no abnormality in HPA axis hormones. Because fatigue, depression rate, sleep disturbance, and mean age of patients affect cortisol levels, these variables should be taken into account in future investigations.

Chronic widespread pain seems to result in either low or high cortisol; the alteration in HPA regulation is the critical determinant rather than a consistent directional pattern. McBeth, Morris, Benjamin, Silman, and Macfarlane (2001) hypothesized that psychological distress and somatization (rather than the pain) might explain HPA dysregulation in FMS. McBeth et al. performed a population study of pain and psychological status in individuals aged 25 to 65 years. Random samples were selected from the following three groups: 131 persons satisfying criteria for chronic widespread pain; 267 free of chronic widespread pain but with strong evidence of somatization ("at risk"); and 56 controls. HPA axis function was assessed by measuring early morning and evening salivary cortisol levels and serum cortisol after physical (pain pressure threshold exam) and chemical (overnight dexamethasone suppression test) stressors. Those in the chronic widespread pain and at risk groups were, respectively, 3.1 and 1.8 times more likely to have a saliva cortisol score in the lowest third. Yet, no psychosocial factors measured were associated with saliva cortisol levels. Furthermore, those in the chronic widespread pain and at risk groups were also more likely to have the highest serum cortisol scores. High poststress serum cortisol was related to high levels of psychological distress. The researchers concluded that this was the first population study to demonstrate that those with and those at risk of chronic widespread pain demonstrate abnormalities of HPA axis function, which is not fully explained by psychological stress.

Van Houdenhove and Egle (2004) proposed that FMS can be understood as a stress disorder in many patients. A genetic predisposition causes hyperresponsiveness to stress, which interacts with adverse developmental experiences, leading to further sensitization of the stress system. Negative affect and poor coping may follow. Accumulating stress caused by role strain, exhaustion, and conflicts can precipitate the condition. They suggest that illness onset may be prodded by a shift from chronic hyperfunction of the stress response to hypofunction, giving rise to chronic disturbance in stress regulation, pain processing, and immune functioning. This would also help to explain why most studies of FMS have found hypocortisolism, yet several have reported hypercortisolism; patients may be at different points on the illness continuum.

Sleep Disturbance

Generalized sleep disturbance is an extremely prevalent feature of FMS. Patients with FMS often report insomnia or light sleep as well as an increase in FMS symptoms after disturbed sleep (Campbell et al., 1983). This is expressed in the common symptoms of awakening unrefreshed with intense muscle stiffness, aching, and fatigue. Molodofsky and colleagues have hypothesized that FMS may be due to nonrestorative deep sleep (Moldofsky, 1993; Moldofsky, Scarisbrick, England, & Smythe, 1975). They found that FMS-like symptoms can be induced in healthy volunteers by depriving them of deep sleep; this was not the case, however, with individuals who exercised regularly (Moldofsky, Scarisbrick, England, & Smythe, 1975). Abnormal amounts of alpha activity on the electroencephalogram (EEG) of FMS patients during deep sleep have been reported (Moldofsky, 1975), but these early EEG findings have not been consistently replicated (Rizzi et al., 2004).

Shaver et al. (1997) found no differences in sleep quality, depth, continuity, efficiency, non–rapid eye movement arousal, or slow wave sleep variables. Yet, women with FMS spent more time in Stage 1 sleep and had a higher number of stage changes. These findings indicate that sleep is lighter and less consolidated in the first half of the night for FMS women. On the stress arousal measure, they found no differences in cardiodynamic stress indicators, catecholamine, or cortisol urine concentrations. A more recent study from this group compared 37 midlife women with FMS and 30 sedentary women without pain on *sleep-spindle* (a burst of brain activity visible on an EEG) incidence (number of spindles per minute of non–rapid eye movement sleep) and spindle wave time, spindle frequency activity, and pain measures (Landis, Lentz, Tsuji, Buchwald, & Shaver, 2004). The FMS group had fewer sleep spindles and reduced spindle frequency compared with the control group. The researchers contended that thalamocortical mechanisms of spindle generation might be impaired in FMS.

Rizzi et al. (2004) investigated the notion that the sleep fragmentation observed in FMS could be due to cyclic alternating pattern. They had 45 patients with FMS and 38 healthy controls undergo polysomnography and found the cyclic alternating pattern rate to be 29% higher in the FMS group relative to controls. As other studies have found, the Rizzi et al. study concluded that the microstructure of sleep is what is affected in FMS and that it is associated with pain. The pain of FMS reduces sleep efficiency and causes more light sleep, more cyclic alternating pattern, more arousals, and breathing irregularities. Collectively, these studies indicate that nonrestorative sleep in FMS is not due to marked abnormalities in sleep architecture but rather a variety of alterations in the microstructure of sleep, most likely secondary to the experience of pain.

Immunological Changes

The dysfunction in pain, mood, and sleep processes could be associated with changes in immune system indicators in FMS. Landis et al. (2004) compared pain, psychological variables, subjective and objective sleep quality, lymphocyte phenotypes and activation markers, and natural killer activity in midlife women (aged 37 to 53 years) with and without FMS. The women had pain pressure tender points assessed, completed a psychiatric interview and questionnaires (BDI, Symptom Checklist, Profile of Mood States, subjective sleep), and underwent polysomnographic assessment for 2 consecutive nights. Compared with controls, women with FMS had lower pain thresholds, more psychological distress, higher depression scores, and reduced subjective and objective sleep quality. Although they had fewer natural killer cells altogether, they had more natural killer cells that expressed the interleukin-2 receptor; these differences were not statistically significant. Landis et al. found little evidence to support the hypothesis that pain, mood, and sleep symptoms are associated with changes in lymphocyte function in FMS. Zurowski and Shapiro (2004) commented that it is possible both that FMS and sleep problems could cause increased stress or that increased stress could contribute to FMS and sleep problems. The only thing they could conclude with certainty is that these symptoms co-occur.

Psychosocial Issues

A contributing factor to FMS is stress; it may be early life stress such as childhood sexual abuse or current stress such as workplace stress. The onset of FMS often follows severe physical or psychological stress, although Cleare (2004) cautioned that stress as a precipitating factor should not be overemphasized.

Childhood Trauma

Goldberg and Goldstein (2000) found that a chronic pain group (including people with FMS) was more likely to have a history of physical, sexual, and verbal abuse than a control group of hospital employees. Although child abuse is reported to be as high as 25% in the general American population, the statistics for chronic pain patients are generally twice as high as in the general population. The risk factors for abuse include age, gender, and early family environment. Finestone et al. (2000) found that women who had experienced childhood abuse reported a greater number of painful body areas, visited health care providers more often, and had more surgeries and hospitalizations than nonabused controls.

Compared with other pain disorders, FMS is associated with a higher prevalence of sexual abuse and childhood illnesses. Goldberg, Pachas, and Keith (1999) examined the relationship between traumatic events in childhood in 91 patients with chronic facial pain, myofascial pain, and fibromyalgia who had been consecutively recruited from the outpatient clinics of a rehabilitation hospital and a general hospital. FMS patients reported the highest rates of abuse (65%). All patient groups had been exposed to a high degree of family violence and alcoholism.

Walker, Keegan, Gardner, Sullivan, Bernstein, and Katon (1997) studied 36 patients with FMS and 33 with rheumatoid arthritis. The participants with FMS had significantly higher rates of victimization, both in childhood and adulthood. Sexual abuse did not have specific effects, whereas experiences of physical assault in adulthood showed a strong and specific relationship with unexplained pain. Trauma severity was correlated significantly with measures of physical disability, psychiatric distress, illness adjustment, personality, and quality of sleep in patients with fibromyalgia but not in those with rheumatoid arthritis.

However, several studies have not found significantly higher rates of sexual abuse in FMS patients compared with healthy controls (Alexander et al., 1998; M. L. Taylor, Trotter, & Csuka, 1995). Ciccone, Elliot, Chandler,

Nayak, and Raphael (2005) attempted to resolve the inconsistent findings on the role of childhood abuse by conducting a community-based study of trauma in FMS. They recruited samples of women from a large community with FMS and major depressive disorder (MDD; $n = 36$) and FMS without MDD ($n = 16$) and compared them with controls with MDD only ($n = 32$) or controls with no physical or psychiatric symptoms ($n = 21$). Women in the FMS group were 3.1 times more likely to report having been raped. FMS and control participants did not differ on the aggregate measure of abuse events. Ciccone et al. did not find exacerbated FMS symptoms in the abused versus nonabused women with FMS, although those in the abused group were more likely to have MDD and have posttraumatic stress disorder (PTSD) symptoms. The risk of FMS in the rape victims was mediated by PTSD; therefore, it is possible that rape and posttraumatic stress are implicated in the etiology of FMS. Ciccone et al. concluded that future studies need to determine whether the effects of specific abuse events (such as rape), which are more violent and life threatening and may be pivotal, are being lost in aggregate measures.

Workplace stress may also contribute to an increased risk of FMS. Kivimaki et al. (2004) conducted a prospective study of 4,791 hospital employees to determine rates of newly diagnosed FMS from 1998 to 2000. The mean age of this sample was 43.3 years, 88% were women, and respondents with FMS at baseline were excluded. High workload, limited decision-making opportunity, and especially being bullied at work were associated with a twofold to fourfold risk of new FMS. These stress exposures did not predict osteoarthritis or sciatica.

Psychiatric Disorders

FMS, headaches, IBS, and CFS share phenotypic and genotypic features with mood disturbances (Goldenberg, 1999; Hudson et al., 2003). A majority of patients with FMS have significant psychiatric illness. Depression is the most common psychiatric disorder associated with FMS (Hawley & Wolfe, 1993; Hudson, Goldenberg, Pope, Keck, & Schlesinger, 1992; Hudson, Hudson, Pliner, Goldenberg, & Pope, 1985; Okifuji, Turk, & Sherman, 2000); explanations for the linkage between the two include the following: (a) FMS is a symptom of depression, (b) FMS causes a reactive depression, and (c) the two conditions share a common pathophysiology (Goodnick & Sandoval, 1993). Psychologic distress is an intrinsic dimension of FMS with a likely bidirectional pathway.

Several studies have concluded that anxiety and depression are more likely to be reactions to the pain and disability imposed by FMS rather than the cause (Dunne & Dunne, 1995; Goldenberg, 1989). Yunus, Ahles, Aldag, and Masi (1991) found that the central features of FMS (e.g., number of pain sites, number of tender points, fatigue, and poor sleep) were independent of psychological status. Meyer-Lindenberg and Gallhofer (1998) suggested that a subgroup of FMS has somatized depression.

A number of psychiatric studies have compared FMS with rheumatoid arthritis patients as well as healthy controls. The rheumatoid arthritis group is meant to control for living with chronic pain in an organically explained condition. Several studies have found no differences between FMS and rheumatoid arthritis in terms of psychopathology, although both were higher than in controls (Ahles, Khan, Yunus, Speigel, & Masi, 1991; Ahles, Yunus, & Masi, 1987; Kirmayer, Robbins, & Kapusta, 1988). Conversely, Hudson et al. (1992) found higher rates of major depression in FMS compared with rheumatoid arthritis patients and healthy controls. Walker, Keegan, Gardner, Sullivan, Katon, and Bernstein (1997) found that 90% of the patients with FMS had a prior psychiatric diagnosis compared with fewer than half of the patients with rheumatoid arthritis.

Studies comparing FMS with a variety of rheumatic diseases have found that depression is higher in FMS. In an analysis of 6,153 consecutive patients of a rheumatic disease outpatient clinic, the rheumatoid arthritis group did not differ from all other clinic patients on depressive symptoms and depression scores. Patients with FMS had significantly more abnormal scores (Hawley & Wolfe, 1993).

Okifuji, Turk, and Sherman (2000) investigated the factors that differentiate FMS patients with and without depressive disorders. A sample of 69 patients with FMS (96% were women) underwent a standardized tender point examination and a semistructured psychological interview and completed a set of self-report inventories; 39 met criteria for depressive disorder, and 30 did not. Those with depression were significantly more likely to live alone, report elevated functional limitations, and display maladaptive thoughts, whereas the nondepressed patients were significantly more likely to have received prior physical therapy than depressed patients. Pain severity, numbers of positive tender points, and pain intensity of tender points and control points did not differentiate the groups. These results indicate that concurrent depression appears to be independent of pain in FMS and, instead, to be related to the cognitive appraisals of the effects of symptoms on daily life and functional activities.

In most of the studies cited above, patients were recruited from rheumatology clinics, but Wolfe and colleagues investigated FMS symptoms in the general population surrounding Wichita, Kansas. In the first report from this survey, they found that depressive symptomatology had a stronger correlation with tender point count than with pain threshold (Wolfe et al., 1995). In the second report from this group, FMS was strongly associated with somatization, anxiety, past or current depression, and family history of depression (Wolfe, Ross, Anderson, Russell, & Herbert, 1995). The researchers concluded that the level of distress seen in FMS in the general population was similar to that of patients seen in specialty clinics. These studies confirm psychologic distress as an intrinsic dimension of FMS.

Although depression is the most common disorder observed in FMS, anxiety may be the most disabling. For instance, S. A. Epstein et al. (1999) sought to determine whether psychiatric comorbidity and psychological variables were predictive of functional impairment in FMS using patients from four tertiary-care centers. Seventy-three individuals were administered the Structured Clinical Interview for *DSM–III–R*, the Rand 36-item Health Survey (SF-36), and multiple self-report measures. The patients with FMS were found to have a high lifetime and current prevalence of major depression and panic disorder. The most common disorders were major depression, dysthymia, panic disorder, and simple phobia. Self-report scales revealed significant elevations in depression, anxiety, neuroticism, and hypochondriasis and severe functional impairment on the SF-36. Multiple-regression analysis found that current anxiety was the only variable that predicted a significant proportion of the variance (29%) in SF-36 physical functioning.

Individuals with FMS and PTSD also have impaired functioning. Sherman, Turk, and Okifuji (2000) examined the prevalence of PTSD in a sample of 93 consecutive FMS patients at an interdisciplinary pain center. They found that 56% of the sample presented with PTSD symptoms. Those with PTSD symptoms reported higher levels of pain, disability, and distress than those without such symptoms. Several explanations are possible: Both FMS and PTSD may be a consequence of poor coping, or alternately, the burden of coping with PTSD increases the danger of a pain condition becoming chronic (Sherman et al., 2000). Although there is likely to be overlap between PTSD and affective distress, PTSD does present with a number of distinct symptoms specific to the traumatic stress response, such as intrusive thoughts, intense fear, racing heart, and agoraphobia.

Brosschot and Aarsse (2001) showed that compared with healthy women, women with FMS showed restrictive emotional processing tendencies and a preponderance of somatic attributions for symptoms at the expense of psychological attributions. Hazlett and Haynes (1992) assessed the correlation between daily stressors, cognitive rumination, and symptoms in 12 FMS patients. Although they found no relationship between previous-day stressors and symptoms, cognitive rumination was associated with symptoms for one third of the patients. Gaston-Johansson, Gustafsson, Felldin, and Sanne (1990) compared 31 individuals with FMS with 30 individuals with rheumatoid arthritis on feelings, behaviors, and attitudes toward their illness. Those with FMS reported more sickness, discussed and experienced pain more often, and received more practical help from others than those with rheumatoid arthritis. They were less satisfied by attention they received, less sure of themselves, and felt that they were mistrusted or viewed as malingering. Those with FMS were significantly less optimistic than rheumatoid arthritis patients regarding relief from pain, improved functioning, and employment prospects.

In a Swedish study, Hellstrom, Bullington, Karlsson, Lindqvist, and Mattsson (1999) conducted qualitative interviews with 19 women and 1 man recruited from local FMS group meetings. Interviews were 30 to 50 minutes long and took place in patients' homes; the interviews started with the open-ended question, "Please tell me a little bit about what it is like to live with fibromyalgia." The dominant themes that emerged were a desire to have their illness validated by physicians and significant others, a feeling that they had been dramatically felled by an incapacitating yet invisible disease, and an attempt to find biomedical explanations. FMS emerged as the sole problem for these individuals; they felt that all would be well in their lives if not for FMS. The researchers speculated that FMS may be a strategy to avoid demands that patients have placed on themselves. This echoes the perfectionism issues documented in CFS—that is, the individual cannot tolerate reduced performance. Patients "choose" illness in order to come to terms with difficult life situations. Hadler (2003) also posited that people choose to become patients because they have exhausted their ability to cope with pain and stress in the context of various psychosocial factors.

Overall, in most studies, persons with FMS exhibited marked functional impairment, high levels of some lifetime and current psychiatric disorders, and significant current psychological distress. Although it appears in many cases to be reactive depression caused by living with chronic pain, the prevalence of psychiatric disorders remains high in subgroups of FMS.

Coping

Psychologically maladaptive responses to stress seem to characterize FMS. Davis, Zautra, and Reich (2001) examined 50 women with FMS and a chronic pain control group of 51 women with osteoarthritis and compared the groups on vulnerability to negative social stress. They found that the FMS group had fewer positive affective resources and used ineffective, avoidant coping strategies to a greater degree than the osteoarthritis group. Those with FMS also had a smaller social network and poorer quality social ties than their osteoarthritis counterparts. Both pain groups had comparable levels of pain and personality dispositions. The women with FMS appeared to be more vulnerable to stress and to have made a poorer adaptation to stress. Studies cited in the pain sensitivity section in this chapter provide evidence that catastrophizing is a particularly poor coping response; it has been consistently associated with heightened pain sensitivity. This could lead to a bidirectional exacerbation of pain experience.

People with FMS recognize that they are coping poorly. Burckhardt and Bjelle (1996) reported that only 13% of patients with FMS believed they were coping successfully compared with 30% of those with rheumatoid arthritis who thought so. In several studies Turk and others have used the West-

Haven Yale Multidimensional Pain Inventory (WHYMPI) and identified three subgroups of FMS patients. One group, labeled *dysfunctional*, had the highest level of pain, emotional distress, and disability. The second group, the *interpersonally distressed*, had significantly lower levels of pain, disability, and marital satisfaction and more negative responses from significant others. *Adaptive copers* made up the third group; they were characterized by lower pain intensity and distress and less interference with daily activities (Turk, Okifuji, Sinclair, & Starz, 1996; Walen, Cronan, Serber, Groessl, & Oliver, 2002). Researchers have also found that type of FMS onset affected coping. Patients with a posttraumatic onset of FMS (following an accident, surgery, or illness) reported significantly higher pain intensity, disability, interference, and distress and lower activity levels than the 53% of patients who could not identify a specific cause for their FMS (Turk, Okifuji, Starz, & Sinclair, 1996).

Thieme, Turk, and Flor (2004) examined the relationship of somatic and psychosocial variables to depression and anxiety in FMS. They also split them into dysfunctional, interpersonally distressed, and adaptive copers according to the WHYMPI. Overall, 75% of the participants had an Axis I disorder, whereas only 8.7% had an Axis II disorder. The dysfunctional subgroup was more likely to have anxiety disorders, PTSD-like symptoms, more sexual and physical abuse, and low levels of depression. They reported more physical symptoms, higher pain intensity and interference, and the most solicitous behaviors by significant others compared with the other two groups. The interpersonally distressed group was most likely to have mood disorders. Thieme et al. also reported fewer physical symptoms, lower pain intensity, higher activity, and more negative behaviors from significant others. The adaptive copers group had little psychiatric comorbidity. Thieme et al. concluded that psychiatric disorders were not directly associated with FMS, but factors such as past trauma, coping, and spousal behaviors seem to mediate the association between FMS symptoms and psychiatric disorder.

Zautra, Fasman, et al. (2005) asked whether in the overemphasis on negative states, investigators have failed to perceive that FMS may entail an inability to mobilize positive affect. They compared 87 FMS patients with 39 osteoarthritis patients from the community. The participants responded to baseline questionnaires on demographic and personality factors and were interviewed weekly for up to 12 weeks regarding pain, affect, fatigue, and stress. The authors found no substantial differences between the groups on neuroticism, depression, anxiety, or negative affect. However, those with FMS did report lower levels of positive affect, joviality, and self-assurance. When reporting more stress, the FMS group could not retain their positive affect as well as the osteoarthritis group did. In an expansion of this study, Zautra, Johnson, and Davis (2005) found that people with greater average positive affect were less likely to show high negative affect during high pain and interpersonal stress weeks. These data are consistent with Zautra and colleagues' dynamic model of affect (Davis, Zautra, & Smith, 2004), which postulates that under conditions of pain and stress there is a strong inverse relationship between positive and negative affect. Evidence is gradually accumulating that indicates that rather than an excess of negative traits such as neuroticism, FMS may involve difficulty in reducing negative affect and mounting a resilient positive affect response. Future research may do well to reduce psychology's traditional emphasis on distress and examine positive features of psychological functioning and resilience resources.

CONCLUSION

FMS provides an exemplar of the biopsychosocial model of illness. A broad, integrative approach that encompasses central sensitization mechanisms affecting pain perception that is associated with cognitive and personality vulnerabilities affords the best approach to understanding FMS (Masi, White, & Pilcher, 2002; Meeus & Nijs, 2007; Shaver et al., 2006). Biological factors such as genetics, central sensitization, lowered pain threshold, sex hormones, and neuroendocrine dysfunction interact with sleep difficulties, stress sensitivity, and psychosocial factors. Psychosocial vulnerabilities found in FMS include trauma history, negative affect, and lack of coping resources. Many of these factors may make women more vulnerable to FMS than men. Negative affect combined with alterations of pain mechanisms may lead to long-term neuroplastic changes that exceed the pain-coping capabilities of people with FMS, resulting in a cycle of increasing pain sensitivity and reduced functioning (Price & Staud, 2005). Meeus and Nijs (2007) have suggested that behavioral and cognitive treatments could affect descending pathways in the spinal cord and reverse these pain pathways.

7

CHRONIC FATIGUE SYNDROME

Chronic fatigue syndrome (CFS) affects people of all ages, racial and ethnic backgrounds, and economic situations, although the typical patient is a woman in her 30s or 40s. CFS is characterized primarily by unexplained chronic fatigue as well as rheumatological, infectious, and neuropsychiatric symptoms. Fatigue represents the chief complaint in 4% to 9% of all visits to primary practice physicians (Manu, Lane, & Matthews, 1992). Fatigue is a common symptom in community-based studies (Cope, 1992; Jason, Jordan, et al., 1999; Lindal, Stefansson, & Bergmann, 2002; Pawlikowska et al., 1994) and among primary care and hospital based studies of fatigue prevalence (Cathebras, Robbins, Kirmayer, & Hayton, 1992; Cope, 1992; Fuhrer & Wessely, 1995; Kroenke, Wood, Mangelsdorff, Meier, & Powell, 1988).

Prins, van der Meer, and Bleijenberg (2006) summarized the myriad controversies surrounding discussion of CFS. Researchers, medical professionals, and patients do not agree on the name, the case criteria, the purported pathophysiology, the utility of further research into physiological etiology, or the effectiveness of various treatment approaches.

DIAGNOSIS

CFS is characterized primarily by unexplained severe, persistent, disabling fatigue lasting for at least 6 months. The diagnosis also includes a number of rheumatological, infectious, and neuropsychiatric symptoms (Fukuda et al., 1994). In addition to unexplained fatigue that results in substantially reduced functioning, an individual must report at least four of the following minor symptom criteria: sore throat, tender lymph nodes, new headaches, myalgias, arthralgias, postexertional fatigue, sleep disturbance, and neuropsychological complaints. It is a diagnosis of exclusion in that the persistent fatigue cannot be accounted for by another medical or psychiatric condition. It has been given numerous labels, including *Epstein–Barr virus infection, chronic mononucleosis, myalgic encephalomyelitis, postviral fatigue syndrome, postinfectious neuromyasthenia, chronic fatigue immune deficiency syndrome,* and *yuppie flu* (Greenberg, 1990; Holmes et al., 1988; Sharpe et al., 1991); the labels tend to reflect current explanatory trends more than research findings.

The first case definition for CFS was developed in 1988 by a number of experts in the field (Holmes et al., 1988), subsequently revised in 1991 (Schluederberg et al., 1992) and again in 1994 (Fukuda et al., 1994; see Table 7.1). The 1988 definition required a history of 6 months of severe fatigue in a previously healthy person (Holmes et al., 1988) and excluded a CFS diagnosis if "chronic psychiatric disease" was present. In 1992, the case definition was modified such that nonpsychotic depression, anxiety, and somatoform disorders could be present (Schluederberg et al., 1992). The 1994 definition was crafted by the joint Centers for Disease Control and Prevention–National Institutes of Health international working group. Conditions that can coexist with a diagnosis of CFS are adequately treated hypothyroidism, Lyme disease, asthma, syphilis, or fibromyalgia (FMS). Goldenberg (1989a) found that most patients with CFS had a tender point examination similar to that of patients with FMS. Concurrent diagnosis of anxiety, panic, somatoform, or nonmelancholic depression is allowed, whereas depression with psychotic or melancholic features, bipolar disorder, schizophrenia, delusional disorder, dementia, anorexia nervosa, or bulimia nervosa would exclude a person from CFS diagnosis. In general, the Fukuda et al. definition is broader than earlier criteria; it reduces the number of symptoms required and includes some concurrent psychiatric diagnoses, resulting in greater heterogeneity in study populations.

Although there are Australian (Lloyd, Wakefield, Boughton, & Dwyer, 1990) and British (Sharpe et al., 1991) case definitions (which use the term *myalgic encephalomyelitis*), the Fukuda et al. (1994) definition has become the standard for clinical practice and research. Jason and others have criticized the development of CFS case criteria by group consensus rather than through empirically derived processes (King & Jason, 2005) and the importance of subtyping on distinguishing characteristics such as severity of postexertional fatigue or neurocognitive impairment (Jason, Corradi, Torres-Harding, Taylor, & King, 2005; S. K. Johnson et al., 1999). Through the International CFS Study Group, Reeves et al. (2003) recommended an empirical case definition using validated instruments to obtain standardized measures of the

TABLE 7.1
Centers for Disease Control and Prevention Case Definitions
for Chronic Fatigue Syndrome

Symptom criteria	1988 case definition (Holmes et al., 1988)	1994 case definition (Fukuda et al., 1994)
Major	New onset of fatigue that results in at least a 50% reduction of daily activities for 6 months Exclusion of other medical conditions that produce similar symptoms	Unexplained persistent or relapsing fatigue that is of new or definite onset that results in a substantial reduction of previous levels of functioning
Minor	Fever	—
	Muscle weakness	—
	Sore throat	Sore throat
	Tender lymph nodes	Tender lymph nodes
	Headaches of new type	Headaches of new type
	Myalgia	Myalgia
	Arthralgia	Arthralgia
	Postexertional fatigue	Postexertional fatigue
	Sleep disturbance	Sleep disturbance
	Neuropsychologic complaints	Neuropsychologic complaints
Physical	Low-grade fever	—
	Nonexudative pharyngitis	—
	Palpable lymph nodes	—

Note. The 1988 definition requires satisfying the major criteria plus eight signs and symptoms to diagnose chronic fatigue syndrome. The 1994 definition requires major criteria plus four symptoms. Dashes in cells indicate no applicable data. From *Fatigue as a Window to the Brain* (p. 138), by J. DeLuca (Ed.), 2005, Cambridge, MA: MIT Press. Copyright 2005 by MIT Press. Reprinted with permission.

major dimensions of CFS. In a study applying this system, Reeves et al. (2005) found that the empirical case definition was less affected by day-to-day fluctuation of the illness and allowed more precision in case ascertainment.

PROGNOSIS

A review of prognosis in CFS (Cairns & Hotopf, 2005) extracted 28 studies (14 studies included individuals with operationally defined CFS, 14 included individuals with CFS and chronic fatigue) and found that for defined CFS the median full recovery rate was 5%, whereas 39.5% had some improvement during follow-up periods. Recovery was more likely in those who did not meet full CFS criteria. The strongest predictors of improved outcome were less severe fatigue at baseline, lack of physical attribution, and less psychiatric disorder (Cairns & Hotopf, 2005). Despite some level of improvement, the majority of persons with CFS remain disabled over time.

Age, comorbid depressive disorders, and somatic attributions are associated with outcomes in CFS. Older age has been associated with better (Bombardier & Buchwald, 1995; Hartz et al., 1999) and worse (Kroenke et al., 1988; Russo et al., 1998; Schmaling, Fiedelak, Katon, Bader, & Buchwald, 2003; Tiersky et al., 2001) outcomes. Depressive disorders have been linked to poorer outcomes in some (Bombardier & Buchwald, 1995; M. R. Clark et al., 1995; Schmaling et al., 2003) but not all (Ciccone, Busichio, Vickroy, & Natelson, 2003; Tiersky et al., 2001) studies. Somatic attributions have been associated with poorer outcomes in longitudinal studies (Hartz et al., 1999; Sharpe et al., 1992; Schmaling, Fiedelak, et al., 2003; Taillefer, Kirmayer, Robbins, & Lasry, 2002; Wilson et al., 1994), and patients who improved over an approximate 3-year period were more likely to endorse both physical and psychological causes than patients whose fatigue persisted, but these differences did not achieve statistical significance (R. R. Taylor, Jason, & Curie, 2002). One U.K. population based incidence study of chronic fatigue found that baseline fatigue score predicted subsequent chronic fatigue, and when controlled for baseline fatigue, subsequent fatigue levels were not predicted by psychological morbidity and somatic attribution (Lawrie, Manders, Geddes, & Pelosi, 1997). Van der Werf, de Vree, Alberts, van der Meer, and Bleijenberg (2002) found that people with a relatively short duration of CFS had a more favorable outcome, whereas those with duration longer than 15 months rarely recovered. More social support and a stronger psychosocial explanation for symptoms also predicted better outcomes. The majority of studies have found that depressive disorders and somatic attributions were associated with poorer outcomes in CFS.

PREVALENCE

Bierl et al. (2004) conducted a random-digit-dialing survey to estimate the prevalence of fatiguing illnesses in diverse areas of the United States. This investigation estimated that nearly 2.2 million American adults suffer from CFS-like illness. Although women had much higher prevalence of chronic fatigue and CFS-like illness than men, the differences between male and female incidence rates were not significant. The prevalence of chronic fatigue was significantly higher in Whites than non-Whites, in the 40- to 69-year-old age group than in the 18- to 29-year-old age group, and in individuals with lower incomes and education.

Only a small minority of patients presenting to their physicians with problematic fatigue receive a diagnosis of CFS. The prevalence of CFS has been estimated to be from 0.24 to 0.4% (Jason et al., 1999; Steele et al., 1998) in community based studies, but these studies had a low participation rate in the clinical examination phase. In a large population based study of members of the Swedish Twin Registry, the preceding 6 months' prevalence rate of CFS was 2.4% (Evengard, Jacks, Pedersen, & Sullivan, 2005). This is closer to the 2.6% prevalence of patients in primary care (Wessely, Chalder,

Hirsch, Wallace, & Wright, 1997). CFS is a heterogeneous condition, fluctuating in terms of symptoms and severity. Although the level of disability varies widely (Carrico, Jason, Torres-Harding, & Witter, 2004; Cox & Findley, 2000), people with CFS have a markedly higher degree of impairment compared with other chronically ill people (Anderson & Ferrans, 1997). In the United States, approximately 400,000 to 900,000 people have CFS (Reeves et al., 2005), and the illness is estimated to cost about $9 billion per year in lost productivity (Reynolds, Vernon, Bouchery, & Reeves, 2004).

NEUROPSYCHOLOGICAL PERFORMANCE

Cognitive complaints are one of the most frequent and debilitating symptoms of CFS (Christodoulou et al., 1998; Komaroff, 1994; Komaroff & Buchwald, 1991). A number of studies have documented objective, albeit modest, neuropsychological impairments in CFS (Tiersky, Johnson, Lange, Natelson, & DeLuca, 1997). The most consistently documented impairments are in the areas of complex information processing speed and efficiency, working memory, and initial learning (Caseras et al., 2006; DeLuca et al., 2004; Michiels & Cluydts, 2001); higher order cognitive abilities are usually intact. Neuropsychological impairments are more likely in CFS persons who do not have a comorbid psychiatric condition or history of a psychiatric condition (DeLuca, Johnson, Ellis, & Natelson, 1997). Objective cognitive impairments appear to be related to functional decline (Christodoulou et al., 1998), employment status (Tiersky et al., 2001), and brain involvement (Lange et al., 1999, 2005; Schmaling et al., 2003).

Emotional factors (Wearden & Appleby, 1996) and self-reported fatigue (Cope et al., 1995; S. K. Johnson, Lange, DeLuca, Korn, & Natelson, 1997; Vercoulen et al., 1998) are related to an increase in subjective report of cognitive difficulty, with little evidence for a relationship between complaints and objective neuropsychological findings (Tiersky et al., 1997; Short, McCabe, & Tooley, 2002). Neither objective impairments nor subjective complaints can be explained by depression or fatigue levels.

ETIOLOGY

A biopsychosocial model is clearly required to explain the etiology of CFS (for reviews, see S. K. Johnson et al., 1999; Sharpe, 1996); CFS clearly is a multidimensional illness experience that cannot be conceptualized as a single diagnostic entity (Afari & Buchwald, 2003; Wessely, 1996). Although some researchers have expressed doubts regarding any biologic basis, there do appear to be neurophysiolological disturbances in a subset of persons with CFS.

Pathophysiology

Several recent studies have attempted to explore the molecular basis of CFS through gene expression analysis. Although these studies are very preliminary, several different laboratories indicate that gene expression profiles show some promise in distinguishing a genetic component of CFS, and genetic analysis may help elucidate pathogenesis of CFS (Fang et al., 2006; Fostel, Boneva, & Lloyd, 2006; Goertzel, Pennachin, de Souza Coehlo, Gurbaxani, et al., 2006).

Many of the symptoms of CFS such as myalgias, sore throat, swollen lymph nodes, and fatigue resemble symptoms seen in viral infections. Immune system abnormalities have been a productive area of research. In reviewing this work, Natelson and Lange (2002) concluded that although the CFS can occur after severe infection, no convincing evidence exists to support an immunologic process in disease maintenance. They proposed several possible etiologic processes: an encephalopathy, an impaired physiological capability to respond to stress, psychological fears about effort exacerbating symptoms, or environmental agents eliciting chronic fatigue states. Glaser et al. (2005) have argued that proinflammatory cytokines may play a role, but heterogeneity produces so much variability that it has been difficult to tell a consistent story. Glaser et al. proposed that a nonstructural Epstein–Barr virus-encoded protein can cause immune dysfunction and symptoms of CFS and may be an etiological agent.

The immune, endocrine, and nervous systems interact, and psychological stress may dysregulate immune responses by affecting these interactions. Hypothalamic–pituitary–adrenal (HPA) axis abnormalities have been widely studied in CFS, and some studies show a mild hypocortisolism of central origin suggesting an altered physiological response to stress. Deficits in cortisol have been linked to lethargy and fatigue in many conditions.

In summarizing studies of basal HPA axis function in CFS, A. J. Cleare (2003) noted that in about half of CFS studies, evidence has been found for lowered cortisol levels. In the pioneering study by Demitrack et al. (1991), low levels of basal cortisol were found in individuals with CFS, possibly because of a deficit in corticotropin-releasing hormone (CRH). Altemus et al. (2001) measured the adrenocorticotropin (ACTH) and cortisol response to infusion of vasopressin in patients with CFS and matched healthy volunteers. Persons with CFS had a reduced ACTH response and a more rapid cortisol response to a vasopressin infusion. They interpreted this as evidence of reduced hypothalamic CRH secretion in patients with CFS.

A study examining endocrine hyporesponsiveness to a maximal treadmill exercise test found that in CFS patients, the stress-responsive hormones were less than half the level of those in sedentary healthy controls 4 minutes after exercise (Ottenweller, LaManca, Sisto, Guo, & Natelson, 1997). Racciatti et al. (2001) found an altered cyclicity of HPA axis hormones (particularly ACTH and prolactin) in a circadian rhythm study.

Glucocorticoids can have an inhibitory effect on serotonin function, and CRH release is modulated by serotonin. Reduced glucocortocoid secretion would therefore result in higher serotonin levels. A number of studies (Bakheit, Behan, Dinan, Gray, & O'Keane, 1992; A. J. Cleare et al., 1995; Vassallo et al., 2001) have provided evidence that serotonin neurotransmission is increased in CFS patients compared with both healthy and depressed individuals.

Several studies have found evidence for subtle abnormalities in HPA function. A. J. Cleare et al. (2001) examined ACTH and cortisol responses to challenge agents in patients with CFS without comorbid psychiatric disorder compared with healthy controls. They found a similar ACTH response to all challenges, suggesting that central control of the HPA axis is intact in CFS, although they did find impaired adrenal response. Gaab, Huster, Peisen, Engret, Heitz, et al. (2002) have suggested that CFS patients are capable of mounting a sufficient cortisol response to a psychosocial stressor, a standardized exercise test, and an insulin tolerance test. Yet, these authors also found moderate HPA axis dysfunction with enhanced sensitivity of the adrenals to ACTH, indicative of secondary or tertiary origin. In a follow-up study, Gaab, Huster, Peisen, Engret, Schad, et al. (2002) found more suppression of salivary free cortisol in CFS patients compared with healthy controls after administration of dexamethasone. This pattern is the opposite of that generally found in depression; depressed patients generally do not suppress cortisol in response to dexamethosone. Rather, this exaggerated suppression of cortisol in response to dexamethasone is similar to what has been reported in posttraumatic stress disorder, chronic pelvic pain, and burnout syndrome (Gaab, Huster, Peisen, Engret, Schad, et al., 2002).

Crofford et al. (2004) studied underreactivity of the HPA axis in CFS patients by assaying blood samples across a 24-hour hormonal cycle. For all patient and control groups, there was an interaction between hormone levels and time period for both ACTH and cortisol. In the early morning periods, there were several hours during which patients with CFS had lower (but not significantly lower) cortisol levels compared with controls. There were no significant differences between patient and control groups for mean ACTH or cortisol over the entire 24-hour period. Jerjes et al. (2006) found that urinary free cortisol levels were significantly lower in CFS across a 3-day time period, whereas indices of cortisol metabolism showed no differences from controls. Future research needs to take into account the circadian cycle that can be seen with cortisol and ACTH. The neuroendocrine patterns in CFS resemble those observed in atypical depression. Van Hoof, Cluydts, and De Meirleir (2003) noted that in persons with CFS attending their clinic, the most common affective disorder diagnosed was atypical depression.

Overall, persons with CFS show subtle abnormalities in the HPA axis function, hormonal stress responses, and serotonin neurotransmission, which are in the opposite direction from the pattern observed in patients with clinical (melancholic) depression. Although dysfunction is mild and is not found consistently in all studies, a blunted HPA stress response is generally observed.

The recurrent stress responses and prolonged activation of cardiovascular and neuroendocrine systems have been termed *allostatic load*. Several studies have found that CFS was associated with a high level of allostatic load (Maloney et al., 2006) and that CFS patients with a high allostatic load had the worst functioning and most severe illness (Goertzel, Pennachin, de Souza Coelho, Maloney, et al., 2006).

Neuroimaging

Numerous studies have used brain imaging technology to examine whether there are structural and functional abnormalities in persons with CFS. Several studies have reported significantly more abnormalities on magnetic resonance imaging (MRI) among CFS patients relative to controls (Buchwald, Cheney, et al., 1992; D. B. Cook, Lange, DeLuca, & Natelson, 2001; Lange et al., 1999; Natelson, Cohen, Brassloff, & Lee, 1993); others, however (Cope, Pernet, Kendall, & Davis, 1995; R. B. Schwartz, Garada, et al., 1994), have not found significant differences. Lange et al. (1999) and Greco, Tannock, Brostoff, and Costa (1997) found brain abnormalities clustered in the nonpsychiatric rather than the psychiatric CFS cases. D. B. Cook, Lange, DeLuca, and Natelson (2001) reported that CFS participants with MRI abnormalities reported significantly more impairments in physical functional activity compared with CFS participants without MRI abnormalities.

Overall, structural MRI studies of the brain in persons with CFS have been inconsistent in demonstrating significant abnormalities. When they do occur, abnormalities are more likely in the subcortical white matter and in persons with CFS who do not have concurrent psychopathology. This is consistent with the neuropsychological data (presented above) suggesting greater neuropsychological impairment in persons with CFS without concurrent psychopathology.

In terms of functional neuroimaging, studies using single photon emission computed tomography (SPECT) technology have also been inconclusive. Some SPECT studies have reported cerebral abnormalities in CFS patients compared with healthy controls. (D. C. Costa, Tannock, & Brostoff, 1995; Ichise et al., 1992; Machale et al., 2000; R. B. Schwartz, Garada, et al., 1994; R. B. Schwartz, Komaroff, et al., 1994). In a co-twin control study of cerebral perfusion on SPECT of monozygotic twins discordant for CFS, no significant difference in cerebral blood flow was observed (D. H. Lewis et al., 2001).

Tirelli et al. (1998) used 18-fluorodeoxyglucose positron emission tomography to study cerebral metabolism and found that both the CFS and depression groups showed significant hypometabolism in the frontal lobes relative to controls. However, CFS patients showed significant brain stem hypometabolism relative to the depression group, a finding consistent with what has been reported in SPECT but not replicated more recently using positron emission tomography (Siessmeier et al., 2003). Regions activated in prior studies (e.g., brain stem [D. C. Costa et al., 1995; Tirelli et al., 1998]; thalamus [Machale et al., 2000]) were not observed by Siessmeier et al. (2003). SPECT findings remain inconclusive, with no consistent pattern of abnormality.

A few studies have attempted to relate neuropsychological performance (or complaints) with cerebral perfusion. Schmaling, Lewis, Fiedelak, Mahurin, and Buchwald (2003) conducted SPECT scans during rest and while performing a complex and speeded working memory task (the Paced Auditory Serial Addition Test [PASAT]). CFS patients showed a pattern of more diffuse regional blood flow compared with a more focal pattern in controls. CFS patients also showed more widespread and diffuse activation in frontal and temporal lobes and thalamus, indicative of increased recruitment of cerebral regions needed to perform the challenging cognitive task. These results were not attributed to group differences in mood, cognitive performance, or effort.

Using blood oxygen level dependent functional MRI (fMRI), Lange et al. (2005) examined persons with CFS without concurrent psychopathology while performing the PASAT. A select group of CFS patients with low PASAT scores displayed more diffuse and bilateral cerebral activation on fMRI while performing the complex working memory task relative to the healthy group. These studies (Lange et al., 2005; Schmaling et al., 2003) suggest that individuals with CFS need additional cerebral resources to perform the same amount of mental work.

Several studies have reported cerebral metabolic dysfunction in CFS using a variety of spectroscopy methods (Chaudhuri & Behan, 2000; Kuratsune et al., 2002; Puri et al., 2002; Tanaka, Matsushima, Tamai, & Kajumoto, 2002). Overall, evidence of brain pathology in CFS continues to accumulate, particularly among persons without comorbid psychiatric disorders. Structural neuroimaging studies show white matter hyperintensities in persons with CFS. Functional neuroimaging shows hypometabolism in the frontal lobes and basal ganglia most consistently in persons with CFS. Collectively, these findings suggest that central nervous system mechanisms may be involved in the pathophysiology of CFS. However, this work needs to be replicated and extended and developed into a cohesive theory (e.g., DeLuca, 2005). Many of the studies cited have a small number of participants and have not been consistently replicated.

Gender and Fatigue

Many studies have examined the role of gender in predicting fatigue. Studies have found gender differences in fatigue, with women tending to be more likely to report having both fatigue and chronic fatigue (Chen, 1986;

Jason, Jordan, et al., 1999; Loge, Ekeberg, & Kaasa, 1998; Nelson et al., 1987; Nisenbaum, Reyes, Mawle, & Reeves, 1998). Lindal et al. (2002) found that 78% of people in a random population study in Iceland who met criteria for CFS were women. Some researchers have also found that women tend to report more severe fatigue (Chen, 1986; Jason, Jordan, et al., 1999; Kroenke et al., 1988; Loge et al., 1998; Nisenbaum et al., 1998; Pawlikowska et al., 1994). In a general practice study, women were more likely to complain of fatigue than men, even after adjustment for psychological distress (Pawlikowska et al., 1994), and the most commonly cited reasons for fatigue were psychosocial (40% of patients). Women are more than twice as likely to seek medical help for their fatigue (Cope, 1992). For example, in one study, two thirds of the people who presented with fatigue in a primary care practice were women (Nelson et al., 1987). However, some primary care and hospital studies have not found statistically significant differences in fatigue according to gender (Cathebras, Robbins, et al., 1992; Kirk, Douglass, Nelson, Jaffee, & Lopez, 1990).

In a population based study of chronic fatigue, Evengard et al. (2005) found that when respondents were asked about the symptom of feeling "abnormally tired" during the past 6 months, there was no gender difference, and after excluding possible medical causes, 17% of the population reported this symptom. As the requirements for a CFS-like illness became more rigorous, however, the gender prevalence became skewed. Using the Fukuda et al. (1994) definition brought the prevalence down to 2.36% of the population; more than 80% were women. This is reminiscent of irritable bowel syndrome (IBS) and FMS in that when more symptoms are included in the diagnostic criteria, the patient population becomes predominantly female. Using the same sample from the Swedish Twin Registry, P. F. Sullivan, Evengard, Jacks, and Pedersen (2005) investigated whether there were differences according to zygosity in chronic fatigue. They found that from a less refined symptom of chronic fatigue to the Fukuda et al. definition, there was no difference in genetic contribution. Using the more restrictive definition did not make the illness more genetic. The modest genetic influences were similar in both genders. Despite differences in prevalence, the relative importance of genes and environment did not differ between genders.

Buchwald, Pearlman, Kith, and Schmaling (1994) examined differences between 348 male and female CFS patients from a university-based referral clinic devoted to chronic fatigue. Clinical variables included symptoms, physical examination findings, and laboratory results. Psychosocial assessment consisted of a structured psychiatric interview; the Medical Outcomes Study Short-Form General Health Survey to assess functional status; the General Health Questionnaire to ascertain psychological distress; the Multidimensional Health Locus of Control; and measures of attribution, social support, and coping. Overall, few gender-related differences were identified. Women had a higher frequency of tender or enlarged lymph nodes and FMS and lower scores on the physical functioning; men more often had pharyngeal inflammation and reported a higher lifetime prevalence of alcoholism. In a subclassification of CFS study, Jason et al. (2003) found that people with high symptom frequencies were more often female and older and had greater disability and more children.

Tseng and Natelson (2004) examined differences in symptom presentation and functional and psychiatric status between 43 men and 78 women with CFS only who were patients at their research center. They found no differences in severity of CFS or functional status, although women had significantly higher endorsement of infectious-type symptoms. There was no significant difference in the rates of lifetime psychiatric disorders, although they were somewhat higher in men (64.3% vs. 47.5%). Collectively, these studies indicate that demographic, clinical, and psychosocial factors do not clearly differ in male and female CFS patients.

Soderlund and Malterud (2005) performed a qualitative interview study of causal attributions in 8 women with CFS. Some gendered factors recurred in the interviews, such as living in a culture where women are overburdened without sufficient relaxation time, having emotional conflicts, having more self-inflicted pressure than men, and having weaker immune systems than men.

Clark (1999) examined gender differences in CFS using qualitative interview methods and found no differences in terms of mode of onset, duration, symptom variability, least and most commonly reported symptoms, and level of activity prior to illness. Women were more likely to attribute their illness to stress, whereas men were more likely to believe the illness resulted from working with chemicals. The biggest differences emerged in the medical encounter. Compared with women, men were more likely to report that their doctors took them seriously and were more likely to be sent to a specialist; women reported more negative experiences with doctors and were more likely to be sent to a psychiatrist.

Abuse

Unlike IBS and FMS, there is little research on the prevalence of abuse history in CFS. R. R. Taylor and Jason (2001) used a randomly selected community sample to compare fatigue groups with healthy controls regarding history of childhood sexual, physical, or death threat abuse. Childhood sexual abuse was significantly associated with idiopathic chronic fatigue and chronic fatigue caused by a psychiatric or medical condition, but it was not associated with CFS. Van Houdenhove et al. (2001) examined emotional, physical, and sexual victimization throughout the life span in patients with CFS or FMS compared with rheumatoid arthritis patients, multiple sclerosis patients, and healthy controls. There were no significant differences in victimization experiences between the CFS and FMS groups. CFS and FMS patients reported more emotional neglect and emotional and physical abuse than rheumatoid arthritis or multiple sclerosis patients or healthy controls. When separated into childhood only, adult only, and lifelong victimization, significantly more CFS and FMS patients belonged to the lifelong victimization group (40.0% vs. 7.6% in the rheumatoid arthritis and multiple sclerosis group and 11.6% in the controls). There were no significant differences in sexual abuse and sexual harassment among groups. The CFS and FMS groups also reported significantly greater emotional impact from emotional neglect, emotional abuse, physical abuse, and sexual harassment compared with the rheumatoid arthritis, multiple sclerosis, and healthy control groups. There was no significant difference in terms of impact of sexual abuse. Van Houdenhove et al. (2001) suggested that CFS and FMS patients remain entangled in problematic relationships, without marshalling protective factors to reduce the emotional impact of these burdens. These studies indicate that sexual abuse is not a specific risk factor for CFS or FMS but rather that victimization takes the form of neglect, violence, chaos, and unpredictable family life.

Psychiatric Disorder

Elevated rates of psychiatric comorbidity or indicators of psychological disorder have been found among chronic fatigue patients in primary care settings (Cathebras et al., 1992). Community based studies have also found that persons suffering from chronic fatigue were more likely to have psychiatric symptoms or to be diagnosed with psychiatric disorders (Lawrie et al., 1997; Pawlikowska et al., 1994).

High levels of somatization in individuals with depression and anxiety suggest that CFS may be a somatic form of depression. Alternatively, high rates of depression and anxiety in CFS may result from overlapping symptomatology, reaction to disability imposed by fatigue, or viral or immune changes affecting the central nervous system. Although CFS patients may meet diagnostic criteria for depressive disorder or score in the depressed range on a self-report inventory, they report significantly lower levels of dysphoria and self-reproach symptoms than clinically depressed patients (S. K. Johnson, DeLuca, & Natelson, 1996a). Patients with CFS are significantly less likely than either depressed individuals, multiple sclerosis patients, or healthy controls to interpret symptoms in terms of negative emotional states (Dendy, Cooper, & Sharpe, 2001). Unlike depressed patients' cognitions, which are dominated by a negative view of the self, CFS patients are primarily preoccupied with symptoms for which they make physical attributions, which helps maintain self-esteem (Moss-Morris & Petrie, 2001).

CFS patients generally demonstrate greater impairment than depressed individuals on various measures of functional disability (Buchwald, Pearlman, Umali, Schmaling, & Katon, 1996; Natelson et al., 1995). Antidepressants have not been efficacious in CFS (Dzurec, 2000; Dzurec, Hoover, & Fields, 2002; Vercoulen et al., 1996). Converging evidence suggests that CFS can be separated from most subtypes of depression, although it resembles atypical depression in neuroendocrine responses. Physiologically and in symptom presentation, CFS looks much more like atypical depression than melancholic depression, but no research to date has addressed these similarities directly by comparing the two patient groups (S. K. Johnson & DeLuca, 2005).

Prevalence of depression in CFS studies spans a wide range, from a low of 5% to as high as 80%. S. K. Johnson, Gil-Rivas, and Schmaling (2006) found that only 5% of patients met criteria for a current depressive disorder. (This was probably attributable to the coding assumptions applied to the psychiatric interview in that study.) Specifically, previous studies (Henningsen, Zimmerman, & Sattel, 2003; Skapinakas, Lewis, & Mavreas, 2003; Skapinakas, Lewis, & Meltzer, 2000; Tiersky et al., 2001) have not adjusted for the symptom overlap between psychiatric disorders and CFS symptoms, potentially overestimating the prevalence of psychiatric disorders among this population. Clearly, it is hard to estimate consistent levels of depression or somatization disorder when there are so many overlapping symptoms that can be attributed to organic or psychiatric causes, depending on coding assumptions made by the researcher or clinician.

Personality Factors

Although early studies of personality in samples of persons with CFS found histrionic and emotional type traits overrepresented compared with their base rates in the population, these studies suffered from methodological flaws (Blakely et al., 1991; C. Millon et al., 1989; Stricklin, Sewell, & Austad, 1988). Studies with improved methodology have also found evidence of personality pathology. The most commonly reported personality disorders have been obsessive–compulsive, histrionic, borderline, and dependent (Henderson & Tannock, 2004; S. K. Johnson, DeLuca, & Natelson, 1996b; Pepper, Krupp, Friedberg, Doscher, & Coyle, 1993). S. K. Johnson et al. (1996b) found that personality dysfunction in the CFS group was accounted for by comorbid depression, whereas Henderson and Tannock (2004) did not find an association.

Thus, across studies, obsessive–compulsive and histrionic personality pathology was most common among persons with CFS, with dependent and borderline features found less consistently. Two studies have examined the association between personality disorders and functioning. Ciccone et al. (2003) found that neither Axis I nor Axis II disorders predicted physical functioning or physical role functioning. Conversely, in a 5-year follow-up study of adolescents with CFS, Rangel, Garralda, Levin, and Roberts (2000) found that adolescents with personality dysfunction were less likely to have recovered from CFS.

Subjectively reported symptoms have been shown to be systematically biased by neuroticism, which is strongly correlated with health complaints but not actual health status (P. T. Costa & McCrae, 1987). S. K. Johnson et al. (1996c) also examined the personality trait of neuroticism, which is associated with a tendency to experience emotional distress, including anxiety, anger, sadness, and other emotions with negative valence (P. T. Costa & McCrae, 1992). In that study, participants with CFS and multiple sclerosis had neuroticism scores that were significantly higher than those of healthy controls yet significantly lower than those of depressed participants. This finding was replicated by Buckley et al. (1999); the sample with CFS scored in between participants who were depressed and healthy controls on the measure of neuroticism.

Neuroticism appears to play a role in poorer prognosis in CFS. Higher neuroticism scores were associated with lower vitality over time (S. K. Johnson et al., 2006). Taillefer, Kirmayer, Robbins, and Lasry (2003) found that neuroticism, somatic attribution, depression, and age contributed to illness worry in CFS. They hypothesized that illness worry leads to restriction of activity and physical deconditioning, contributing to the chronicity of fatigue, consistent with S. K. Johnson et al.'s (2006) finding of increased suppression of competing activities being associated with worse functioning. Likewise, the cognitive–behavioral model of CFS posits a vicious cycle of suppressing and avoiding activity that results in deconditioning, further reduction of activity, and illness perpetuation (Surawy, Hackman, Hawton, & Sharpe, 1995).

A Belgian study found that CFS patients described themselves as significantly more "action-prone" premorbidly than comparison groups (Van Houdenhove, Onghena, Neerinckx, & Hellin, 1995), and a later study found that this was not due to idealistic appraisal of premorbid traits (Van Houdenhove et al., 2001). Clinical observations of more than 100 CFS patients revealed a typical premorbid characterization of perfectionism, high achievement orientation and work performance standards, high valuation of the opinions of others, and suppression of emotions (Surawy et al., 1995). White and Schweitzer (2000) found that CFS patients had higher perfectionism and lower self-esteem scores than did healthy controls, although they did not differ on a measure of emotional control. The results obtained by Wood and Wessely (1999) did not support the view of CFS sufferers as perfectionists with more negative attitudes toward psychiatry compared with a rheumatoid arthritis group.

Indications of defensiveness among persons with CFS were reported by Creswell and Chalder (2002) using the Emotional Stroop Test to determine whether participants with CFS were different from those with diabetes and a healthy group in "covert" self-esteem. Individuals with CFS were slower to name negative words than positive words compared with the other two groups. The authors maintained that this result reveals higher levels of self-esteem than expected from the level of depression, anxiety, and self-esteem that was overtly reported. In another study the same authors found participants with CFS frequently used "defensive high anxious" coping styles (Creswell & Chalder, 2001). The low levels of overt psychopathology suggest defensiveness regarding psychological contributions to illness.

In a prospective design, Kato, Sullivan, Evengard, and Pedersen (2006) investigated the relationship between self-perceived stress, extraversion, and emotional instability assessed from 1972 to 1973 and chronic fatigue assessed from 1998 to 2002 in 19,192 twins from the population based Swedish twin registry. Kato et al.'s analysis showed strong support for premorbid stress and emotional instability to predict chronic fatigue several decades later. The role of emotional instability in chronic fatigue was found to be mediated by genetic and family environment factors, whereas stress had exogenous, direct effects on the later appearance of chronic fatigue.

CONCLUSION

CFS can be conceptualized as a stress disorder along the same lines as FMS. Stressful life events, infectious illness, autonomic and HPA axis functioning, and cognitive biases interact at the biopsychosocial level and initiate symptoms of fatigue, myalgias, and sleep difficulties. Research on brain pathology and genetic abnormalities are ongoing, but a consistent story has yet to emerge. Women may be more vulnerable to CFS because of pressure from role expectations, stressful experiences, and neuroendocrine vulnerabilities; further research is needed to explore these possible explanations for the greater prevalence of the condition in women.

8

MULTIPLE CHEMICAL SENSITIVITY

Multiple chemical sensitivity (MCS) is a syndrome in which multiple disabling symptoms are reported in response to low-level chemical exposure. MCS has been described by a number of labels: *environmental illness, chemical hypersensitivity syndrome, universal reactor syndrome, universal allergy, total allergy syndrome, 20th century disease, chemical AIDS,* and *ecologic illness* (Graveling, Pilkington, George, Butler, & Tannahill, 1999; Kroll-Smith & Floyd, 1997; Mooser, 1987; Simon, Katon, & Sparks, 1990). Some have proposed calling the condition *idiopathic environmental intolerance* (IEI) because *multiple chemical sensitivity* implies that the cause of these disorders is known, even though no relation between exposure and symptoms has thus far been substantiated (Wiesmuller, Ebel, Hornberg, Kwan, & Friel, 2003, p. 420). However, because *multiple chemical sensitivity* is the term most widely used in the scientific literature, I use it in this chapter. In discussions of specific studies, however, I use the nomenclature used by the study authors.

Of the medically unexplained illnesses (MUIs) discussed in this volume, MCS is the most controversial and the least recognized by the medical profession. The U.S. government has directed little research attention toward chemical sensitivities or toward adverse effects associated with toxic chemicals in general. There is considerable scientific skepticism regarding the existence of MCS as a distinct disorder. For example, the *Journal of the*

American Medical Association and the *New England Journal of Medicine* publish articles on chronic fatigue syndrome (CFS), irritable bowel syndrome (IBS), and fibromyalgia (FMS), but they have not published studies investigating MCS (Zavestoski et al., 2004). Zavestoski et al. (2004) commented that there is really no better understanding today of the physiological dysfunction and prevalence of MCS than when it was first identified.

DEFINING MULTIPLE CHEMICAL SENSITIVITY

A growing number of individuals have presented with symptoms of MCS since the 1980s. A range of symptoms are reportedly precipitated and then exacerbated by exposure to commonly occurring chemical substances such as petroleum products, synthetics, and food additives. The most common symptoms of MCS appear to be headache; shortness of breath; dizziness; weakness; pain in joints, muscles, back, or abdomen; neuropsychological problems; fatigue; congestion; sore throat; and nausea or vomiting (Fiedler, 1996; Ziem & McTamney, 1997). No group of core symptoms that are common to all individuals with MCS has been identified (Wiesmuller et al., 2003).

The term *chemical* in MCS is used broadly to refer to a range of natural and man-made chemical agents, some of which have multiple chemical constituents. The most commonly reported substances that elicit MCS symptoms are perfumes and colognes, spray paint, perfumes in cosmetics, cigarette smoke, gasoline, garage fumes, diesel exhaust, hair spray, restroom deodorizer, and air fresheners (Fiedler, 1996). This list is notable for the predominant presence of everyday substances rather than industrial chemicals or pollutants. The toxic responses of MCS sufferers are occurring at extremely low (generally considered safe) levels.

Clearly, there is the potential for large costs to be incurred by industry if a direct connection could be made between manufactured chemicals and serious illness. The economic and regulatory implications of accepting MCS as a medical disorder caused by common chemicals and the built environment are enormous. News media have generally portrayed people with MCS as histrionic and psychologically disturbed rather than legitimately sick from chemical products; this view downplays the effects of pollutants and toxins on health (Lipson, 2004). MCS sufferers and their advocates maintain that people with MCS may be akin to "canaries in a coal mine"; that is, only the most sensitive harbingers of a toxic industrial environment that may eventually affect the health of the general population. More than with other MUIs, people with MCS request that other people modify their behaviors to accommodate them. People with MCS may require coworkers, friends, and family to avoid scents, soaps, and cleaners to avoid exacerbating the MCS symptoms (Kroll-Smith & Floyd, 1997).

The broad and baffling array of symptoms associated with sensitivity to chemicals has made many doctors wary of treating MCS patients. Indeed, many in the medical community see MCS as a faulty set of beliefs rather than a disease. In MCS, the biomedical model does not allow patients to assume the sick role and the doctor to assume the expert healer role (Kroll-Smith & Floyd, 1997). As a consequence, doctor shopping occurs because patients are not taken seriously by doctors. However, a group of physicians, formerly called *clinical ecologists* and now called *environmental medicine physicians*, specialize in MCS. These specialists tend to cast a wide net and attribute many diseases such as cancer, arthritis, and vasculitis to chemical exposures (Fiedler & Kipen, 1997). The specialty of clinical ecology is not recognized by conventional medicine.

The first definition of MCS was developed by Cullen (1987), and it described the following characteristics: Initial symptoms are acquired from identifiable environmental exposure, symptoms involve more than one organ system, symptoms occur and abate in response to predictable stimuli, symptoms are elicited by low-level exposures, and symptoms cannot be explained through standard medical testing. Known organ system dysfunction and disease are excluded from Cullen's definition. Ashford and Miller (1997) have postulated that MCS develops through a two-stage process of sensitization and triggering. Sensitization occurs as the result of one massive exposure or following low-level chronic exposures to common toxins, such as in sick building syndrome. Symptoms are then triggered by a variety of chemicals and, in some individuals, electromagnetic exposures, foods, light, sound, or natural substances such as pollen or molds.

Other researchers have noted that no consensus exists regarding case criteria; some studies include patients with gradual onset of symptoms, rather than requiring an identifiable initial exposure. The lack of agreement on an empirically validated symptom profile prevents standardized diagnostic recommendations (Fiedler, 1996; Lacour, Zunder, Schmidtke, Vaith, & Scheidt, 2005). Lacour et al. (2005) performed a systematic literature review of 1,429 MEDLINE references of MCS-related terms and found 36 articles, which included symptom profiles, clinical overlap with other conditions, quality of life indices, and diagnostic procedures. From this review, Lacour et al. concluded that central nervous system complaints, such as headaches, fatigue, and cognitive deficits, were the most frequently reported symptoms, followed by musculoskeletal and gastrointestinal complaints. They recommended that diagnostic procedures exclude any diseases that might account for nonspecific central nervous system symptoms, as is done in CFS. Food or alcohol intolerance is not an exclusion for MCS (i.e., they may coexist with it). Lacour et al. also found significant overlap of MCS, CFS, and FMS.

In their review of MCS, Graveling et al. (1999) used a broad definition of MCS, requiring symptoms in more than one organ system elicited by various chemicals at very low levels of exposure. Like Kipen and Fiedler (2002), they conceded that MCS raises many questions about the nature of illness. Some have suggested that MCS is an olfactory preference to be protected from noxious scent and not a pathological condition. There appears to be no resolution to this debate, partly because of the paucity of funding and peer-reviewed research on this topic. Because MCS often occurs with other MUIs, it is unclear whether MCS is a distinct malady. This question continues to be debated (Fiedler, Maccia, & Kippen, 1992).

PREVALENCE

Very little research into the prevalence of MCS has been attempted, largely because there is no consensus definition. Fiedler and Kipen (1997) summarized the literature on patients who report a symptomatic intolerance for low-level chemical exposures, express symptoms in multiple organ systems, and have no other medical illnesses. Fiedler and Kipen found 10 studies meeting these criteria. Despite some discrepancies in selection criteria, they found striking consistencies in the demographic profiles. The ratio of women to men was 8:2. The average age was mid-40s, and the average educational level was at least 2 years of college.

Kreutzer, Neutra, and Lashuay (1999) conducted a population-based telephone survey of 4,046 people in California and found that 15.9% reported being allergic or unusually sensitive to everyday chemicals, and an even more astounding 6.3% were diagnosed with "environmental illness" or MCS by their physician. Hispanic ethnicity was associated with physician-diagnosed MCS. Female gender was associated with individual self-reports of sensitivity. Marital status, employment, education, geographic location, and income were not predictive of reported chemical sensitivities or diagnosis of MCS. Kreutzer et al. believed that the homogeneity of responses across ethnicity, geography, education, and marital status was compatible with a physiologic response or with widespread societal apprehensions in regard to chemical exposure.

Caress and Steinemann (2003, 2004b) found that MCS affected 12.6% of the population, and 3.1% of these had been diagnosed medically in a randomly selected sample from the Atlanta, Georgia, metropolitan area. In follow-up questioning of the respondents who reported hypersensitivity, the most commonly reported triggers for the onset of symptoms were pesticides and solvent exposure. Only 1.4% reported experiencing depression, anxiety, or other emotional problems before the onset of their symptoms, yet 38% said they experienced these problems after developing hypersensitivity (Caress & Steinemann, 2004b).

In another study, Caress and Steinemann (2004a) conducted a telephone survey of 1,054 randomly selected individuals within the continental United States to determine the prevalence of chemical hypersensitivity and the medical diagnosis of MCS in the U.S. population. They found that 11.2% of Americans reported an unusual hypersensitivity to common chemical products such as perfume, fresh paint, pesticides, and other petrochemical-based substances, and 2.5% reported that they had been medically diagnosed with MCS. Additionally, 31.1% of those sampled reported adverse reactions to perfumed products, and 17.6% experienced breathing difficulties and other health problems when exposed to air fresheners. Although chemical hypersensitivity was more common in women, it affected individuals in all demographic groups studied. Although only based on self-reports, it does appear that an MCS-like condition that impairs quality of life is common in the general U.S. population.

One might wonder why MCS does not appear more often in groups that are occupationally exposed to petrochemicals and pesticides. It is possible that self-selection and reporting biases play a role. Reid et al. (2002) performed an epidemiological health survey of U.K. military personnel, which included an assessment of chemical sensitivities. They received responses from 3,531 veterans of the Gulf War, 2,614 veterans in active service but not deployed to the Gulf, and 2,050 veterans from Bosnian peacekeeping operations. Most demographic profiles show MCS as occurring predominantly in females and do not measure occupational exposures, so the fact that the sample was 92% male and included occupational exposures such as diesel fumes and pesticides that have been frequently reported in military cohorts makes this survey different from previous studies. Sensitivity to at least one common chemical was reported by 28% of the Gulf War veterans, 14% of those not deployed to the Gulf, and 13% of the Bosnian conflict group. These results show, rather surprisingly, that a significant proportion of U.K. veterans appeared to have sensitivity to various chemicals, although they were clearly not typical of the MCS demographic profile.

C. S. Miller (1999) described diverse demographic groups with MCS-like conditions, ranging from radiology workers exposed to X-ray developer solution, Environmental Protection Agency employees exposed to carpet building materials, German log home owners exposed to pentachlorophenol wood preservative, sheep dippers in Great Britain exposed to organophosphate pesticides, and Gulf War veterans exposed to a variety of substances during military service.

PROGNOSIS

Black, Okiishi, and Schlosser (2001) performed a 9-year follow-up on 18 persons with MCS from an original sample of 26. Overall, there was little change in psychological and functional status, and the individuals remained strong in their illness conviction and resistant to psychological explanations. Eighty-five percent of the sample met criteria of the *Diagnostic and Statistical Manual of Mental Disorders* (4th ed. [DSM–IV]; American Psychiatric Association, 1994) for Lifetime Mood Disorder, 56% for Lifetime Anxiety, and 56% for Lifetime Somatoform Disorder. Other than this report, there are few data on longitudinal outcomes for people with MCS.

OVERLAP WITH OTHER MEDICALLY UNEXPLAINED ILLNESSES

Several studies have documented the co-occurrence of MCS with CFS and FMS according to self-reports of symptoms (Buchwald & Garrity, 1994; Kipen & Fiedler, 2002); about 30% to 50% of individuals with one illness also met criteria for one of the others. MCS also has substantial overlap with Gulf War illness (Kipen, Hallman, Kang, Fiedler, & Natelson, 1999). In their population-based study, Caress and Steinemann (2003, 2004b) found that 26% of those with MCS also reported gastrointestinal problems, 22% said they also had FMS, and 19% reported CFS.

One of the important distinctions between MCS and other MUIs is that MCS purportedly results from a chemical insult. Therefore, toxic exposures in the environment are a more prominent issue, both for theoretical explanations of this illness and for clinical management. As with other MUIs, rates of disability and functional impairment are very high in MCS. People with MCS often significantly alter their behavior in an attempt to avoid presumed precipitants of symptoms. They often withdraw from activities, friends, and family in an attempt to eliminate chemical exposures. In a study of 35 patients with occupationally related MCS evaluated in an occupational medicine clinic (Lax & Henneberger, 1995), 97% of the patients had stopped activities outside the home, 91% had limited travel, 89% had limited their contact with friends, and 77% had left their jobs. Additionally, many patients changed their home life drastically: 97% had stopped using cleaning compounds, 69% removed home furnishings, and 63% limited their contact with family members. In their personal care, 94% stopped using fragrances, 91% changed their diet, and 86% changed the type of clothing they wore. As with other MUIs, MCS results in significant disruption of everyday life and a heavy burden of disability.

GENDER

As with the other MUIs explored in this book, gender is a consistent, robust predictor of MCS. Middle-aged, educated women make up 60% to 80% of samples in clinical studies (Black, 2000; Fiedler & Kipen, 1997). Bell, Baldwin, and Schwartz (2001) have suggested that "chemical intolerance" may be more sensitizable in some individuals, driven by differences in genetic and gender-related vulnerability of various target organs and the prevailing environmental context. We have seen the evidence for increased life stress and childhood trauma in various MUIs. Bell et al. suggested that these stressors could provide an initiating stimulus for sensitization that subsequent stressors such as low-level chemical exposure could later elicit. Allostatic load from adapting to amplified stress reactivity should lead to chronic health problems sooner in more sensitizable than in less sensitizable individuals. Middle age may be the point where allostatic load impairs adaptability. Bell et al. also suggested that women who have a family history of substance abuse have inherited an enhanced capacity for sensitization, one that leads to chemical intolerance and food cravings and intolerances.

Mooser (1987) noted that the most common statistical finding in MCS is female predominance and speculated that this may be due to innate heightened allergic sensitization and food sensitivities in females. There is also evidence that women of reproductive age have enhanced sensitivity to odors; women's olfactory sensitivity increases faster and to a significantly greater degree than that of men (Dalton, Doolittle, & Breslin, 2002). This sensitivity may be hormone mediated; it was not found in girls (ages 8 to 10 years) or postmenopausal women. Dalton et al. (2002) suggested that this enhanced sensitivity may account for the greater prevalence of MCS in women, although there may be adaptive benefits conferred on reproductive age women in increased ability for olfactory-based kin recognition and mother–infant bonding. Lipson (2004) speculated that MCS is more prevalent in reproductive age women because their hormonal systems may be more vulnerable to the large number of endocrine-disrupting chemicals in pesticides and plastics that mimic estrogen. Estrogen load may be one reason that females (both human and animal) are more susceptible than males to metabolic disorders, sensitization, and MCS.

Compared with men, women appear to have more health concerns about the effects of toxins, pollutants, and dangerous chemicals such as pesticides. Petrie et al. (2005) found that worries about modernity, including concerns about the health effects of toxins, pollution, tainted food, and radiation, predicted symptom complaints after a pesticide-spraying program in New Zealand. In this study, Petrie et al. assessed worries about modernity before the spraying program and found that higher levels of modern health worries and baseline symptoms were associated with a higher number of symptoms being attributed to the spray program. Petrie et al. corroborated previous findings that modern health worries are associated with increased somatic complaints and medical utilization and that such concerns and complaints are more common in women (S. K. Johnson & Blanchard, 2006; Kaptein et al., 2005). Kaptein et al. specifically reported in samples of medical students from New Zealand and Holland that modern health worries were related to the use of health care services and that the relationship was mediated by subjective health complaints.

ETIOLOGY

A number of theories have been articulated to explain MCS symptomatology. The earliest theory of MCS proposed immune dysfunction; this theory is most popular among clinical ecologists who posit a chemical overload–induced immune dysregulation. Clinical ecologists believe that chemical exposure causes the development of allergy to low levels of many chemicals, not just the initiating one. Although some abnormalities have been found in patients with MCS, there are many problems with these tests, such as wide natural variation in the test results, few reference standards to determine what is statistically "normal," and lack of reproducibility (Magill & Surada, 1998). Controlled studies have not supported any consistent pattern of immune dysfunction or deficiency (Graveling et al., 1999; Simon, Daniell, Stockbridge, Claypoole, & Rosenstock, 1993).

Although much MCS research has focused on an immune system mechanism, most MCS symptoms cannot be immune system mediated because they occur too quickly on exposure. With the exception of a histamine response and some IgE-mediated responses such as anaphylactic shock, the immune system is not generally capable of reacting as quickly as the symptoms appear. This has led some researchers to look at central nervous system responses, which would be consistent with the time frame most patients report. The proposed mechanism is that affected persons develop increasing neurologic sensitivity to the adverse effects of chemicals (Bell, 1994; Bell et al., 2001).

Bell and her colleagues have published a number of reports supporting a neurogenic mechanism for MCS wherein connections between the olfactory nerve, limbic structures (particularly amygdale and hippocampus), and hypothalamus develop sensitization. The neurological phenomenon known as *time-dependent sensitization* (TDS), which has been studied primarily in animals for the last 20 years, has shown some similarity to MCS. TDS is the progressive amplification of response to intermittent exposure to stimuli. Animals repeatedly exposed to seizure-inducing chemicals or electrical stimulation have been found to develop lower thresholds for seizure induction than the thresholds observed before exposure. With other stimuli, animals have been found to have an amplification of the response to the stimulus over time, as well as cross-sensitization to unrelated chemicals (Bell, 1994; Bell, Miller, Schwartz, Peterson, & Amend, 1996; Friedman, 1994). TDS may explain how the brain becomes sensitized to low-level chemical exposures and the role that stress plays in adverse reactions. Cross-sensitization can turn chemical sensitivity into a progressive condition. After a person is sensitized to one chemical, the sensitivity can spread to include other unrelated compounds. Then repeat exposures reduce the body's tolerance level by an as yet unknown mechanism, so the body becomes more easily reactive to more and more chemicals at lower and lower levels until it finally reaches the point where the person is sick all the time. Besides animal models, Bell has studied cacosmic college students (*cacosmia* is a negative response and illness from common chemical odors) and found evidence for increased sensitivity in some individuals (Bell et al., 1996).

A related theory involves altered function of respiratory passages, a neurogenic inflammation (Bascom et al., 1997). Meggs (1995) has proposed a reactive upper airway dysfunction syndrome, essentially a chronic rhinitis developing from inhalation exposure to a toxic substance. Meggs (1999) has also argued that allergy and chemical sensitivity are closely related disorders in which environmental exposures produce inflammatory reactions. Both the allergic and chemical irritant responses may be subjected to conditioning so that the response is triggered by other stimuli and becomes chronic. The problem with neurogenic theories is that they cannot account very well for the multisystem nature of MCS symptoms.

The finding that some MCS sufferers have increased urinary coproporhyrin levels led to speculation that MCS is an acquired form of porphyria (Donnay & Ziem, 1995). The *porphyrias* are a group of rare metabolic, enzyme deficiency disorders involving the production of *heme* (a component of blood) and liver or bone marrow damage; some of the symptoms are similar to those for MCS. Disorders of porphyrinopathy have also been claimed for people with CFS, FMS, amalgam problems, and silicone implants. This theory has been widely disseminated by advocates for MCS patients but has not held up under scientific scrutiny (Hahn & Bonkovsky, 1997; McDonagh & Bissell, 1998).

Claudia Miller (1999) has proposed a mechanism called *toxicant induced loss of tolerance* to explain MCS. This mechanism involves two steps:

1. Exposure to certain chemicals causes vulnerable individuals to lose their previous tolerance for common chemicals, food, or drugs.
2. Previously tolerated exposures trigger symptoms in sensitive individuals at everyday low levels.

Controlled exposure studies allow an empirical approach to determining the concentrations of substances that produce symptoms. Fiedler and colleagues (Fiedler, 2000; Fiedler et al., 2004; Fiedler & Kipen, 2001) maintained a controlled environment facility where they tested different chemically sensitive groups. They found that MCS and individuals sensitive to methyl tertiary butyl ether (MTBE) do not consistently respond with symptoms differently from healthy controls. Individuals with MCS responded differently from controls only to suprathreshold levels of a rose-scented chemical (phenyl ethyl alcohol) but not to a noxious odorant (pyridine). MTBE-sensitive individuals responded symptomatically to gasoline with 15% MTBE but not to gasoline alone or gasoline with 11% MTBE. Controlled exposure studies also found that chemically sensitive individuals did not detect or identify odors better than healthy controls. However, in a single, controlled diesel vapor exposure that Fiedler et al. (2004) conducted with chemically sensitive Gulf War veterans compared with healthy Gulf war veterans, the chemically sensitive veterans reported significantly increased symptoms of disorientation, dizziness, reduced end-tidal CO_2, respiratory discomfort, and malaise as exposure increased. Fiedler et al. concluded that both psychologic and physiologic mechanisms contribute to symptomatic responses in ill Gulf War veterans.

Staudenmayer, Binkley, Leznoff, and Phillips (2000) reviewed toxicogenic theories of MCS to determine whether such explanations held up, using Bradford Hill's (1965) nine criteria for causation (strength, consistency, specificity, temporality, biological gradient, biological plausibility, coherence, response to intervention, and analogy). Staudenmayer et al. concluded that toxicogenic theories do not meet any of the nine criteria, rendering such theories invalid. This skepticism and lack of scientifically validated etiologic evidence help explain why MCS remains a controversial diagnosis.

Psychological Factors

Because the relationship between chemical exposures and symptoms in MCS does not fit well into current toxicological paradigms for such relationships, the psychiatric explanation for symptoms has been investigated more than any other. Lipson (2004) commented on the "psychologization" of MCS as a women's disease. Except in the cases of a defined toxically exposed cohort, close to 80% of those with MCS are women. As in the other MUIs, patients are often told that their medical tests are normal and that their illness must be caused by stress or depression. Lipson referred to this biomedical viewpoint, which finds that female-predominant illnesses are disproportionately attributed to psychiatric causes, as male oriented.

Fiedler and Kipen (1997) summarized the early psychiatric explanations of MCS, which tended to emphasize an anxiety response; typical or atypical posttraumatic stress disorder; or modern expressions of anxiety, depression, or somatization. Numerous studies have found elevated rates of depression and anxiety traits in MCS; about one half of the patients in various studies have met the criteria for depressive and anxiety disorders (Fiedler et al., 1992; Simon, 1994)

Simon et al. (1990) examined plastics workers at an aerospace manufacturing plant who reported symptoms attributed to chemical exposure in the workplace. Thirty-seven workers filed compensation claims. Subsequently, Simon et al. measured the development of "environmental illness" with a four-item survey and found 13 individuals with high scores—in other words, they could be considered cases—and compared them with 13 noncases. The 13 cases scored higher on all measures of psychiatric symptoms, particularly on prior history of anxiety and depressive disorder and of medically unexplained symptoms before exposure.

Fiedler, Kipen, DeLuca, Kelly-McNeil, and Natelson (1996) found a significantly higher rate of psychiatric disorders in individuals who did not report a date of onset for their chemical sensitivities. This same finding has been reported in CFS (DeLuca, Johnson, & Natelson, 1997)—that is, individuals who developed CFS after an acute flu-like illness had lower rates of psychiatric disorder than those who reported a gradual onset of symptoms.

Caccappolo-van Vliet, Kelly-McNeil, Natelson, Kipen, and Fiedler (2002) compared 30 individuals with MCS according to Cullen's (1987) criteria with 19 individuals with asthma and 31 healthy controls on psychiatric disorders and personality traits associated with symptom reporting. Relative to controls, individuals with MCS and asthma demonstrated a significantly greater proportion of lifetime anxiety disorders. In terms of current psychiatric disorders, a higher proportion of those with MCS met criteria for depression and somatization disorder than either individuals with asthma or controls. There were no significant differences on alexithymia, but individuals with MCS and asthma reported significantly higher anxiety sensitivity than controls. As in many similar studies, approximately 50% of individuals with MCS did not meet criteria for any psychiatric disorder.

A Japanese study compared 46 individuals with MCS meeting Cullen's (1987) criteria with a control group with various opthalmologic diseases using the State–Trait Anxiety Inventory, the Self-Rating of Depression scale, and the Hamilton Depression Scale. They found higher levels of current anxiety and depression among the MCS group than the controls (Tonori et al., 2001).

Bell, Peterson, and Schwartz (1995) conducted a study of women with cacosmia, some of whom also had MCS and some of whom did not, and compared them with healthy controls on medical and psychological measures. The MCS group reported high rates of disability and much more extensive medical histories than the other two groups; the MCS group also had increased psychopathology on the Symptom Checklist–90—Revised.

Black (2000) summarized the reported prevalence of psychiatric disorder in published studies as ranging between 42% and 100%. Mood, anxiety, somatoform, and personality disorders are the most commonly diagnosed conditions. He also made the interesting point that substance use disorders are rarely linked with MCS, which appears to be true of other MUIs as well. Black suggested that personality factors or health beliefs of people predisposed to MCS might preclude the development of substance abuse.

Anxiety disorders and symptoms appear to be very prevalent psychiatric problems in MCS. Several groups have looked specifically at inducing panic attacks in individuals with MCS. Poonai et al. (2000) compared responses in 36 individuals with MCS (according to Simon criteria; Simon et al., 1990) with those of 37 healthy controls. Although individuals with MCS had to be free of psychiatric history and medication use, 71% of them met criteria for a panic attack after CO_2 inhalation compared with 26% of controls. In another study of the same cohort (Poonai et al., 2001), MCS patients also scored significantly higher than controls on self-report measures of anxiety and agoraphobia. Tarlo, Poonai, Binkley, Anthony, and Swinson (2002) observed that not all individuals with MCS experience panic responses to CO_2 challenges. The symptoms of MCS have been called a "toxic agoraphobia," with panic attacks and avoidance behavior manifested through confinement to clean, safe environments and avoiding contact with any situation that might involve toxins (Black, 2000; Simon, Katon, & Sparks, 1990).

Bailer's group in Germany has investigated the association between MCS, somatization, and somatoform disorders to explore the possibility that MCS could be conceptualized as an atypical somatoform disorder. Bailer, Rist, Witthöft, Paul, and Bayerl (2004) compared individuals with moderate and high MCS intensity with nonsensitive controls. The high-MCS group scored significantly higher than the other two groups on depression and somatoform scales and on diagnosed somatoform disorder; it also reported significantly more trait anxiety, chemical triggers, avoidance behavior, doctor visits, sensitivity to chemical substances and environmental stimuli, and dysfunctional beliefs about environmental threat than the other two groups. In another study, Bailer, Witthöft, Paul, Bayerl, and Rist (2005) examined four comparison groups using the Structured Clinical Interview for *DSM–IV*: IEI only, IEI and somatoform disorder, somatoform disorder only, and a nonsomatoform control group. Although 57% of the individuals with IEI met the *DSM–IV* criteria for at least one somatoform disorder, the medically unexplained symptoms attributed by the participants to environmental chemicals were counted by the interviewer as somatoform symptoms. This explains the high percentage of somatoform diagnoses. The people who met criteria for both IEI and somatoform disorders had a more severe type of IEI; they had more symptom complaints and more doctor visits. The IEI-only group still had multiple unexplained symptoms, but the symptoms were less likely to cause significant distress or impairment. All groups were higher on depression, anxiety, and self-reported allergic diseases than the control group.

Gupta and Horne (2001) assessed 85 patients in a tertiary clinic who were exposed to chemicals that included pesticides, wood preservatives, volatile organic compounds, metals, and gases. Fifty-seven patients reported moderate to severe symptoms following the exposure, whereas 26 patients did not suffer from physical symptoms. There were no differences between the groups on meeting criteria for depression, MCS, or CFS. Furthermore, the researchers did not find any differences in beliefs about chemicals. This suggests that patients who suffer from documented and validated chemical exposures do not appear to show psychological complications.

Bornschein, Hausteiner, Konrad, Forstl, and Zilker (2006) examined psychiatric disorders and toxic burden through blood and urine samples in

309 outpatients with IEI compared with 59 semiconductor workers. Psychiatric disorders were significantly higher in individuals with IEI than the controls (75% vs. 24%), particularly in somatoform, mood, and anxiety disorders. Furthermore, the industry workers had higher metal and solvent concentrations in their blood and urine samples. This is further evidence that objective measures of chemical exposure are not closely linked to IEI, whereas psychiatric morbidity is high.

Associative Learning

Schottenfeld (1987) proposed a learning model in which patients believe that their nonspecific symptoms are the result of disease. These patients become increasingly anxious about being diseased, experience more symptoms, and consequently become more anxious and more entrenched in disease conviction. Some investigators have posited an associative learning process contributing to MCS symptoms. The initial toxic exposure is the unconditioned stimulus that results in symptoms (the unconditioned response). The odorous context becomes the conditioned stimuli, and conditioned responses are symptoms elicited by subsequent exposures at lower levels. Through stimulus generalization, completely different odors can also become conditioned stimuli leading to the same conditioned response systems (Bolla-Wilson, Wilson, & Bleeker, 1988).

Winters et al. (2003) investigated whether warnings about environmental pollution would produce symptoms in 32 healthy volunteers, regardless of the noxiousness of the smell. Half of the study participants received a leaflet describing the "widespread chemical pollution of our environment" (p. 334) as a potential cause for MCS and a MCS case description. Then they received ammonia mixed with CO_2 or with room air, or *niaouli* (a pleasant smell) mixed with CO_2 or with room air. The researchers found that the group that read the leaflet prior to exposure learned symptoms in response to both odors more readily than the group that did not receive information. These results echo Petrie et al.'s (2005) findings in regard to pesticide spraying reported above: People who are primed to believe in the dangers of chemicals (i.e., have more modern health worries) report more symptoms after exposure.

Bailer et al. (2005) proposed a cognitive–behavioral model of IEI. People predisposed to develop IEI possess the characteristic of hypersensitivity to common chemical agents. IEI develops when an interaction occurs between this predisposition and environmental stress (trauma, stressful life events, overwhelming hassles); physiological changes caused by asthma or allergy; beliefs about the harm from chemicals; and other traits such as negative affectivity, suggestibility, or a schema of sickliness. IEI is then maintained by a self-perpetuating cycle of increased attention to exposures and sensations, which are interpreted as symptoms of IEI.

Lipson (2004) performed an ethnographic interview study of 36 people with MCS to try to understand the experiences and beliefs of people with MCS. Most participants had become chemically sensitive from remodeling, sick buildings, or workplace exposures. Lipson found that economic, medical, and social contexts increase the stigma experienced in MCS, such as corporate motives to delegitimize MCS and the hyperindividualistic values of wearing scents even if they harm others. The social suffering often exceeds the physical suffering.

In a qualitative study, Gibson, Placek, Lane, Brohimer, and Lovelace (2005) asked 178 women and 25 men with MCS an open-ended question about how MCS had affected their identities. The themes that emerged included loss of stable personality, loss of self-positioning, emotional suppression, redesigning plans, forced growth, struggling with support, discovering the spiritual self, and identity reconsolidation. The difficulties encountered by those with MCS are shared with other delegitimized illnesses and include negative effects on employment, finances, social relations and roles, mental health, and quality of life (Gibson et al., 2005).

CONCLUSION

MCS sits at the lower rungs of the credibility ladder compared with the other MUIs examined in this volume. Although a variety of theories favor a pathophysiological etiology, that etiology remains elusive. It may be that beliefs, expectations, and poor coping responses are more viable explanations for MCS than toxic insult. The more likely explanation is that a heightened sensitivity to toxins combined with psychosocial factors contribute to the development of MCS in vulnerable individuals. The lack of sufficient research on this condition makes it difficult to develop consistent explanatory theories.

III

GENERAL TREATMENT ISSUES IN MEDICALLY UNEXPLAINED ILLNESS

In this section, several general themes are addressed that are relevant to treatment for all medically unexplained illnesses (MUIs). Symptoms such as pain and fatigue can arise from multiple sources, and biopsychosocial factors can cause these symptoms become chronic. There is a delicate balance between overemphasis on medicalization of symptoms and dismissing the patient's experience as psychosomatic. Excessive, unwarranted medical testing and prescribing of numerous pharmaceuticals can encourage iatrogenic symptoms. Conversely, dismissive attitudes that label every symptom as benign or imagined can damage the relationship between patient and therapist or miss symptoms that require medical attention. Patients with MUIs should be encouraged to ask questions of their providers and advocate for themselves when necessary.

Numerous investigators (Barsky & Borus, 1999; Kirmayer, Robbins, & Paris, 1994; Kroenke et al., 1997; Manu, 2004) have argued that somatizing processes pervade the MUIs, yet people with MUIs are wary of psychological approaches and are wedded to somatic attributions. People with MUIs are sensitive to terms such as *somatization* and *somatoform disorders*, and applying these labels is not helpful for these individuals. Somatization remains a demeaning diagnosis, and this is not likely to change. Although resistance to psychological explanations of MUIs may be a function of defensiveness and denial, it may also reflect a realistic perception of the stigma of psychiatric labels (Kirmayer et al., 1994). Kirmayer, Groleau, Looper, and Dao (2004) made the valid point that unexplained symptoms are a threat to medical competence, and clinicians may deflect this threat by attributing these symptoms to psychological traits or states of the patient.

Patients with strong organic disease convictions may resist the suggestion that psychological factors influence pain or fatigue and misinterpret the involvement of a psychologist as a sign that their illness is illegitimate (D. A. Williams, 2003). The psychologist must recognize and overcome this view. Therapists generally need to focus on helping clients live their lives as best they can given the challenges of their illness and not present a direct challenge to their interpretation of symptoms. It may be difficult for some MUI clients to acknowledge the effects of emotional pain. As trust builds, clients may be more comfortable confronting psychosocial issues and come to focus less on the physical symptoms.

Kirmayer et al. (2004) described the miscommunication that often occurs between physicians and patients because physicians assume that psychological factors explain MUIs, yet psychological explanations often do not effectively address patient concerns and may lead patients to reject treatment or referral because of potential stigma. Physicians also may not fully appreciate that psychogenic causation, somatization, and somatic amplification cannot fully explain MUIs. A biopsychosocial model can provide sociosomatic explanations linking problems in family and social situations with bodily distress.

Most MUI patients are not actually averse to biopsychosocial explanations (R. M. Epstein et al., 2006) but rather to the dismissive nature of assertions that "it's all in your head." When acknowledgement of suffering is validated, most patients accept that stress, social conditions, and emotions have an effect on their illness state. The stigma of an MUI abetted by lack of medical legitimization may be somewhat assuaged by conceptualizing MUIs as stress disorders. The concept of stress has physiological as well as psychological bases and is accepted as such by most patients (Van Houdenhove & Egle, 2004).

Stressful life events and difficulty coping with stress can clearly influence outcomes and severity of MUIs (Monnikes et al., 2001; Whitehead, Bosmajian, Zonderman, Costa, & Schuster, 1988). Stress can also interfere with successful treatment (E. J. Bennett, Tennant, Piesse, Badcock, & Kellow, 1998). An emphasis on stress provides an entree for applying strategies of cognitive–behavioral therapy and psychotherapy to address the psychosocial factors that contribute to the chronicity of and disability inflicted by MUIs.

A number of psychosocial factors can contribute to chronicity of symptoms and disability in MUI. The burden of ongoing fatigue and pain are exacerbated by depression, anxiety, catastrophic thinking, somatic hypervigilance, and sleep problems. A number of other factors are common to MUIs: physical deconditioning, social withdrawal, amplification, secondary gain issues, and medicolegal disputes may also perpetuate symptoms and disability (Van Houdenhove & Egle, 2004). The patient who has considerable comorbid depression or anxiety or the patient who has suffered physical or sexual abuse is much more likely to have refractory symptoms and also to be especially responsive to psychological approaches (Creed, Guthrie, et al., 2005).

Misinformation abounds in controversial disorders, so patient education is critical. Cognitive–behavioral therapy generally informs the patient about the illness but also teaches techniques to assist with daily activities and to dispel feelings of helplessness and hopelessness. This type of therapy effectively strengthens individuals' beliefs in their own abilities and teaches them to develop tools for dealing with stress. A specific goal of cognitive therapy is to change the idea that patients are helpless in the face of their symptoms.

Cognitive–behavioral treatment is usually not used independently but rather in combination with other treatment modalities, particularly medications and exercise. Treatment is directed at changing MUI-related cognitions and behaviors specific to that particular disorder. Although conclusive research on factors that initiate and facilitate MUIs is lacking, there is a body of evidence on perpetuating factors. Perpetuating factors generally involve strong somatic attributions, focus on bodily symptoms, feelings of helplessness and futility regarding symptoms, and avoidance of activities for fear of symptom aggravation (Bleijenberg, Prins, & Bazelmans, 2003; Prins et al., 2001; Vercoulen, Hommes, et al., 1998). Cognitive–behavioral treatment usually consists of three phases: (a) the educational phase, familiarizing the client with the biopsychosocial model; (b) the skills training phase; and (c) the real-world application phase. The educational phase involves making clients aware of perpetuating factors and how they can be manifested in automatic thoughts. The therapist explains that rather than searching fruitlessly for causes of symptoms, it is more useful to focus on ways to resolve them. Some of the skills that have been shown to be effective are time-based graded activity, wherein activities are limited to time periods that patients can tolerate; scheduling pleasant activities into their routine; problemsolving strategies to attain a greater sense of control; relaxation training; sleep hygiene; and attributional change (D. A. Williams, 2003).

Among the important issues that require addressing in MUI therapy are perfectionistic beliefs, need for approval, social desirability, anger, and control (Toner et al., 1998; Toner, Koyama, Garfinkel, Jeejeebhoy, & Gasbarro, 1992). Women with MUI have often internalized the sex role message that they need to be both productive and nurturant, putting other's needs above their own. Yet, they may not be attuned to their own psychological and emotional needs and how bodily reactions are affected until the symptoms of MUI become prominent (Brosschot & Aarse, 2001; Toner, 1994). Thus, therapeutic approaches should emphasize understanding of mind–body interactions and greater emotional flexibility. Brosschot and Aarsse (2001) found that women with FMS showed restrictive emotional processing. A helpful tactic in therapy would be helping them to better differentiate emotional and physiological bodily reactions.

Malterud (2000) advocated empowering MUI patients by using communication strategies that acknowledge the experience of the patient. These could include stating the role of the patient as a source of important information, using open-ended questions, legitimizing the patient's language by using his or her own words, and problem solving as a cooperative endeavor between patient and clinician. Such approaches can help assuage the history of misunderstanding that may have accrued from numerous, often humiliating medical encounters.

Although many treatment approaches in MUI emphasize changing thoughts, behaviors, beliefs, emotions, and perceptions, a new approach that has recently gained attention may prove to be a fruitful alternative. Acceptance and commitment therapy and mindfulness-based cognitive therapy seek to change the individual's relationship to psychological events through such approaches as acceptance, mindfulness, and cognitive defusion (Hayes, Luoma, Bond, Masuda, & Lillis, 2006; Masuda, Hayes, Sackett, & Twohig, 2004).

Future studies should examine whether it may be useful to frame the treatment of MUIs in terms of acceptance and change. People with MUIs may be helped by learning to accept some level of symptoms and pain to reduce self-defeating struggles. With acceptance, change efforts may be directed toward actions that are personally meaningful and satisfying (McCracken, Carson, Eccleston, & Keefe, 2004). Rather than attempting to change the content of thoughts and behaviors as in cognitive–behavioral treatment, the emphasis is on changing "awareness of and relationship to thoughts" (Segal, Teasdale, & Williams, 2004, p. 47).

9

TREATMENT APPROACHES TO IRRITABLE BOWEL SYNDROME

Recent developments have led to improvement in the care of irritable bowel syndrome (IBS). If a patient meets Rome II criteria for IBS and does not have alarm factors, treatment should be initiated as soon as possible. There is evidence for differential response to treatment in subtypes of IBS. In some studies, individuals with diarrhea-predominant IBS responded better to treatment with tricyclic antidepressants (Whitehead, 1999). Interpersonal psychotherapy is also more effective for the diarrhea and pain symptoms of IBS, presumably because therapy helps patients understand the connection between stress and gastrointestinal symptoms and helps them control stress (Guthrie, Creed, Dawson, & Tomenson, 1993). A connection between stress and constipation symptoms is not as obvious.

In treating IBS, it is important to remember that IBS represents a spectrum of symptoms that tend to fluctuate over time. An IBS patient with an alternating pattern of constipation and diarrhea may be treated for diarrhea only to have the symptom pattern shift to constipation, making drug treatment unhelpful. This suggests that symptom-directed treatment may not be useful as a global approach to the problem. Additionally, because IBS is often a chronic condition, medication should be used cautiously and temporarily. This chapter summarizes the findings regarding both drug and psychological treatments for IBS, recognizing that multimodal therapy will be the most effective approach for most patients.

DRUG TREATMENTS

Several reviews have evaluated the efficacy of various drug treatments for IBS (Brandt et al., 2002; Jailwala, Imperiale, & Kroenke, 2000). A meta-analysis of antispasmodic medications found that they were superior to placebo as treatment for IBS (Poynard, Regimbeau, & Benhamou, 2001). The American College of Gastroenterology task force reviewed the available evidence for the usefulness of bulking agents, such as wheat bran, corn fiber, and psyllium, and found that they were no more effective than placebos at relieving overall IBS symptoms, although they could be helpful specifically for constipation (Brandt et al., 2002). The antidiarrheal agent loperamide was found to be helpful in relieving IBS-related diarrhea, but it was no better than placebo at relieving global symptoms of IBS (Efskind, Bernklev, & Vatn, 1996).

Antidepressants' impact on anticholinergic, serotonergic, and noradrenergic receptors that affect gastrointestinal motility makes these drugs good candidates for the treatment of IBS (Clouse & Lustman, 2005; Talley, 2003). However, a systematic review performed by the American College of Gastroenterology concluded that evidence did not support the effectiveness of tricyclic antidepressants in ameliorating global IBS symptoms (Brandt et al., 2002). SSRIs appear to have a more efficacious profile. Evidence suggests that both desipramine (Drossman et al., 2003) and paroxetine (Creed et al., 2003) may be more effective than standard medical treatment in IBS.

The presence of a significant number of 5-HT$_3$ receptors in the gut has led to the development of a number of agents specific to this receptor site. Antagonism of the 5-HT$_3$ receptor causes significant slowing in colonic transit and a decrease in visceral sensation and should help the diarrhea-predominant form of IBS. The first agent developed in this class was alosetron, which has been found effective in relieving abdominal pain, discomfort, and rectal urgency and improving well-being in patients with IBS (Camilleri, 2001; Camilleri et al., 1999). Viramontes et al. (2001) found that the reduction in colonic transit was significantly greater in women than in men. Alosetron was withdrawn from the market in November 2000 because a small number of patients experienced severe constipation and ischemic colitis. The drug was re-released by the U.S. Food and Drug Administration under a restricted prescribing program for women with severe diarrhea-predominant IBS who did not respond to conventional IBS therapy. Careful patient education and monitoring can reduce adverse events associated with this agent (Camilleri, 2001; Camilleri et al., 1999).

Stimulation of the 5-HT$_4$ receptors in the gut appears to increase the rate of intestinal colonic transit, reduce the firing rate of colonic visceral afferent nerves, and in turn, to reduce visceral sensitivity. The 5-HT$_4$ partial agonist tegaserod is the only drug in this class approved by the U.S. Food and Drug Administration. Currently approved for the treatment of IBS with constipation in women, this drug has been shown in trials, when compared with a placebo, to increase the number of bowel movements, decrease bloating, reduce abdominal pain or discomfort, and improve stool frequency and consistency (Camilleri, 2001; Muller-Lissner et al., 2001).

To summarize the findings for prescription drug treatment for IBS, some antidepressants and antispasmodic agents are more effective than placebos for treating IBS, although the studies are small and poorly designed. There are no randomized controlled trials examining the efficacy of laxatives for managing IBS. Gender appears to play an important role in the serotonin receptor specific drugs; research reveals that they are significantly more effective in women than in men. Tegaserod is more effective than placebo at improving global IBS symptoms in women with non-diarrhea-predominant IBS. Alosetron is more effective than placebo in women with diarrhea-predominant IBS, although its use should be limited to patients who have not improved with conventional therapy because of its adverse event profile (Schoenfeld, 2005; Talley, 2003).

No single drug therapy has proved to be beneficial for the majority of people with IBS (Tan, Corydon Hammond, & Gurrala, 2005). There is a clear trend in the literature showing that behavioral treatment of IBS, as well as "combined treatment" consisting of medical management, psychological treatment, and judicious use of antidepressants, can be more effective than standard medical treatment alone in treating such patients, particularly patients with severe IBS symptoms (Brandt et al., 2002).

DIETARY ISSUES

Recent studies suggest that although individual patients may have "food triggers," there is no definitive evidence that food allergies or food intolerance to large food groups, such as meats or grains, are associated with either the development or the exacerbation of IBS symptoms. Dietary triggers reported include caffeine, citrus, corn, dairy lactose, wheat, and wheat gluten. Lactose and caffeine may be associated with diarrhea-predominant IBS (H. R. Mertz, 2003). Patients should be encouraged to eat a healthful diet and to avoid foods that can trigger their symptoms. Extensive testing for gut-based food allergies is usually nonproductive in IBS patients, although Zar, Kumar, and Benson (2001) have argued that a subgroup of IBS could benefit from therapeutic dietary manipulation. For example, increasing dietary fiber has long been recommended as a treatment for constipation-predominant

IBS (Floch & Narayan, 2002). A systematic review of 13 randomized controlled trials found no convincing evidence that bulking agents relieve global symptoms of IBS (Brandt et al., 2002); another systematic review (Jailwala et al., 2000) found significant improvement in the ease of stool passage and in general satisfaction with bowel movements. Using fiber is reasonable for constipation-predominant patients. Partially hydrolyzed guar gum has reportedly been successful in alleviating constipation. A nonblinded randomized controlled trial found that symptoms of IBS were improved equally by diets supplemented with fiber or guar gum, but more patients preferred guar gum (Parisi et al., 2005).

Monsbakken, Vandvik, and Farup (2005) advocated a general therapeutic approach in the management of IBS and documented its effect. They assessed the abdominal symptoms, musculoskeletal pain, and mood disorders of 65 individuals with IBS identified in a public screening. A doctor presented IBS as a positive diagnosis and offered information, reassurance, and lifestyle advice but no pharmacotherapy. A dietician gave dietary advice. At 6-month follow-up, 20 individuals (31%) had satisfactory relief of symptoms. Dietary advice was effective only in those with diarrhea-predominant IBS. Previous consultations for the complaints, visits for psychiatric disorders, and presence of mood disorders were predictors of persistent complaints. Although this study reported significant relief of symptoms after 6 months, those with psychological comorbidity were not as responsive as the others. The sections that follow describe approaches that may benefit individuals with treatment-resistant IBS.

STRESS REDUCTION

Stressful life events and difficulty in coping with stress play important roles in MUIs, and IBS is paradigmatic of this connection (Monnikes et al., 2001; Sagami et al., 2004). Although not a direct cause of illness, stress can clearly influence outcomes and severity of IBS (Whitehead, Bosmajian, Zonderman, Costa, & Schuster, 1988) and interfere with treatment. E. J. Bennett, Tennant, Piesse, Badcock, and Kellow (1998) prospectively examined the relation of chronic life stress threat to IBS symptom intensity over time in a sample of 117 consecutive outpatients who satisfied the modified Rome criteria for IBS (66% with one or more concurrent functional disorder syndromes) participated. The life stress and symptom intensity measures were determined 6 months prior to study entry and at 6 and 16 months after entry; these measures assessed the potency of chronic life stress threat during the prior 6 months or more and the severity and frequency of symptoms during the following 2 weeks. Chronic life stress was a powerful predictor of subsequent symptom intensity, explaining 97% of the variance on this measure over 16 months. No patient exposed to even one chronic highly threatening stressor improved clinically (by 50%) over the 16 months; all patients who improved did so in the absence of such a stressor. This shows the importance of identifying and managing stressors in a patient's life.

Developing more effective coping strategies and relaxation training can be key to improving symptomatology. Patients who can make a clear association between their symptoms and stress or anxiety benefit the most from stress management and relaxation training (Palsson & Drossman, 2005). Shaw et al. (1991) randomized 35 patients with IBS to receive treatment either in a stress management program or with the antispasmodic drug Colpermin. The stress management program involved a median of six 40-minute sessions with a physiotherapist, during which patients were helped to understand the nature of their symptoms and the relationship of those symptoms to stress and were taught relaxation exercises. Two thirds of those in the stress management program found it effective in relieving symptoms and experienced fewer attacks of less severity. This benefit was maintained for at least 12 months. The drug group reported no benefit.

Keefer and Blanchard (2001) used a relaxation response meditation program group compared with a wait-list control group (symptom monitoring only) in a 6-week crossover design. IBS patients were paired on the basis of presence of Axis I disorders, primary IBS symptoms, age, and gender. One member of the pair was randomly assigned to either treatment or wait list. Both groups were required to monitor symptoms in a daily diary. Relaxation group members met once a week for 30 minutes, and they were instructed to practice relaxation techniques twice a day for 15 minutes. Most participants managed to practice only once per day. Immediately after treatment, 77% of the relaxation group members had improved. At 3-month follow-up, improvement was maintained. The control group also received treatment after 6 weeks of wait list, but in the wait-list condition, only 28% improved. Relaxation is often an important component of other psychological treatments such as cognitive–behavioral therapy, hypnotherapy, and meditation.

PSYCHOLOGICAL APPROACHES

The literature supporting the efficacy of psychological approaches to treating IBS is positive. Psychosocial treatments have generally been found to be more effective than medication alone or various control conditions. Cognitive–behavioral therapy, hypnosis, pure cognitive therapy, and relaxation therapy have all been effectively applied to the treatment of IBS, especially in patients with severe symptoms (Blanchard, Schwarz, & Neff, 1988; Drossman et al., 2003; Galovski & Blanchard, 1998).

Behavioral treatments are based on a biopsychological model of IBS. The biological disturbance in gut sensitivity or motility interacts with emotional regulation problems and disturbed central nervous system processing.

Emotional disturbance or early encoded childhood traumas might increase ascending visceral signals, thus producing more intense pain experiences. Psychological interventions or antidepressant drugs can intervene with these stimulus pathways and decrease the pain experience (Halpert & Drossman, 2005). Psychological treatments can help individuals regulate emotions more adaptively and develop coping skills that can affect central processing, which in turn reduces gastrointestinal and other symptoms.

Because such varied psychological approaches have yielded positive results, they all have some key factors in common. The critical factor addressed by all of these treatments is the patient's belief system: providing the patient with a more thorough understanding of the disorder and an enhanced sense of control by learning new coping approaches. Teaching the individual that IBS is a biobehavioral disorder, illuminating the role of stress and coping in symptom maintenance, teaching positive self-management strategies, and discouraging excessive health care seeking behaviors are critical (Naliboff, Chang, Munakata, & Mayer, 2000). Naliboff et al. (2000) recommended a psychoeducational approach that alters the patient's beliefs and understanding of the disorder so that he or she can benefit from a variety of approaches.

As in other MUIs, organic disease conviction can be tenacious in IBS. Toner and Akman (2000) have suggested that the feminine gender role can affect illness attributions. This disease conviction could come from focusing on others' needs, which leads to neglect of self, and lack of self-nurturance exacerbates stress. The distressing symptoms of IBS cannot be ignored, but IBS patients who go to specialists tend to selectively attend to physiological symptoms and are less likely to acknowledge stress than those who do not see gastrointestinal specialists (Toner, 1994). Strong disease convictions also contribute to high levels of doctor shopping. Thus, the cognitions may go something like this: "I have it all under control, I'm doing just fine, but please cure my embarrassing symptoms with some medication or procedure." Examples of dysfunctional cognitions typical of IBS are presented in Exhibit 9.1. These cognitions do not help patients to cope with chronic symptoms and must be addressed through cognitive–behavioral therapy. Toner and Akman (2000) have noted that bowel functioning is more of a source of embarrassment for women than for men. For women with IBS, the shame associated with bowel function may contribute to feelings of isolation.

Greene and Blanchard (1994) laid out an intensive cognitive therapy system that consisted of ten 1-hour individual sessions. Cognitions were emphasized as the determining factors in IBS symptoms. Treatment was aimed at increasing patients' awareness of the association between stress, thoughts, behaviors, and bowel symptoms; training patients in the identification and modification of appraisals of situations, thoughts, and behaviors; and changing dysfunctional schemas. The researchers randomized 20 people with IBS to either cognitive therapy or a symptom monitoring condition in a crossover design. Of those receiving cognitive therapy, 80% experienced clini-

EXHIBIT 9.1
Cognitive Scale for Functional Bowel Disorders

Theme	Example of statements endorsed
Bowel performance anxiety	"I worry there might not be a toilet available."
Pain	"I often feel this abdominal pain will never go away."
Control	"My bowel symptoms make me feel out of control."
Self-efficacy	"I feel my bowel symptoms are too much for me to handle."
Embarrassment/shame	"I worry that other people will hear my stomach noises."
Anger/frustration	"I am constantly frustrated by my symptoms."
Disease conviction	"I feel I am always sick with my bowel symptoms."
Perfectionism	"It's important to do my absolute best at everything."
Social approval	"I hate the thought of making a fool of myself."
Social rules/norms	"The idea of being late upsets me."
Self-nurturance	"I often give up my own wishes to make others happy."

Note. Statements are rated on a scale that ranges from 1 (*strongly disagree*) to 7 (*strongly agree*). Adapted from "Cognitive Change in Patients Undergoing Hypnotherapy for Irritable Bowel Syndrome," by W. M. Gonsalkorale, B. B. Toner, and P. J. Whorwell, 2004, *Journal of Psychosomatic Research, 56,* p. 273. Adapted with permission from Elsevier.

cally significant improvement compared with only 10% in the symptom monitoring condition. Payne and Blanchard (1995) sought to extend these findings by using a support group condition to control for patient expectations and therapist contact. They randomized 34 people to three conditions: cognitive therapy, self-help support, or wait list (controls). The support group met weekly with a therapist who led discussions of IBS issues such as stress and diet. All three groups kept gastrointestinal symptom diaries for 8 weeks. The wait-list control was contacted at 4 weeks to check on diary keeping. Results replicated Greene and Blanchard's, with an average reduction in primary gastrointestinal symptoms of 67% in the cognitive therapy condition, compared with 31% for the support group condition and 10% for the wait-list condition. This improvement was sustained at 3 months posttreatment. Boyce, Gilchrist, Talley, and Rose (2000) assessed 8 participants undergoing cognitive–behavioral therapy for IBS. They found significant improvement in the distress and disability associated with bowel symptoms and alleviation of anxiety and depression. Frequency of bowel symptoms remained unchanged.

Payne and Blanchard (1995) indicated that in cognitive therapy, participants learned to alter their distorted thinking and change fundamental beliefs and to reduce behavioral avoidance and physiological reactivity. They argued that the crucial ingredient is interrupting the cognitive pathway that links the physiological, behavioral, and cognitive aspects of IBS.

Heymann-Monnikes et al. (2000) compared behavioral treatment with drug treatment alone in patients consulting a tertiary gastrointestinal referral center. IBS outpatients were randomly assigned to the combination of standardized multicomponent behavioral therapy plus standard medical treatment or standard medical treatment alone. The behavioral treatment group received IBS information and education, progressive muscle relaxation, training in illness-related cognitive coping strategies, problem solving, and assertiveness training in 10 sessions over 10 weeks. Standard medical treatment included symptom-oriented medical treatment and regular visits to a gastroenterologist every 2nd week. Follow-ups were conducted at 3- and 6-month intervals. Compared with the group receiving standard medical treatment alone, the behavioral treatment group showed significantly greater IBS symptom reduction and improved quality of life and overall well-being as measured by daily symptom diaries. Heymann-Monnikes et al.'s data provide evidence that medical treatment alone is not especially effective, whereas the combination of medical treatment plus multicomponent behavioral treatment is superior in the therapy of IBS. Although all of these studies involved relatively small numbers of participants, they show consistently that cognitive–behavioral approaches are effective in IBS.

Boyce, Talley, Balaam, Koloski, and Truman (2003) randomized 105 people recruited from gastroenterology clinics and advertisements to three treatment arms. All participants received routine clinical care, and the other two groups received weekly sessions of either relaxation or cognitive–behavioral therapy for 8 weeks. Only individuals with no psychiatric diagnosis and with gastroenterologist-diagnosed IBS were included. Routine care consisted of three 15- to 30-minute sessions with a gastroenterologist, during which individuals received recommendations for a high-fiber diet along with the bulking agent psyllium husk in a standard dose. The relaxation treatment consisted of 30-minute instructional sessions using a variety of relaxation techniques. Cognitive–behavioral therapy sessions consisted of strategies to manage anxiety, incorporate realistic symptom appraisal, enhance coping strategies, teach relaxation skills, and restructure cognition. Participants were assessed at baseline and at 4, 8, 26, and 52 weeks. All three groups demonstrated significant improvement over time in IBS severity, anxiety, depression, and quality of life. Gender was not associated with outcome. There was a high attrition rate in the treatment groups. Although this study might indicate that good clinical care and support are sufficient for many individuals with IBS, these findings have limited generalizability because Boyce et al. (2003) excluded those with psychiatric disorder.

A randomized study of 431 women with moderate to severe functional bowel disorders (including IBS, functional abdominal pain, painful constipation, and unspecified functional bowel disorder) compared cognitive–behavioral therapy, education, desipramine, and placebo in a multicenter treatment trial (Drossman et al., 2003). Cognitive–behavioral therapy consisted of 12 weekly hour-long sessions aimed at modifying the influence of attention, appraisal, gender-related cognitive schemas, and illness attribution related to participants' gastrointestinal symptoms to develop more effective coping strategies. Examples of gender-related cognitions include the belief that girls and women must always be in control of bodily functions and that they must always be fresh, clean, and socially desirable; that bodily functions must be kept hidden and private; and that social approval can be secured by pleasing others. The education control sessions were conducted with the same therapist over the same time frame but consisted of reviewing symptom diaries and reading and discussing educational materials. The remaining participants were randomized to desipramine or placebo and visited a nurse weekly over the 12 weeks for monitoring. Outcome measures were satisfaction with treatment, well-being, diary card scores, and quality of life. Cognitive–behavioral therapy was significantly more effective than education on a composite outcome measure. Desipramine was more effective than placebo but only in secondary analysis. Participants in the placebo drug group had a higher response rate than those in the education control group. Drossman et al. (2003) also found that desipramine was more effective for those with less severe illness and a history of abuse, whereas cognitive–behavioral therapy was effective regardless of those factors. Surprisingly, participants with depression were not more likely to benefit from active treatment than those who were not depressed.

Given that cognitive–behavioral therapy has proved effective for IBS, Kennedy et al. (2006) sought to determine whether it could be delivered by primary care nurses to patients with moderate or severe IBS that was resistant to the antispasmodic drug mebeverine. They concluded that this type of therapy had more benefit than mebeverine for up to 6 months, but that after 12 months, most of the benefit had dissipated.

A systematic review of the effectiveness of psychological interventions in patients with IBS, chronic fatigue syndrome (CFS), and chronic back pain was conducted to determine whether psychological treatment was as efficacious in a primary care setting as in specialty settings (Raine et al., 2002). They identified 61 randomized controlled studies and two meta-analyses; 20 of these studies assessed patients in primary care. Although cognitive–behavioral therapy and cognitive treatments were generally effective for CFS and IBS, greater improvements were seen in the specialty settings. Raine et al. cautioned that their conclusions are qualified because of many methodological weaknesses in the studies reviewed. Patients in specialty care tended to be sicker, had longer treatment times, and had more supervised interventions than patients in primary care, which may explain the greater improvements in specialty care settings. Raine et al. also reported that although antidepressants were not helpful in CFS, they were found to be effective for IBS in both primary and specialty care settings.

Toner, Segal, et al. (1998) discussed the usefulness of group cognitive–behavioral therapy in IBS. A group setting helped reduce the stigma of the condition, and participants gained support from others experiencing the same difficulties. Clinicians often endorse same-gender groups, because women may be more willing to disclose shame-related issues or sexual and physical abuse in same-gender groups. The common themes that emerge and should be addressed in group therapy are associations between thoughts, feelings, and bowel symptoms; the specific cognitions associated with bowel symptoms; pain management; and "bowel performance" anxiety. Important issues that commonly require addressing in therapy with IBS are perfectionistic beliefs, need for approval, social desirability, anger, and control (Toner, Koyama, Garfinkel, Jeejeebhoy, & Gasbarro, 1992; Toner, Segal, et al., 1998).

Below are several therapy excerpts from Karen,[1] a 32-year-old married woman, that exemplify several common themes addressed by Toner et al. (1992; Toner, Segal, et al., 1998). Karen had no children and worked as an accountant, a job she enjoyed but found "pretty stressful." She had had IBS symptoms for 3 years and described the embarrassment of unpredictable diarrhea and the loss of libido affecting sexual activity. These were her most troubling presenting symptoms.

> I just finished having a huge array of tests to confirm IBS as a diagnosis. My sex drive was huge before I got this, and now I have nothing, and simply make an effort for [my] husband's sake, but not as often as he would like. He is really understanding, but if I can't stop how bad I'm feeling enough to get back to a relatively normal life (I'm still coming to terms with diagnosis) then how long will he continue to put up with this? We had been married for five years before my symptoms started, but I feel so bad for him. I'm afraid I'll have an accident if I lose control during sex. I just feel disgusting and disgusted about it.

There is an emphasis on her partner's needs and on letting him down by not being an enthusiastic sexual partner. After several months of cognitive–behavioral therapy, a theme of acceptance arose in the therapy dialogue with Karen. Her therapist worked with her on relaxation techniques and avoiding self-blame. Another important theme was accepting that embarrassing events will occur but avoiding a catastrophizing response.

> Things are going much better now. Part of this involved my journey to accepting that I had a chronic illness. And realizing eventually that if I waited [to have sex] till I felt "well" or even "good" . . . it just wouldn't happen most of the time. And once I realized that sometimes it actually made me feel better. And once I had a few positive experiences, and a few negative ones and my husband didn't leave the room running or screaming . . . nor did he love me any less . . . things improved a lot.

Karen reported that using relaxation techniques helped reduce the intensity of some of her symptoms. The last several sessions of therapy focused on not letting IBS control her life yet accepting that she may have to live with the symptoms. Karen was still having difficulty moving toward acceptance.

---

[1]This case study is a fictionalized amalgam of typical patients.

I know that it's best to just keep on keeping on, I definitely don't freak out and obsess about my symptoms as much as I used to. . . . I think I am still having trouble accepting I have this illness, and am always hoping I will wake up one day and be cured . . . but I'm not letting it overrun my life.

HYPNOTHERAPY

Hypnosis has emerged as an especially effective treatment for IBS. Galovski and Blanchard (1998) randomly assigned 6 matched pairs of IBS patients to either a gut-directed hypnotherapy condition or to a symptom monitoring wait-list control condition. Those assigned to the control condition were later crossed over to the treatment condition. Patients were matched on concurrent psychiatric diagnoses, susceptibility to hypnosis, and various demographic features. Results from the entire treated sample indicate that the individual symptoms of abdominal pain, constipation, and flatulence improved significantly. State and trait anxiety scores were also seen to decrease significantly. Results at the 2-month follow-up point indicated good maintenance of treatment gains. A positive relationship was found between the incidence of psychiatric diagnosis and overall level of improvement.

Gonsalkorale, Houghton, and Whorwell (2002) established a hypnotherapy unit devoted to IBS in the United Kingdom. The technique involved hypnotic induction using relaxation procedures to deepen the hypnotic state, followed by suggestions and imagery tailored to each individual, such as induced warmth in the patient's abdomen aimed at controlling and normalizing gut function. Hypnotherapy consisted of weekly 1-hour sessions for 12 weeks, and people were required to practice techniques between sessions. They were able to audit 250 patients who participated in this hypnotherapy treatment and found marked improvement in IBS symptoms, anxiety, depression, and quality of life, with 71% responding favorably. Only gender was significantly associated with responder status; men with diarrhea-predominant IBS were the least likely to respond. The authors speculated that these nonresponsive men may have had somewhat lower imaginative abilities or differing pathophysiologic mechanisms that made them less suited to a hypnotherapeutic approach. Gonsalkorale, Miller, Afzal, and Whorwell (2003) then followed up with these patients to determine whether improvement was maintained as much as 6 years after the original hypnotherapy treatment. They found that 81% of responders maintained their improvement over time. Responders also reported a reduction in medical consultation rates and medication use.

Palsson, Turner, Johnson, Burnett, and Whitehead (2002) were interested in determining the mechanism for the success of hypnosis treatment for severe IBS. They examined whether hypnosis was effective by normalizing interpretation of aversive intestinal stimuli, reducing rectal smooth muscle tone, reducing autonomic arousal, and reducing somatizing. They found that hypnosis was effective in reducing symptoms of IBS, replicating previous studies. However, hypnosis treatment did not change rectal pain thresholds, rectal muscle tone, or cardiovascular responses. The only physiological response that improved was skin conductance, which could reflect a slight reduction in sympathetic autonomic activity after hypnosis. Conversely, somatization and general distress were significantly reduced. Palsson et al. hypothesized that hypnosis may improve IBS symptoms by altering the patient's attentional and belief systems about the meaning of sensations arising from the gastrointestinal tract.

Gonsalkorale, Toner, and Whorwell (2004) were interested in determining whether the cognitive changes were related to the success of hypnotherapy. They assessed 78 patients with IBS who underwent a course of hypnotherapy. As in other studies, hypnotherapy significantly reduced IBS symptoms and improved psychological well-being and quality of life. IBS-related cognitions were assessed with the Cognitive Scale for Functional Bowel Disorders, which yields a total cognitive score (Toner, Stuckless, et al., 1998). The score was made up of statements derived from diaries of IBS patients. Exhibit 9.1 summarizes the themes and statements found on the scale. The total cognitive score was associated with symptom severity and interference. These cognitions improved after hypnotherapy, and this change was correlated with improvement in symptoms. In particular, bowel-related cognitions improved after hypnotherapy, but there was less change in cognitions relating to perfectionism, self-nurturance, and social norms.

Tan et al. (2005) reviewed 14 studies of the efficacy of hypnosis in treating IBS. They concluded that hypnosis consistently produces improvement in IBS symptoms as well as in psychological states and quality of life and that these improvements last over a number of years. They summarized the possible mechanism of action for hypnotherapy as improving abnormal pain perception, normalizing rectal sensitivity, altering electroencephalogram activity, or, alternatively, working through psychological mechanisms by reducing somatization and distress or increasing placebo analgesia. Tan et al. found that hypnosis for IBS qualifies for the highest level of acceptance; they noted that the Clinical Psychology Division of the American Psychological Association guidelines regard hypnosis as both efficacious and specific for this condition.

PSYCHOTHERAPY

The effectiveness of psychotherapy in patients with chronic, refractory IBS was demonstrated by Guthrie, Creed, Dawson, and Tomenson (1993), who conducted a randomized controlled trial of psychotherapy versus supportive listening with a sample of 102 patients. Physical and psychological assessments were carried out at the beginning and end of the 12-week trial. For women, psychotherapy was found to be superior to supportive listening in terms of improving both physical and psychological symptoms. There was a similar trend for men, but this did not reach significance. Following completion of the trial, patients in the control group were offered psychotherapy; 33 accepted and after treatment experienced a marked improvement in their symptoms; 10 declined. At 1-year follow-up, those patients who had received psychotherapy remained well, patients who had dropped out of the trial were unwell with severe symptoms, and most of the controls who declined psychotherapy had relapsed. This study shows that psychotherapy is effective in the majority of IBS patients with chronic symptoms unresponsive to medical treatment.

Individuals with IBS who have a history of being physically or sexually abused or are patients with psychiatric disorders such as depression or panic disorder often benefit from psychotherapy. Not surprisingly, it is individuals with the greatest psychological comorbidity who appear to benefit the most from psychological approaches. These patients may be more motivated. Creed, Guthrie, et al. (2005) found that the association between abuse history and impaired functioning was mediated by somatization tendencies. In a 15-month trial of psychotherapy and paroxetine, Creed et al. (2003) found the greatest beneficial response in those with abuse history, particularly those with a reported history of rape. Psychotherapy allowed the patients to discuss and resolve previous and current interpersonal difficulties, which argue for a treatable component in functioning with IBS. Somatization processes were also decreased after psychotherapy (Creed et al., 2003).

New pharmacological treatments may hold some promise for treating IBS, but it appears likely that multimodal approaches are more likely to be the most effective. This chapter has presented evidence that in controlled trials approaches that incorporate stress reduction, relaxation, imagery, and more effective coping techniques have significantly improved IBS symptoms. Psychotherapy is also helpful, particularly to patients with an abuse history. The most well-researched and impressive improvements in symptoms and quality of life come from trials of cognitive–behavioral therapy and hypnotherapy. Cognitive–behavioral therapy that includes strategies to manage anxiety, learning realistic symptom appraisal, enhancing coping strategies and relaxation skills, and restructuring cognitions has proven effective in IBS. Similarly, hypnotherapy works to improve coping and to change maladaptive cognitions and shows great promise for treating IBS.

10

TREATMENT APPROACHES
TO FIBROMYALGIA

Fibromyalgia (FMS) treatment must be guided by the biopsychosocial model. The interaction between neurally mediated nociceptive activity, anxiety, depression, catastrophizing, and decreases in physical activity level can result in increased pain experiences. Some patients experience significant relief of symptoms after treatment, some find moderate improvement, and others report little or no relief. Only about 5% of FMS patients become symptom free. Most treatment regimens include medication, lifestyle changes, exercise, physical therapy, and behavior modification (Millea & Holloway, 2000). R. M. Bennett (1996) recommended multidisciplinary group programs to treat FMS patients, including physiatrists, psychologists, and rheumatologists.

Successful management of FMS is more likely if patients have sufficient information and skills to deal with it. In randomized clinical trials, educating FMS patients about their condition resulted in improvements in pain, sleep, fatigue, self-efficacy, quality of life, and exercise ability (Burckhardt & Bjelle, 1994). Most education trials range from 6 to 17 weekly sessions, but even a 1½ day multidisciplinary education program was found to be successful (Pfeiffer et al., 2003).

MEDICATION

No medical therapies have been specifically approved by the U.S. Food and Drug Administration for the management of FMS. Antidepressants appear to be the most effective class of medications used. In addition to their potential side effects, their analgesic effect has been demonstrated in many chronic pain disorders and may be related to increasing the spinal concentrations of serotonin and norepinephrine. Tricyclic antidepressants are one of the few classes of medications proven to be effective in randomized clinical trials (Arnold & Keck, 2001; O'Malley et al., 2000; Rao & Bennett, 2003). Another class of antidepressants used in FMS is that of the SSRIs, which tend to improve mood but not physical symptoms. These inhibitors have been effective as monotherapy (Arnold et al., 2002) or in combination with tricyclic antidepressants in FMS (Goldenberg, Mayskiy, Mossey, Ruthazer, & Schmid, 1996).

Trigger point injections involve injecting a local anesthetic into a tender point. Local anesthetic increases blood flow to the muscle, and corticosteroids reduce inflammation. Although the injections are used commonly in clinical practice, few studies of their efficacy have been conducted. The injections can be painful and take several days to show results. However, because of the complicated nature of pain management in some patients, injections should not be ruled out as an alternative treatment. Further study of this treatment is warranted (Goldenberg, Burckhardt, & Crofford, 2004).

The negatives of drug treatments are that they treat only certain symptoms, their long-term benefits have not been well established, and improvement with drugs seems to fade over time. Because FMS is usually a chronic disorder, a multimodal approach with lifestyle changes is likely to confer the most benefit.

REVIEWS OF TREATMENT STUDIES

A number of reviews and meta-analyses have examined treatment efficacy in FMS. A meta-analysis of 49 FMS treatment outcome studies assessed the efficacy of pharmacological and nonpharmacological treatment across four types of outcome measures: physical status, self-report of FMS symptoms, psychological status, and daily functioning (Rossy et al., 1999). Antidepressant drugs resulted in improvements on physical status and self-report of symptoms, whereas nonpharmacological treatments were associated with significant improvements in all four categories of outcome measures, with the exception that physically based treatment (primarily exercise) did not significantly improve daily functioning. Additionally, nonpharmacological treatment appeared to be more efficacious in improving self-reported FMS symptoms than pharmacological treatment alone. This meta-analysis suggests that optimal intervention for FMS would include nonpharmacological treatments, specifically exercise and cognitive–behavioral therapy, with appropriate medication management only as needed for sleep and pain symptoms.

Goldenberg, Burckhardt, and Crofford (2004) used the major citation indexes to identify and review 505 randomized controlled trials and meta-analyses of randomized controlled trials of FMS. Although they noted major limitations to the FMS literature, with many trials compromised by short duration and lack of controls, they found support for the efficacy of low-dose tricyclic antidepressants, cardiovascular exercise, cognitive–behavioral therapy, and patient education. Goldenberg et al. recommended a stepwise program emphasizing education, certain medications, exercise, cognitive–behavioral therapy, or a multimodal combination of all four.

Several reviews have specifically examined nonpharmacological and complementary and alternative medicine (CAM) approaches to FMS treatment (Hadhazy, Ezzo, Creamer, & Berman, 2000; Holdcraft, Assefi, & Buchwald, 2003; Rossy et al., 1999). Holdcraft et al. (2003) performed a database citation review using the National Institutes of Health classification of complementary and alternative medicine. They found evidence of the efficacy for these therapies: acupuncture, some herbal and nutritional substances (e.g., magnesium, S-adenosyl-L-methionine), and massage therapy. Limited evidence (at least one randomized controlled trial) supports relaxation, biofeedback, and *chorella* (green algae; Holdcraft et al., 2003).

Hadhazy et al. (2000) reviewed mind–body therapies and found 13 controlled trials involving 802 participants (92% women, 8% men). Therapies included biofeedback, exercise, education, relaxation, stress management, and hypnotherapy. According to these authors, mind–body therapies did not significantly improve pain and function over wait-list or treatment as usual conditions, although when combined with exercise, they were moderately more effective. These therapies were most successful in enhancing self-efficacy and quality of life. People who responded to these therapies tended to have shorter disease duration, less depression, and higher premorbid activity levels, suggesting that mind–body therapies should be initiated early to be effective. Illness behaviors may become less amenable to change as FMS progresses. This is in contrast to the meta-analysis by Rossy et al. (1999), which found that nonpharmacological treatments were generally superior to pharmacological treatment.

Sim and Adams (2002) built on the review of Rossy et al. (1999) by reviewing 25 randomized controlled trials of nonpharmacological interventions, including exercise, education, relaxation, cognitive–behavioral therapy, acupuncture, and hydrotherapy. They concluded that most studies were of low methodological quality and underpowered and that no single intervention was especially effective. Aerobic exercise did emerge as the most efficacious intervention, and the authors suggested that exercise should be incorporated into any management strategy for FMS.

EXERCISE

Exercise has been one of the most consistently robust and effective treatments for FMS. Exercise has also been shown to decrease the perception of central pain, which appears to be high in FMS patients. Routine low-impact aerobics and strength-building exercise may help reduce pain, tender point counts, depression, and sleep disturbance. Exercise increases time spent in deep sleep, perhaps a mechanism for its therapeutic effect.

Several of the reviews cited above indicated that exercise combined with other treatments improved outcomes. Aerobic exercise has consistently led to improvements in FMS symptoms and function as well as in physical fitness (Burckhardt, Mannerkorpi, Hedenberg, & Bjelle, 1994; Mannerkorpi, Ahlmen, & Ekdahl, 2002; Mannerkorpi, Nyberg, & Ekdahl, 2000; McCain, Bell, Mai, & Halliday, 1988). Busch, Schacter, Peloso, and Bombardier (2002) identified 16 controlled trials of exercise interventions and found that participants experienced significant improvements in aerobic performance, reduced tender point pain thresholds, and decreased pain reports relative to controls. However, these studies were plagued by poor descriptions of exercise programs; insufficient information regarding the intensity, duration, frequency, and mode of exercise; and adverse events. Sufficient descriptions of measures and outcomes would make them more useful to clinicians.

Gowans et al. (2001) described an intensive 3-day-per-week aerobic exercise regime over 23 weeks that ameliorated depression (measured by Beck Depression Inventory) and improved physical function (measured by 6-minute walk distances). P. T. Costa et al. (2001) evaluated self-reported activity and depression in 70 Canadian women with FMS at baseline and 3 years later. Women who engaged in more physical activity reported lower depressed mood at follow-up after controlling for baseline depression, socioeconomic status, age, and changes in daily functioning.

Still, not all studies have found that exercise is effective. Van Santen et al. (2002) randomized 143 women with FMS into three groups: a fitness program, biofeedback training, or no active treatment control. The women were assessed at baseline and at 24 weeks for pain, tender points, myalgia, physical fitness, functioning, distress, and fatigue. No significant differences in change scores were found for any of the groups.

Because most exercise intervention studies show benefits from exercise, FMS patients should attempt to exercise if it is not contraindicated (Mannerkorpi & Daly Iverson, 2003). Exercise should be introduced gradually and incrementally, targeting at least 30 minutes of cardiovascular fitness training three times each week. Daily, gentle, low-impact aerobic exercise appears to be of central importance in the treatment of FMS (McCain et al., 1988), but too much or the wrong kind of exercise may exacerbate FMS symptoms. Patients who are deconditioned should start out with just 3 to 5 minutes of exercise every day and gradually increase as tolerated, usually up to 20 to 30 minutes a day. The benefit of the exercise seems to be from its systemic effects rather than any direct effect on the exercised muscles (Sim & Adams, 2002). Patients should choose an exercise program they enjoy and stick with it, because exercise must be routine to be beneficial. Recommended methods of exercise and pain control are cardiovascular fitness training and muscle strengthening and stretching (Gowans & deHueck, 2004; Quisel, Gill, & Walters, 2004). Multidisciplinary programs using cognitive–behavioral therapy in combination with exercise have been the most effective (Karjalainen et al., 2000).

FMS patients often respond to physical modalities including physical therapy, massage, tissue manipulation, soft-tissue injections, and acupuncture (B. M. Berman, Ezzo, Hadhazy, & Swyers, 1999) or chiropractic (Blunt, Rajwani, & Guerriero, 1997). Tender point thresholds have been increased with exercise and external muscle stimulation through massage (Hadhazy, Bausell, Berman, Creamer, & Ezzo, 2005) and spa therapy (Evcik, Kizilay, & Gokcen, 2002). Therefore, a consultation with a rehabilitation team, including physiatrists and physical therapists, can be a helpful adjunct to treatment.

COGNITIVE–BEHAVIORAL THERAPY

A specific goal of cognitive–behavioral therapy in FMS treatment is to change the idea that patients are helpless against their pain (Turk, 2003). Gaston-Johansson et al. (1990) found that individuals with FMS were significantly less optimistic than rheumatoid arthritis patients regarding relief from pain, improved functioning, and employment prospects. Cognitive rumination and pessimism reported in FMS (Gaston-Johansson et al., 1990; Hazlett & Haynes, 1992) have implications for treatment. Catastrophizing is common in women with FMS and chronic pain conditions and appears to contribute to poorer outcomes (I. Jensen et al., 1994). Catastrophizing responses and other dysfunctional cognitions can be addressed in cognitive therapy.

Patients' initial beliefs about the success of treatment can have an important influence on the treatment outcome. Goosens, Vlaeyen, Hidding, Kele-Snijders, and Evers (2005) examined the extent to which treatment expectancy predicts the short-term and long-term outcomes of cognitive–behavioral treatment of chronic pain. This study used the data of two pooled randomized clinical trials evaluating the effectiveness of cognitive–behavioral interventions for 171 patients with FMS and chronic low back pain. Pretreatment and posttreatment expectancy were measured by a short questionnaire before and after the intervention and at 12-month follow-up. Patients with higher treatment expectancies were significantly less fearful and received less disability compensation. Pretreatment expectancy significantly predicted outcome measures immediately after treatment as well as at

12-month follow-up. This study corroborates the importance of evaluating treatment expectation before attempting cognitive–behavioral intervention with FMS patients.

I. Jensen, Bergstrom, Ljungquist, Bodin, and Nygren (2001) evaluated the outcome of behavioral approaches compared with a treatment-as-usual control group in chronic pain patients on sick leave in Sweden. The results showed that the risk of full-time early retirement was significantly lower for women in behavior-oriented physical therapy and cognitive–behavioral therapy compared with the control group during the 18-month follow-up period. However, the total absence from work in days over the 18-month follow-up period was not significantly different in the control group compared with the treatment groups. On the Short Form–36 (SF-36), women receiving cognitive–behavioral therapy either exclusively or in conjunction with physical therapy reported a significantly better health-related quality of life than women in the control group at the 18-month follow-up. No significant differences for men were found on the SF-36 scales. The results revealed gender differences in the outcome of the treatments and that the components of behavioral programs yielded results as effective as the comprehensive program. The authors speculated that the women may have benefited more than the men from pain management techniques because women have a greater need for the specific coping strategies presented or are able to apply the strategies more effectively. Because many women have a higher total workload than men (paid plus unpaid work), they may be able to apply more effective coping strategies to their home environment (I. Jensen et al., 2001).

Behavior modification is an important component of cognitive–behavioral therapy. Behavior modification involves learning coping skills, relaxation exercises, and self-hypnosis. Nielson and Jensen (2004) examined the relationship between changes in coping and treatment outcome after a multicomponent treatment. The treatment program was a 5-day-a-week, 4-week outpatient program aimed at improving pain management and physical and psychological functioning. It included cardiovascular, strengthening, and stretching exercises; a graded activity program; group cognitive–behavioral therapy; assertiveness and relaxation training; group pain education; and tapering of pain medications. Regression analyses revealed that the following beliefs and coping strategies were most likely to be associated with improved outcomes at 3- and 6-month follow-up: increased sense of control and belief that FMS is not disabling and that pain is not necessarily a sign of damage, decreased guarding, increased exercise, seeking support, activity pacing, and use of coping self-statements.

Disclosure writing has shown benefits in chronic illness groups such as rheumatoid arthritis and cancer as well in psychological disorders (R. S. Campbell & Pennebaker, 2003). Broderick, Junghaenel, and Schwartz (2005) investigated the effect of written emotional expression in FMS. Ninety-two women were randomized to a trauma writing group, a control writing group that wrote about time management, or a usual care control group. At the 4-month follow-up, pain and fatigue measures were significantly lower in the trauma writing group compared with the control groups, and there was a slight improvement in psychological well-being. However, at the 10-month follow-up, none of the measures reflected that improvement.

The problem of not sustaining benefits in FMS treatment is not surprising given the high level of attrition and nonadherence to regimes. Meaningful improvement rarely occurs without active participation by patients in their treatment (Clauw & Crofford, 2003). It may be more efficacious for treatment to be tailored to subgroups within FMS. For example, dysfunctional patients might benefit from an operant behavioral approach to reduce the solicitous behaviors of significant others, whereas interpersonally distressed patients might benefit from interpersonal problem-solving and communication skills and treatment for depression. The adaptive coper group may benefit the most from exercise regimes (Thieme, Turk, & Flor, 2004; Turk, Okifuji, Sinclair, & Starz, 1998).

CASE STUDY

This case study[1] illustrates a fairly typical picture of an FMS patient beginning cognitive–behavioral therapy. Well illustrated here is the tortuous route toward obtaining a diagnosis of FMS, which, although providing some validation, does not provide any efficacious treatment avenues.

Abigail was a 39-year-old mother of 8-year-old twins. She had been amicably divorced for 3 years, although her ex-husband had moved 350 miles away so saw the children only for vacations. She had her 72-year-old parents living with her. She had trouble enjoying family life because of constant pain and exhaustion. When she arrived for psychological therapy, she seemed pleasant and soft-spoken yet somewhat anxious as she told her therapist that she had had headaches all her life. Abigail was also struggling with sleeplessness, depression, nervousness, panic attacks, and constant exhaustion, all while trying to raise her family and tend to her parents' needs. Her mother was in good health but her father had suffered a stroke and had many health problems. Pain would wake Abigail two to three times a night. She was taking St. John's wort for depression.

Along with her health, her personal freedom and family life were deteriorating. "I was really irritable with my Mom and Dad for anything, and with the kids. I would get really upset over anything." Ordinary daily activities like driving caused great distress and pain. She described headaches causing tension that

> pulled my muscles so much that it was painful to stretch my arms or to
> turn my head. I would do an aerobics class and get a strong headache.

---

[1]This case study is a fictionalized amalgam of typical patients.

Eventually I stopped exercising completely because I didn't even have the energy to go.

Abigail didn't know what was wrong with her. One doctor told her she had tension headaches; another, muscle spasms. Subjecting herself to many tests and treatments, she still didn't get a clear answer or any relief.

Abigail described one visit to her primary care physician:

> He put me in a dark room and gave me a shot in the arm. We waited for 10 minutes to see if my headache would go away, but I still had it. The doctor told me I'm not suffering from migraines. Then they put iodine in the vein to find out if I had some kind of brain tumor. A CAT scan was negative.

Her doctor prescribed Tylenol with codeine and then Valium. The pain returned. After 3 days on a higher dose, still in pain, she decided to stop taking the drug because it didn't seem to be helping. He referred her to an orthopedic physician, who reported a narrowing of the spaces in the cervical spine, but the MRI came back negative for abnormalities. For pain relief and muscle spasms, the doctor performed an infiltration of the spine with pain medication and corticosteroids. Abigail didn't like taking the steroid shots. She knew it wasn't a cure. "With the shots, I felt so scared. I knew he wasn't on the right track."

Visits to a chiropractor and a massage therapist provided pain relief for only an hour or so. Going from doctor to doctor to try to find a cure, with minimal results, Abigail lamented, "I felt afraid because I didn't know what was going on with me. I didn't know if the problems were from allergies, age, or my hormone system. I thought it could be my thyroid or too much stress." When she went back to her primary care physician, he decided she was suffering from FMS. He told her there was no real treatment for it except antidepressant drugs and muscle relaxants. He suggested that she see a psychologist and referred her to a clinician who specialized in patients with MUIs.

The psychologist explained to Abigail that when positive states of mind are restored, the physical body responds. Troublesome feelings such as fear, frustration, loss, anger, anxiety, sadness, depression, and hopelessness often chronically surround a physical illness and hamper healing, undermining the ability to feel in control of the outcome. Abigail understood the limits of biomedical treatment for her FMS, and she expressed willingness to try cognitive–behavioral therapy. Her therapist outlined the goals of treatment as follows:

> The primary goals of [cognitive–behavioral therapy] in FMS are to change distorted perceptions and self-defeating behaviors. Using specific tasks and self-observation, you will learn to think of pain as something other than a negative factor that dominates your life. Over time, the idea that you are helpless against pain will recede and you will learn that you can manage your FMS.

Cognitive therapy is especially helpful in defining and setting limits—a behavior that is extremely important for FMS patients. Abigail, you are like many FMS patients who are trying to do everything for everyone. People with FMS often doggedly push themselves past the point of endurance until they collapse and withdraw. This inevitable backlash reverses their self-perception, and they then view themselves as complete failures, unable to cope with the simplest task. One important aim of cognitive–behavioral therapy is to help you find a middle route, where you can prioritize your responsibilities and drop some of the less important tasks or delegate them to others. Learning these coping skills can eventually lead to a more manageable life and to less of an absolutist perspective on yourself and others.

Abigail's therapy lasted for 16 sessions, 1 hour each week. She was also given homework: keeping a diary, attempting tasks that she had been avoiding, and practicing relaxation. Her program included the following tasks:

- Keeping a diary: A diary is often a key component of cognitive therapy. The diary serves as a general guide for setting limits and planning activities. Patients use the diary to track any stress factors, such as a job or a relationship that may be making the pain worse or better.
- Cognitive restructuring of negative thoughts: Abigail was taught to challenge and reverse negative beliefs ("e.g., I'm not good enough to control this condition, so I'm a total failure") to using coping statements ("Where is the evidence that I cannot control this illness?").
- Graded activation and setting limits: Limits are designed to keep both mental and physical stress within a manageable framework so that patients do not get discouraged by forcing themselves into situations in which they are likely to fail. For example, tasks and exercise are broken down into small, incremental steps, and patients focus on one at a time.
- Seeking out pleasurable activities: List a number of enjoyable low-energy activities that can be conveniently scheduled.
- Prioritizing: Learn to drop some less critical tasks or delegate them to others.
- Relaxation training: Abigail was taught several relaxation techniques to use throughout the day.
- Accepting relapses: Accomplishing too much too soon can often cause a relapse of symptoms. Patients should respect these relapses and back off. They should not consider them a sign of treatment or self-failure.

Abigail's beliefs in her ability to control pain were strengthened as she gained success in using self-management skills. She was exercising for 20 minutes every other day, and her mood was considerably improved. She was no longer taking St. John's wort, because she didn't believe that it had helped her. Beliefs in her ability to control pain also appeared to be stable; a follow-up visit 4 months after the end of therapy revealed that she had maintained her progress. Cognitive–behavioral therapy assumes that beliefs in control evolve from successful use of cognitive skills, and Abigail's case provides a clear example of this principle.

Because FMS involves a range of symptoms, different treatment modalities that target different symptoms are required. Exercise can help reduce hypersensitivity to pain and improve mood. Low-dose antidepressants may improve sleep and reduce pain. Cognitive–behavioral therapy can help modify maladaptive thoughts and improve depressed mood, activity levels, and social relationships. A person-centered multimodal approach tailored toward the individual's most pressing needs should enhance the patient–provider relationship and help prioritize patients' goals (Masi et al., 2002). Although FMS is difficult to treat, the studies reviewed in this chapter indicate that tailored approaches, often involving a team of health professionals, can be effective in reducing suffering and disability.

11

TREATMENT APPROACHES TO CHRONIC FATIGUE SYNDROME

Given the diagnostic evolutions and heterogeneity of the chronic fatigue syndrome (CFS) population, it is hardly surprising that there are no firmly established treatment recommendations for CFS. This chapter reviews some of the approaches that have been studied with this population.

PHARMACOLOGICAL APPROACHES

A number of pharmacological approaches have been attempted without notable success. Many pharmacological treatments, including antivirals, immune modifiers, essential fatty acids, antifungal agents, vitamins, and minerals, have been reported anecdotally to be helpful, but they have not demonstrated efficacy in double-blind, placebo-controlled clinical trials (Blondel-Hill & Shafran, 1993). A randomized, placebo-controlled, double blind, multicenter study of a ribonucleic acid drug—Poly(I):Poly(C12U), Ampligen—with antiviral and immunomodulatory properties was conducted on 92 participants with severe CFS (Strayer et al., 1994). After 24 weeks of treatment, participants receiving Ampligen reported a significantly reduced disability score, enhanced ability to perform activities of daily living, and reduced cognitive impairment, and they were able to tolerate a greater workload during treadmill testing. However, Ampligen has not yet been approved for use in treating CFS. Despite frequent use of antidepressants for fatigue, Dzurec (2000; Dzurec, Hoover, & Fields, 2002) concluded that antidepressants provide little long-term amelioration of fatigue for patients with normal laboratory values. In a double-blind, placebo-controlled study, fluoxetine had no beneficial effect in patients with CFS, with and without depression (Vercoulen et al., 1996).

Given that hypocortisolism has been found in some persons with CFS, treatment with hydrocortisone has been attempted. Cleare et al. (1999) found that CFS patients reported significant reductions in self-rated fatigue and disability compared with a placebo group after 28 days of treatment with low-dose hydrocortisone, which led to a rise in circulating cortisol. A group using a higher dose found adrenal suppression indicating that risks outweighed benefits (McKenzie et al., 1998). Cleare et al. (2001) found that about 28% of CFS patients responded to hydrocortisone treatment with reduced fatigue levels (similar to the percentage found in the previous two studies). In those who responded to treatment, there was a corresponding normalization of the blunted cortisol response to human corticotropin-releasing hormone challenge. Although molecular biology advances are promising, pharmaceutical approaches do not appear to offer significant benefits to the majority of individuals with CFS.

Beliefs and Coping Styles

Several studies have found that people with CFS have negative coping styles such as escape–avoidance and denial (Blakely et al., 1991; Cope, Mann, Pelosi, & David, 1996). Similarly, people with CFS tend to make external attributions for their illness, maintaining organic illness convictions over psychological explanations (Cope et al., 1996; S. K. Johnson, Lange, Tiersky, DeLuca, & Natelson, 2001; R. Powell, Dolan, & Wessely, 1990; Schweitzer, Robertson, Kelly, & Whiting, 1993; Surawy, Hackman, Hawton, & Sharpe, 1995); only one study has found that psychological morbidity and physical attribution were not risk factors for chronic fatigue (Lawrie et al., 1997). In a study of Gulf War veterans with CFS, Fiedler et al. (2000) found that life stressors after the war, environmental exposures, neuroticism, defensiveness, and negative coping style were predictors of low physical functioning on the Short Form-36.

S. K. Johnson, Gil-Rivas, and Schmaling (2006) found that the use of instrumental social support, which includes seeking information, advice, and assistance, was negatively associated with vitality. Although it may seem counterintuitive, studies have found that membership in a self-help group is a robust predictor of poor treatment response to a graded exercise trial (Bentall,

Powell, Nye, & Edwards, 2002) and poor outcomes over time (Sharpe et al., 1992). Involvement in self-help groups may represent illness conviction and stronger attachment to the illness as well as involve information and advice seeking, which may be counterproductive in CFS. Similarly, religious involvement has usually been associated with positive health outcomes (L. H. Powell, Shahabi, & Thoresen, 2003) but greater CFS symptom severity. The COPE scale items tapping religious coping are turning to God, praying, and finding comfort in religion, which imply a passive, internal process that might involve more rumination than being engaged in religious activities; seen in this light, it is perhaps not surprising that religious coping techniques are used by the more symptomatic and disabled participants. These studies indicate that addressing beliefs and coping styles could improve outcomes in CFS.

COGNITIVE–BEHAVIORAL THERAPY

Cognitive–behavioral therapy is designed to alter a patient's cognitive focusing on bodily symptoms and somatic attribution. This type of therapy designed for CFS patients usually consists of challenging fatigue-related cognitions, diminishing strong somatic attributions, improving sense of control over symptoms, and facilitating increased levels of physical activity (Prins et al., 2001; Sharpe et al., 1996). Cognitive–behavioral therapy and graded exercise therapy are the primary interventions that have been found to be effective in CFS (Prins, van der Meer, & Bleijenberg, 2006). Surawy et al. (1995) have proposed that although infection and/or severe stress are precipitating factors, cognitive and behavioral factors are central in perpetuating illness. Thus, effective approaches need to break the cycle of deconditioning, avoidance, and depression through graded activity and cognitive restructuring. The therapist's goal should be recovery, which means that the client with CFS strives to discard the "patient label" (Prins, Bleijenberg, & van der Meer, 2002). This does not mean that the client returns to premorbid functioning, which was often an extremely active life. Rather, individuals with CFS must accept limitations but work toward lifestyle goals that make them feel healthier.

Before considering cognitive–behavioral therapy, therapists should assess a CFS patient's complaints. Responses to the following questions (adapted from Bleijenberg, Prins, & Bazelmans, 2003) can be illuminating:

How does the patient spend the day?
What are the patient's views on the causes of complaints?
Does the patient have a tendency to catastrophize the complaints?
Is the patient afraid to undertake activities?
What effects do the patient's complaints have on his or her social
environment?

Has their work situation been affected by CFS?

Typical problematic cognitions encountered in therapy with CFS patients include statements along these lines:

"I'll never get better."
"I used to be able to do it all. I'd be cleaning the kitchen floor
   while watching *Late Night with David Letterman*."
"I hate to have to ask others to do things for me. I've always been
   the one doing for other people."

These themes of interference with previous high-activity levels or nurturant roles, a reversal of the caregiving role, can result in guilt-tinged cognitions, especially for women with CFS. It is important for the therapist to guide their patients into more accepting and adaptive cognitions:

"I don't have to be perfect; everyone has limits."
"I can still achieve some goals; I have to set realistic limits."

Several early cognitive–behavioral therapy studies reported benefits in improving disability outcomes (Bonner, Ron, Chalder, Butler, & Wessely, 1994; Butler, Chalder, Ron, & Wessely, 1991), whereas others have not (Freidberg & Krupp, 1994; A. Lloyd et al., 1993). Bonner et al. (1994) conducted a 4-year follow-up study of 47 patients diagnosed with CFS and offered cognitive–behavioral therapy and found that 87% of the 23 participants who successfully completed therapy remained well 4 years later. In a nonblind, nonrandomized study, Butler et al. (1991) found that 70% of participants who started treatment rated themselves as "better" or "much better" at the end of treatment and remained better at 3-month follow up. From their initial pool of 50 patients who were offered cognitive–behavioral therapy, 18 declined and 5 withdrew after the start of treatment. Conversely, a randomized, double-blind comparison of treatment and routine clinic attendance found neither cognitive–behavioral therapy alone or in combination with immunologic therapy of dialyzable leukocyte extract provided any benefit greater than nonspecific treatment (A. Lloyd et al., 1993). However, cognitive–behavioral therapy in this study comprised only six sessions over 10 weeks and may not have been intensive enough to sustain improvement. Freidberg and Krupp (1994) found that cognitive–behavioral therapy (their intervention emphasized coping skills) benefited only those individuals with both CFS and depression; fatigue severity remained unaffected, although catastrophic thinking, stress, and symptom magnification were reduced.

Deale, Chalder, Marks, and Wessely (1997) performed a study that controlled for nonspecific treatment factors such as therapist time, attention, support, and homework practices by using a relaxation comparison group. They found that 70% of CFS patients showed improvement (on a physical functioning scale) after 13 sessions over 4 to 6 months, whereas only 19% of a relaxation group improved. A total of 21% of eligible participants either declined participation or dropped out before the 4 months were complete. In a follow-up interview 5 years later (Deale, Kaneez, Chalder, & Wessely, 2001), 68% of the patients who received cognitive–behavioral therapy and 36% of those who received relaxation therapy rated themselves as "much improved" or "very much improved." Significantly more patients who received cognitive–behavioral therapy met criteria for complete recovery, were free of relapse, and experienced symptoms that had steadily improved or were consistently mild or absent since treatment ended; they also worked significantly more hours per week. Another randomized controlled trial of 16 weekly sessions of cognitive–behavioral therapy showed that 73% improved to a level of normal daily functioning compared with 27% of those given only medical care (Sharpe et al., 1996). Only 2 out of 62 refused to participate, and all participants completed treatment. At 12-month follow-up, work status had improved for 63% of the cognitive–behavioral therapy group but for only 20% of the control group.

Prins et al. (2001) compared cognitive–behavioral therapy with guided support groups and a no-intervention control in a multicenter randomized trial. Ninety-three individuals with CFS were randomly assigned the cognitive–behavioral treatment (administered by 13 therapists trained in this technique for CFS), 94 were assigned the support-group approach, and 91 the control group. At 8 months, 83 in the treatment group, 80 in the support group, and 78 in the no-intervention group had complete data. At 14 months, cognitive–behavioral therapy was significantly more effective than both control conditions for fatigue severity and for functional impairment measures. Support groups were not more effective for CFS patients than the no-intervention condition. Among the cognitive–behavioral group, clinically significant improvement was seen in fatigue severity for 20 of 58 (35%), in Karnofsky performance status[1] for 28 of 57 (49%), and in self-rated improvement for 29 of 58 (50%). Those who improved with cognitive–behavioral therapy had a higher sense of control, whereas a passive activity pattern and focusing on bodily symptoms predicted less improvement.

EXERCISE

Graded exercise has shown effectiveness in CFS. Treatment should be gradual, starting at a low level of activity or exercise and increasing incrementally under controlled conditions (Sharpe & Wessely, 1998). In a randomized controlled trial of graded aerobic exercise compared with flexibility

---

[1]The Karnofsky Performance Status Scale has the following anchors: 0 = *Dead*; 50 = *Requires considerable assistance and medical care*; and 100 = *Normal, no complaints, no evidence of disease* (Mor, Laliberte, Morris, & Weiman, 1984).

and relaxation treatment, CFS participants reported significantly greater improvements in fatigue, functional capacity, and fitness after exercise treatment (Fulcher & White, 1997). Wearden et al. (1998) performed a 6-month prospective randomized placebo and therapist-contact-time controlled trial with allocation to one of four treatment conditions: exercise and 20 milligrams of fluoxetine, exercise and placebo, appointments with a therapist and 20 milligrams fluoxetine, and appointments and placebo. Results showed that exercise was effective in reducing fatigue and improving health perception 6 months after the intervention, although patients were more likely to drop out of exercise than nonexercise treatment and disability levels remained unaffected. Fluoxetine had a significant effect on depression at Week 12 only but had no effect on fatigue or disability.

P. Powell, Bentall, Nye, and Edwards (2004) performed an educational intervention designed to encourage graded activity. At 2-year follow-up, 63 of the treated patients (55%) no longer fulfilled trial criteria for CFS. This was similar to the percentage at 1-year follow-up and showed that the benefits of the intervention were maintained. Wallman, Morton, Goodman, Grove, and Guilfoyle (2004) also performed a randomized controlled trial of graded exercise with pacing (32 patients) compared with relaxation–flexibility therapy (29 patients) performed twice a day over 12 weeks. Following the graded exercise intervention, scores were improved for resting systolic blood pressure, work capacity, perceived exertion after exercise, net blood lactate production, depression, and performance on a modified Stroop color–word test. No such changes were observed in the relaxation–flexibility condition. The authors suggested that improvements may be associated with the abandonment of avoidance behaviors.

Moss-Morris, Sharon, Tobin, and Baldi (2005) were interested in determining the mechanism underlying effectiveness of graded exercise therapy. Do individuals with CFS improve with exercise interventions because of improved physical fitness, which reduces symptoms caused by deconditioning, or does an exercise program increase patients' sense of control, reduce focus on symptoms, and alter fears about the consequences of exercise? Forty-nine CFS patients were randomized to a 12-week graded exercise program or to standard medical care. At the end of treatment, the exercise group rated themselves as significantly more improved and less fatigued than the control group. The authors concluded that a decrease in focus on symptoms rather than an increase in fitness mediated the treatment effect.

Bleijenberg et al. (2003) recommended different approaches for relatively active versus low-active CFS patients. Relatively active patients need help in building up their activity levels in a graded fashion without exacerbating symptoms. Low-active patients have fears that any activity may aggravate symptoms. These patients typically spend a lot of time in supine positions and daytime napping. For these patients, the following cognitions should be encouraged:

"I need to stop looking for explanations and do something about my symptoms."

"I know I will feel bad when I exercise, but my body needs to get used to being active."

Graded activity with low-active patients should start with about six exercise bouts per day for 1 minute each, and then they should be increased by 1 minute each day. The therapist needs to reassure the patient that it is all right to feel tired. Social support that maintains the patient's complaints must be curtailed.

These studies present evidence that both graded exercise and cognitive–behavioral therapy may be effective through reducing avoidance behavior, decreasing symptom focusing, and increasing efficacy through increased functioning and return to work, supporting the validity of a biopsychosocial model of CFS. Some have argued that cognitive–behavioral therapy or graded exercise would benefit only subgroups of CFS who attend tertiary clinics, because they tend to have greater functional impairment and more psychological disorder (Jason, Richman, et al., 1997). On the other hand, exercise treatment may be limited to a high functioning subgroup of individuals with CFS. Risdale, Darbishire, and Seed (2004) addressed these issues by randomizing primary care patients with unexplained fatigue for 3 months or longer to 6 weeks of either cognitive–behavioral therapy or exercise treatment. They found that the two treatments were roughly equivalent in reducing fatigue scores. However, fewer patients took up the offer of graded exercise therapy, and more dropped out of that treatment arm. Overall, Risdale et al. found cognitive–behavioral therapy to be more palatable to these primary care patients. Fairly high refusal and drop-out rates for cognitive–behavioral therapy and exercise also indicate that one treatment will not fit all cases, and the heterogeneity of CFS requires individualized treatment programs.

Treatment strategies should focus on strategies such as effective coping skills and reducing catastrophic thinking as well as addressing deconditioning effects through increasing activity, all of which have been shown to increase levels of functioning. To be effective, treatment must be collaborative and consistent with the explanatory models relevant to the individual with CFS. Future research should determine what individual characteristics predict success for various interventions and what treatments are most cost-effective and efficient in improving health outcomes and reducing disability in CFS.

12

TREATMENT APPROACHES TO MULTIPLE CHEMICAL SENSITIVITY

There is little research examining the efficacy of treatment for multiple chemical sensitivity (MCS). Yet, many of the approaches shown to be effective for other medically unexplained illnesses (MUIs) should be helpful in MCS as well. Therapists must consider the pain, loss, and estrangement of a debilitating chronic illness that is not explained and often not recognized by the medical profession. Somatization processes can result in amplification of bodily sensations to the point where symptoms are painful and disabling. It then becomes difficult to separate effects induced by beliefs from physiologic responses. For the therapist who wants to help an individual with MCS achieve better functioning and quality of life, it is important to understand the patient's belief system. This can help elucidate irrational cognitions that may be amenable to change through cognitive–behavioral therapy.

Because individuals with MCS generally encounter a high degree of skepticism from the medical community, they are likely to develop defensive responses to direct questioning. Appreciation for this defensive posture led Gomez, Schvaneveldt, and Staudenmayer (1996) to develop an indirect route to understanding beliefs surrounding MCS using the Pathfinder networking scaling algorithm. They examined persons with allergies, persons with MCS, asymptomatic controls, and allergists. The participants were given a list of 14 MCS symptoms and 10 causal factors and asked to rate every possible pairwise combination on a 9-point relatedness scale. They found marked differences in the network organization, with the MCS group placing multi-chemical exposure at the center of their belief system and all other groups placing multichemical exposure at the periphery.

An issue for individuals with any MUI, but perhaps even more so in MCS, is the perceived illegitimacy of the illness. The lack of medical and cultural validation increases a sense of stigma (Chircop & Keddy, 2003). People will challenge biomedical precepts because conventional medicine cannot explain their body's reduced ability to function in the face of chemical exposures. There is often an antipsychological stance in people with MCS. Individuals with MCS and other MUIs are often hostile to any theories that include psychological causation. In Poonai et al.'s (2001) study of the 26 individuals who had panic responses, only one was agreeable to a referral to a psychologist or psychiatrist.

Although psychological approaches have been shown to be effective in various MUIs, it is worth considering evidence of selection bias in these studies. It is likely that people who are amenable to cognitive–behavioral approaches are only a subset of the MUI patient populations; they may be those who are more flexible in their attitudes and more open to change.

Haller (1993) described inpatient psychiatric treatment for 3 women who had been severely disabled by MCS. Each improved significantly from a nonjudgmental, comprehensive approach and tapering off of aggressive medications. The women reported that their experiences were validated in the hospital, and they substantially reduced their symptoms and described improved ability to cope.

Desensitization training has been reported to be effective anecdotally, but few studies have examined this approach. Guglielmi, Cox, and Spyker (1994) described cognitive–behavioral treatment of phobic avoidance in 3 women with severe MCS. They hypothesized that the incapacitating severity of MCS is similar to agoraphobia. Some evidence in their cases was a significant increase in electrodermal activity during a review of chemical exposure and description of the test exposure, whereas actual exposure to stimuli described by the patient as particularly noxious produced a decrease in physiological arousal. Thus, all 3 patients exhibited anticipatory anxiety. The cases were treated with an intensive desensitization program consisting of biofeedback-assisted relaxation training, in vivo exposure to a hierarchy of the offending chemicals, and cognitive restructuring. All 3 patients showed significant improvement; 1 woman returned to work and continued to do well, but the others were lost to follow-up.

Although approaches such as behavioral desensitization, cognitive–behavioral therapy, cognitive therapy, and psychotropic medications can be useful, Staudenmayer (2000) warned that the greatest challenge in treatment is to overcome the patient's disabling belief in a toxicogenic etiology for symptoms. Many of the recommendations of clinical ecologists to avoid all chemicals even to the point of remodeling the home or moving to cleaner locales may be counterproductive, because they further insulate the individual with MCS and encourage avoidance. This will likely increase phobic behaviors. Approaches that emphasize increasing activity and decreasing symptom focusing are probably the most effective in treating individuals with MCS.

13

CONCLUSION: UNDERSTANDING MEDICALLY UNEXPLAINED ILLNESS

This book has presented a vast amount of information about the most common medically unexplained illnesses (MUIs). Although diagnostic technology has become increasingly sophisticated, MUIs still remain largely unexplained by organic factors. There are many reasons for this: heterogeneity of groups, fairly recent case definitions, inconsistent research findings, and an etiology that appears to be multidetermined. The biopsychosocial model helps illuminate a contextual perspective to account for the interaction of biological, psychological, social, and cultural factors. Biopsychosocial components play a role in disease perception, symptom generation, and health care seeking (Mayer, 1999).

Biological vulnerabilities may encompass genetics, hypothalamic–pituitary–adrenal axis dysregulation, neuronal sensitization and hyperexcitability, visceral hypersensitivity, immune suppression, and autonomic dysregulation. These vulnerabilities are aggravated by psychosocial stress, including childhood abuse, work, role strain, and interpersonal stress. Cognitive factors that increase the experience of symptoms are hypervigilance, catastrophizing, and amplification. All of these processes are bidirectional (Wilhelmsen, 2005). The pathophysiology of MUIs is heavily influenced by

185

psychosocial factors, particularly chronic stress. Much of the research reviewed in this volume suggests that the physiological systems of people with MUIs do not respond normally to physical and psychological stresses.

It is well established that virtually all of the MUIs are much more common in women. So, what more have we learned about MUI by focusing on gender? Women's symptoms are more likely to be multidetermined than men's symptoms, and because the most-established finding regarding MUIs is that they are multidetermined, it is not surprising that MUIs are more prevalent in women. Factors that occur more commonly in women—abuse, neglect, role strain, depression, anxiety, and emotional coping styles—have been shown to influence the precipitation and chronicity of MUIs. Women have lower thresholds for perceiving symptoms and are more likely to seek help for symptoms than men. Much of this is due to gender role expectations and social learning wherein women are allowed to complain about symptoms and seek help.

Psychopathologies, such as depression and anxiety, contribute to vigilance regarding symptoms. Nonetheless, many studies have found that close to half of individuals with MUIs have no significant psychiatric pathology. However, other psychosocial factors, such as premorbid perfectionism, overactivity, emotional rigidity, neuroticism, and poor coping mechanisms, have been shown to increase risk for MUIs. An example of an important psychosocial stressor that appears to make women more vulnerable to MUIs is susceptibility to abuse. Although boys and men suffer sexual and physical abuse as well, it appears to be more common in girls and women. Because it is such a difficult area to study, relying on notoriously subjective self-report, the true prevalence of such abuse may never be understood. There is no question that a trauma history accompanied by a lack of protective factors, whether these be personality factors, psychological resilience, social support, or physiology (genetic fitness), contribute to a greater risk of MUI.

What is the best approach for psychologists confronting people with MUIs? Early diagnosis and management can help reduce disability. Sharpe and Carson (2001) proposed a paradigm shift in which unexplained symptoms become "remedicalized" around the notion of a functional disturbance of the nervous system. They proposed that integrating psychological treatment into general medical care would improve the care of individuals with MUIs. Certainly, the treatment evidence in this volume indicates that psychological approaches are generally more efficacious than drug therapies. Others (Heath, 1999; Wilhelmsen, 2005) have argued that normalizing rather than pathologizing unexplained symptoms with an emphasis on acceptance is the best approach. Is medicalization of MUIs helpful to patients in that it legitimizes their complaints, or is it more helpful to encourage coping with symptoms and reducing reliance on fruitless medical visits? This is where health psychologists must step up to the plate and advocate for a biopsychosocial approach to patients with MUIs, rather than treatments guided by "either–or" explanations.

Future research ought to avoid reductionism and biological primacy and examine the contributions of interdependent mechanisms. MUIs may defy efforts to be simplified, just as individuals with MUIs cannot be lumped into a single category. Malterud (2000) warned against this "universalist lumping trap" and the tendency to stereotype women with MUIs as a homogenous group. The complexity of MUIs calls for more dynamic models to better apportion variance among multiple factors (Hamilton & Gallant, 1993). Emphasizing the role of stress in MUIs, Van Houdenhove, Egle, and Luyten (2005) exhorted researchers to use "multiwave data to investigate recursive interactions" between past and current stressors and personality variables and how these interactions initiate or perpetuate MUIs (p. 367). This volume has laid out the evidence for multiple factors and for the complex and dynamic interaction of biopsychosocial factors. It is the task of future researchers to illuminate gender factors more fully in searching for explanations of MUIs.

REFERENCES

Aaron, L. A., & Buchwald, D. (2001). A review of the evidence for overlap among unexplained clinical conditions. *Annals of Internal Medicine, 134,* 868–881.

Aaron, L. A., & Buchwald, D. (2003). Chronic diffuse musculoskeletal pain, fibromyalgia and co-morbid unexplained clinical conditions. *Best Practice & Research. Clinical Rheumatology, 17,* 563–574.

Aceves-Avila, F. J., Ferrari, R., & Ramos-Remus, C. (2004). New insights into culture driven disorders. *Best Practice & Research. Clinical Rheumatology, 18,* 155–171.

Afari, N., & Buchwald, D. (2003). Chronic fatigue syndrome: A review. *American Journal of Psychiatry, 160,* 221–236.

Ahles, T. A., Khan, S. A., Yunus, M. B., Speigel, D. A., & Masi, A. T. (1991). Psychiatric status of patients with primary fibromyalgia, patients with rheumatoid arthritis, and subjects without pain: A blind comparison of DSM–III diagnoses. *American Journal of Psychiatry, 148,* 1721–1726.

Ahles, T. A., Yunus, M. H., & Masi, A. T. (1987). Is chronic pain a variant of depressive disease? The case of primary fibromyalgia syndrome. *Pain, 29,* 105–111.

Alagiri, M., Chottiner, S., Ratner, V., Slade, D., & Hanno, P. M. (1997). Interstitial cystitis: Unexplained associations with other chronic disease and pain syndromes. *Urology, 49*(Suppl. 5A), 52–57.

Alexander, R. W., Bradley, L. A., Alarcon, G. S., Triana-Alexander, M., Aaron, L. A., Alberts, K. R., et al. (1998). Sexual and physical abuse in women with fibromyalgia: Association with outpatient health care utilization and pain medication usage. *Arthritis Care Research, 11,* 102–115.

Ali, A., Richardson, D. C., & Toner, B. B. (1998). Feminine gender role and illness behavior in irritable bowel syndrome. *Journal of Gender, Culture, and Health, 3,* 59–65.

Ali, A., Toner, B. B., Stuckless, N., Gallop, R., Diamant, N. E., Gould, M. I., & Vidins, E. I. (2000). Emotional abuse, self-blame, and self-silencing in women with irritable bowel syndrome. *Psychosomatic Medicine, 62,* 76–82.

Allen, L. A., & Escobar, J. I. (2005). Fatigue and somatization. In J. DeLuca (Ed.), *Fatigue as a window to the brain* (pp. 173–183). Cambridge, MA: MIT Press.

Aloisi, A. M. (2003). Gonadal hormones and sex differences in pain reactivity. *Clinical Journal of Pain, 19,* 108–174.

Alonso, C., Loevinger, B., Muller, D., & Coe, C. (2004). Menstrual cycle influences on pain and emotion in women with fibromyalgia. *Journal of Psychosomatic Research, 57,* 451–458.

Altemus, M., Dale, D. K., Michelson, D., Demitrack, M. A., Gold, P. W., & Straus, S. E. (2001). Abnormalities in response to vasopressin infusion in chronic fatigue syndrome. *Psychoneuroendocrinology, 26,* 175–188.

American Psychiatric Association. (1952). *Diagnostic and statistical manual of mental disorders.* Washington, DC: Author.

American Psychiatric Association. (1968). *Diagnostic and statistical manual of mental disorders* (2nd ed.). Washington, DC: Author.

American Psychiatric Association. (1980). *Diagnostic and statistical manual of mental disorders* (3rd ed.). Washington, DC: Author.

American Psychiatric Association. (1987). *Diagnostic and statistical manual of mental disorders* (3rd ed., rev.). Washington, DC: Author.

American Psychiatric Association. (1994). *Diagnostic and statistical manual of mental disorders* (4th ed.). Washington, DC: Author.

American Psychiatric Association. (2000). *Diagnostic and statistical manual of mental disorders* (4th ed., text revision). Washington, DC: Author.

Anderberg, U. M. (2000). Comment on: Johns and Littlejohn, The role of sex hormones in pain response. *Pain, 87,* 109–111.

Anderberg, U. M., Lui, Z., Berglund, L., & Nyberg, F. (1998). Plasma levels on nociceptin in female fibromyalgia syndrome patients. *Zeitschrift für Rheumatologie, 57,* 77–80.

Anderberg, U. M., Lui, Z., Berglund, L., & Nyberg, F. (1999). Elevated plasma levels of neuropeptide Y in female fibromyalgia patients. *European Journal of Pain, 3,* 19–30.

Anderberg, U. M., Marteinsdottir, I., Hallman, J., & Backstrom, T. (1998). Variability in cyclicity affects pain and other symptoms in female fibromyalgia syndrome patients. *Journal of Musculoskeletal Pain, 6,* 5–22.

Anderberg, U. M., Marteinsdottir, I., Hallman, J., Ekselius, L., & Backstrom, T. (1999). Symptom perception in relation to hormonal status in female fibromyalgia syndrome patients. *Journal of Musculoskeletal Pain, 7,* 21–38.

Anderson, J. S., & Ferrans, C. E. (1997). The quality of life of persons with chronic fatigue syndrome. *Journal of Nervous and Mental Disease, 185,* 359–367.

Arias, I. (2004). The legacy of child maltreatment: Long-term health consequences for women. *Journal of Women's Health, 13,* 468–473.

Arnold, L. M., Hess, E. V., Hudson, J. I., Welge, J. A., Berno, S. E., & Keck, P. E., Jr. (2002). A randomized, placebo-controlled, double-blind, flexible-dose study of fluoxetine in the treatment of women with fibromyalgia. *American Journal of Medicine, 15,* 191–197.

Arnold, L. M., Hudson, J. I., Hess, E. V., Ware, A. E., Fritz, D. A., Auchenbach, M. B., et al. (2004). Family study of fibromyalgia. *Arthritis and Rheumatism, 50,* 944–952.

Arnold, L. M., & Keck, P. E. (2001). Antidepressant treatment of fibromyalgia: A meta-analysis and review. *Psychosomatics, 41,* 104–113.

Asbring, P., & Narvanen, A. L. (2002). Women's experiences of stigma in relation to chronic fatigue syndrome and fibromyalgia. *Qualitative Health Research, 12,* 148–160.

Ashford, N. A., & Miller, C. S. (1997). *Chemical exposures: Low levels and high stakes*. New York: Van Nostrand Reinhold.

Assefi, N. P., Coy, T. V., Uslan, D., Smith, W. R., & Buchwald, D. (2003). Financial, occupational, and personal consequences of disability in patients with chronic fatigue syndrome and fibromyalgia compared to other fatiguing conditions. *Journal of Rheumatology, 30*, 804–808.

Bailer, J., Rist, F., Witthöft, M., Paul, C., & Bayerl, C. (2004). Symptom patterns, and perceptual and cognitive styles in subjects with multiple chemical sensitivity (MCS). *Journal of Environmental Psychology, 24*, 517–525.

Bailer, J., Witthöft, M., Paul, C., Bayerl, C., & Rist, F. (2005). Evidence for overlap between idiopathic environmental intolerance and somatoform disorders. *Psychosomatic Medicine, 67*, 921–929.

Bakheit, A. M. O., Behan, P. O., Dinan, T. G., Gray, C. E., & O'Keane, V. (1992). Possible upregulation of hypothalamic 5-hydroxytryptamine receptors in patients with postviral fatigue syndrome. *British Medical Journal, 304*, 1010–1012.

Barnett, R. C. (1997). How paradigms shape the stories we tell: Paradigm shifts in gender and health. *Journal of Social Issues, 53*, 351–364.

Barsky, A. J., & Borus, J. F. (1995). Somatization and medicalization in the era of managed care. *Journal of the American Medical Association, 274*, 1931–1934.

Barsky, A. J., & Borus, J. F. (1999). Functional somatic syndromes. *Annals of Internal Medicine, 130*, 910–921.

Barsky, A. J., & Wyshak, G. (1990). Hypochondriasis and somatosensory amplification. *British Journal of Psychiatry, 157*, 404–409.

Bascom, R., Meggs, W. J., Frampton, M., Hudnell, K., Killburn, K., Kobal, G., et al. (1997). Neurogenic inflammation: With additional discussion of central and perceptual integration of nonneurogenic inflammation. *Environmental Health Perspectives, 105*(Suppl. 2), 531–537.

Beard, G. (1880). *A practical treatise on nervous exhaustion (neurasthenia)*. New York: William Wood.

Becker, D. (2005). *The myth of empowerment: Women and the therapeutic culture in America*. New York: New York University Press.

Bell, I. R. (1994). Neuropsychiatric aspects of sensitivity to low-level chemicals: A neural sensitization model. *Toxicology and Industrial Health, 10*, 277–312.

Bell, I. R., Baldwin, C. M., & Schwartz, G. E. (2001). Sensitization studies in chemically intolerant individuals: Implications for individual difference research. In B. A. Sorg & I. R. Bell (Eds.), *Annals of the New York Academy of Sciences: Vol. 933. The role of neural plasticity in chemical intolerance* (pp. 38–47). New York: New York Academy of Sciences.

Bell, I. R., Miller, C. S., Schwartz, G. E., Peterson, J. M., & Amend, D. (1996). Neuropsychiatric and somatic characteristics of young adults with and without self-reported chemical odor intolerance and chemical sensitivity. *Archives of Environmental Health, 51*, 9–21.

Bell, I. R., Peterson, J. M., & Schwartz, G. E. (1995). Medical histories and psychological profiles of middle-aged women with and without self-reported illness from environmental chemicals. *Journal of Clinical Psychiatry, 56,* 151–160.

Bennett, E. J., Evans, P., Scott, A. M., Badcock, C. A., Shuter, B., Hoschl, R., & Tennant, J. E. (2000). Psychological and sex features of delayed gut transit in functional gastrointestinal disorders. *Gut, 46,* 83–87.

Bennett, E. J., Tennant, C. C., Piesse, C., Badcock, C. A., & Kellow, J. E. (1998). Level of chronic life stress predicts clinical outcome in irritable bowel syndrome. *Gut, 43,* 256–262.

Bennett, R. M. (1996). Multidisciplinary group programs to treat fibromyalgia patients. *Rheumatic Disease Clinics of North America, 22,* 351–367.

Bennett, R. M. (2005). Fibromyalgia: Present to future. *Current Rheumatology Reports, 7,* 371–376.

Bentall, R. P., Powell, P., Nye, F. J., & Edwards, H. T. (2002). Predictors of response to treatment for chronic fatigue syndrome. *British Journal of Psychiatry, 18,* 248–252.

Benyami, Y., Leventhal, E. A., & Leventhal, H. (2000). Gender differences in processing information for making self-assessments of health. *Psychosomatic Medicine, 62,* 354–364.

Berman, B. M., Ezzo, J., Hadhazy, V., & Swyers, J. P. (1999). Is acupuncture effective in the treatment of fibromyalgia? *Journal of Family Practice, 48,* 213–218.

Berman, S., Munakata, J., Naliboff, B. D., Chang, L., Mandelkern, M., Silverman, D., et al. (2000). Gender differences in regional brain response to visceral pressure in IBS patients. *European Journal of Pain, 4,* 157–172.

Bhagwagar, Z., Hafizi, S., & Cowen, P. J. (2005). Increased salivary cortisol after waking in depression. *Psychopharmacology, 182,* 54–57.

Bierl, C., Nisenbaum, R., Hoaglin, D. C., Randall, B., Jones, A. B., Unger, E. R., et al. (2004). Regional distribution of fatiguing illnesses in the United States: A pilot study. *Population Health Metrics, 2,* 1–5.

Binder, L. M., & Campbell, K. A. (2004). Medically unexplained symptoms and neuropsychological assessment. *Journal of Clinical and Experimental Neuropsychology, 26,* 369–392.

Black, D. W. (2000). The relationship of mental disorders and idiopathic environmental intolerance. *Occupational Medicine, 15,* 557–570.

Black, D. W., Okiishi, C., & Schlosser, S. (2001). The Iowa follow-up of chemically sensitive persons. In B. A. Sorg & I. R. Bell (Eds.), *Annals of the New York Academy of Sciences: Vol. 933. The role of neural plasticity in chemical intolerance* (pp. 48–56). New York: New York Academy of Sciences.

Blakely, A. A., Howard, R. C., Sosich, R. M., Murdoch, J. C., Menkes, D. B., & Spears, G. F. S. (1991). Psychiatric symptoms, personality and ways of coping in chronic fatigue syndrome. *Psychological Medicine, 21,* 347–362.

Blanchard, E., Keefer, L., Galovski, T. E., Taylor, A. E., & Turner, S. M. (2001). Gender differences in psychological distress among patients with irritable bowel syndrome. *Journal of Psychosomatic Research, 50,* 271–275.

Blanchard, E., Keefer, L., Lackner, J., Galovski, T., Krasner, S., & Sykes, M. (2004). The role of childhood abuse in Axis I and Axis II psychiatric disorders and medical disorders of unknown origin among irritable bowel syndrome patients. *Journal of Psychosomatic Research, 56*, 431–436.

Blanchard, E., Schwarz, S. P., & Neff, D. (1988). Two-year follow-up of behavioral treatment of irritable bowel syndrome. *Behavior Therapy, 19*, 67–73.

Bleijenberg, G., Prins, J., & Bazelmans, E. (2003). Cognitive behavioral therapies. In L. A. Jason, P. A. Fennell, & R. R. Taylor (Eds.), *Handbook of chronic fatigue syndrome* (493–526). New York: Wiley.

Blondel-Hill, E., & Shafran, S. D. (1993). Treatment of the chronic fatigue syndrome. *Drugs, 46*, 639–651.

Blunt, K. L., Rajwani, M. H., & Guerriero, R. C. (1997). The effectiveness of chiropractic management of fibromyalgia patients: A pilot study. *Journal of Manipulative and Physiological Therapeutics, 20*, 389–399.

Boissevain, M. D., & McCain, G. A. (1991a). Toward an integrated understanding of fibromyalgia: I. Medical and pathophysiological aspects, *Pain, 45*, 227–238.

Boissevain, M. D., & McCain, G. A. (1991b). Toward an integrated understanding of fibromyalgia: II. Psychological and phenomenological aspects. *Pain, 45*, 239–248.

Bolla-Wilson, K., Wilson, R. J., & Bleeker, M. L. (1988). Conditioning of physical symptoms after neurotoxic exposure. *Journal of Occupational Medicine, 30*, 684–686.

Bombardier, C. H., & Buchwald, D. (1995). Outcome and prognosis of patients with chronic fatigue versus chronic fatigue syndrome. *Archives of Internal Medicine, 155*, 2105–2110.

Bonner, D., Ron, M., Chalder, T., Butler, S., & Wessely, S. (1994). Chronic fatigue syndrome: A follow up study. *Journal of Neurology, Neurosurgery, and Psychiatry, 57*, 617–621.

Borglin, G., Jakobsson, U., Edberg, A. K., & Hallberg, I. R. (2005). Self-reported health complaints and their prediction of overall and health-related quality of life among elderly people. *International Journal of Nursing Studies, 42*, 147–158.

Bornschein, S., Hausteiner, C., Konrad, F., Forstl, H., & Zilker, T. (2006). Psychiatric morbidity and toxic burden in patients with environmental illness: A controlled study. *Psychosomatic Medicine, 68*, 104–109.

Bose, M., & Farthing, M. J. G. (2001). Irritable bowel syndrome: New horizons on the path of physiology and treatment. *British Journal of Surgery, 88*, 1425–1426.

Boyce, P., Gilchrist, J., Talley, N. J., & Rose, D. (2000). Cognitive–behaviour therapy as a treatment for irritable bowel syndrome: A pilot study. *Australian and New Zealand Journal of Psychiatry, 34*, 300–309.

Boyce, P. M., Talley, N. J., Balaam, B., Koloski, N. A., & Truman, G. (2003). A randomized controlled trial of cognitive behavior therapy, relaxation training, and routine clinical care for the irritable bowel syndrome. *American Journal of Gastroenterology, 98*, 2209–2218.

Brandt, L. J., Bjorkman, D., Fennert, M. B., Locke, G. R., Olden, K., Peterson, W., et al. (2002). Systematic review on the management of irritable bowel syndrome in North America. *American Journal of Gastroenterology, 97*(Suppl.), S7–S26.

Bremner, J. D. (2005). Effects of traumatic stress on brain structure and function: Relevance to early responses to trauma. *Journal of Trauma and Dissociation, 6,* 51–68.

Bremner, J. D., Randall, P., Vermetten, E., Staib, L., Bronen, R., Mazure, C., et al. (1997). Magnetic resonance imaging–based measurement of hippocampal volume in posttraumatic stress disorder related to childhood physical and sexual abuse—A preliminary report. *Biological Psychiatry, 41,* 23–32.

Bremner, J. D., Vermetten, E., Vythilingam, M., Afzal, N., Schmahl, C., Elzinga, B., & Charney, D. (2003). Neural correlates of the classic color and emotional Stroop in women with abuse-related posttraumatic stress disorder. *Biological Psychiatry, 55,* 612–620.

Bremner, J. D., Vythilingam, M., Vermetten, E., Southwick, S., McGlashan, T., Nazeer, A., et al. (2003). MRI and PET study of deficits in hippocampal structure and function in women with childhood sexual abuse and posttraumatic stress disorder. *American Journal of Psychiatry, 160,* 924–932.

Bremner, J. D., Vythilingam, M., Vermetten, E., Southwick, S., McGlashan, T., Staib, L., et al. (2003). Neural correlates of declarative memory for emotionally valenced words in women with posttraumatic stress disorder related to early childhood sexual abuse. *Biological Psychiatry, 53,* 879–889.

Breuer, J., & Freud, S. (1987). *Studies on hysteria* (J. Strachey, Ed. & Trans.). New York: Basic Books. (Original work published 1895)

Brewin, C. (2005). Systematic review of screening instruments for adults at risk of PTSD. *Journal of Traumatic Stress, 18,* 53–62.

Broderick, J. E., Junghaenel, D. U., & Schwartz, J. E. (2005). Written emotional expression produces health benefits in fibromyalgia. *Psychosomatic Medicine, 67,* 326–334.

Brosschot, J. F., & Aarsse, H. R. (2001). Restricted emotional processing and somatic attribution in fibromyalgia. *International Journal of Psychiatry in Medicine, 31,* 127–146.

Buchwald, D. P. R., Cheney, P. I., Peterson, B., Henry, B., Wormsley, S. B., Geiger, A. A., et al. (1992). A chronic illness characterized by fatigue, neurologic and immunologic disorders, and active herpesvirus Type 6 infection. *Annals of Internal Medicine, 116,* 103–113.

Buchwald, D., & Garrity, D. (1994). Comparison of patients with chronic fatigue syndrome, fibromyalgia, and multiple chemical sensitivity. *Archives of Internal Medicine, 154,* 2049–2053.

Buchwald, D., Goldenberg, D. L., Sullivan, J. L., & Komaroff, A. L. (1987). The chronic, active Epstein–Barr virus infection syndrome and primary fibromyalgia. *Arthritis and Rheumatism, 30,* 1132–1136.

Buchwald, D., Pearlman, T., Kith, P., & Schmaling, K. (1994). Gender differences in patients with chronic fatigue syndrome. *Journal of General Internal Medicine, 9,* 397–401.

Buchwald, D., Pearlman, T., Umali, J., Schmaling, K., & Katon, W. (1996). Functional status in patients with chronic fatigue syndrome, other fatiguing illnesses, and healthy individuals. *American Journal of Medicine, 101*, 364–370.

Buckley, L., MacHale, S. M., Cavanagh, J. T. O., Sharpe, M., Deary, I. J., & Lawrie, S. M. (1999). Personality dimensions in chronic fatigue syndrome and depression. *Journal of Psychosomatic Research, 46*, 395–400.

Burckhardt, C. S., & Bjelle, A. (1994). Education programmes for fibromyalgia patients: Description and evaluation. *Baillière's Clinical Rheumatology, 8*, 935–955.

Burckhardt, C. S., & Bjelle, A. (1996). A comparison of women with fibromyalgia, rheumatoid arthritis, and systemic lupus erthematosus. *Scandinavian Journal of Rheumatology, 25*, 300–306.

Burckhardt, C. S., Mannerkorpi, K., Hedenberg, L., & Bjelle, A. (1994). A randomized, controlled clinical trial of education and physical training for women with fibromyalgia. *Journal of Rheumatology, 21*, 714–720.

Burke, H. M., Davis, M. C., Otte, C., & Mohr, D. C. (2005). Depression and cortisol responses to psychological stress: A meta-analysis. *Psychoneuroendocrinology, 30*, 846–856.

Busch, A., Schacter, C. L., Peloso, P. M., & Bombardier, C. (2002). Exercise for treating fibromyalgia syndrome. *Cochrane Database of Systematic Reviews, 3*, CD003786. Available from http://www.cochrane.org

Buskila, D., & Neuman, L. (2005). Genetics of fibromyalgia. *Current Pain and Headache Reports, 9*, 313–315.

Buskila, D., Neumann, L., Alhoashle, A., & Abu-Shakra, M. (2000). Fibromyalgia syndrome in men. *Seminars in Arthritis and Rheumatism, 30*, 47–51.

Butler, S., Chalder, T., Ron, M., & Wessely, S. (1991). Cognitive behavior therapy in the chronic fatigue syndrome. *Journal of Neurology, Neurosurgery, and Psychiatry, 54*, 153–158.

Caccappolo-van Vliet, E., Kelly-McNeil, K., Natelson, B., Kipen, H., & Fiedler, N. (2002). Anxiety sensitivity and depression in multiple chemical sensitivities and asthma. *Journal of Occupational and Environmental Medicine, 44*, 890–901.

Cairns, R., & Hotopf, M. (2005) A systematic review describing the prognosis of chronic fatigue syndrome. *Occupational Medicine, 55*, 20–31.

Camilleri, M. (2001). Review article: Tegaserod. *Alimentary Pharmacology & Therapeutics, 15*, 277–289.

Camilleri, M., Mayer, E., Drossman, D., Heath, A., Dukes, G. E., McSorley, D., et al. (1999). Improvement in pain and bowel function in female irritable bowel syndrome patients with alosetron, a 5HT3 receptor antagonist. *Alimentary Pharmacology & Therapeutics, 13*, 1149–1159.

Campbell, R. S., & Pennebaker, J. W. (2003). The secret life of pronouns: Flexibility in writing style and physical health. *Psychological Science, 14*, 60–65.

Campbell, S. M., Clark, S., Tindall, E. A., Forehand, M. E., & Bennett, R. M. (1983). Clinical characteristics of fibrositis: I. A "blinded" controlled study of symptoms and tender points. *Arthritis and Rheumatism, 26*, 817–824.

Cannon, J. G., & St. Pierre, B. A. (1997). Gender differences in host defense mechanisms. *Journal of Psychiatric Research, 31*, 99–113.

Caress, S. M., & Steinemann, A. C. (2003). A review of a two-phase population study of multiple chemical sensitivities. *Environmental Health Perspectives, 111*, 1490–1497.

Caress, S. M., & Steinemann, A. C. (2004a). A national population study of the prevalence of multiple chemical sensitivity. *Archives of Environmental Health, 59*, 300–305.

Caress, S. M., & Steinemann, A. C. (2004b). Prevalence of multiple chemical sensitivities: A population-based study in the southeastern United States. *American Journal of Public Health, 94*, 746–747.

Carrico, A. W., Jason, L. A., Torres-Harding, S. R., & Witter, E. A. (2004). Disability in chronic fatigue syndrome and idiopathic chronic fatigue. *Review of Disability Studies, 1*, 79–88.

Carrion, V., Weems, C., Eliez, S., Patwardhan, A., Brown, W., Ray, R., & Reiss, A. (2001). Attenuation of frontal asymmetry in pediatric posttraumatic stress disorder. *Biological Psychiatry, 50*, 943–951.

Caseras, X., Mataix-Cols, D., Giampetro, V., Rimes, K. A., Brammer, M., Zolyaya, F., et al. (2006). Probing the working memory system in chronic fatigue syndrome: A functional magnetic resonance imaging study using the n-back task. *Psychosomatic Medicine, 68*, 947–955.

Cately, D., Kaell, A., Kirschbaum, C., & Stone, A. (2000). A naturalistic evaluation of cortisol secretion in persons with fibromyalgia and rheumatoid arthritis. *Arthritis Care and Research, 13*, 51–61.

Cathebras, P. J., Robbins, J. M., Kirmayer, L. J., & Hayton, B. C. (1992). Fatigue in primary care: Prevalence, psychiatric comorbidity, illness behavior, and outcome. *Journal of General Internal Medicine, 7*, 276–286.

Celentano, D. D., Linet, M. S., & Stewart, W. F. (1990). Gender differences in the experience of headache. *Social Science & Medicine, 30*, 1289–1295.

Chang, L., Berman, S., Mayer, E. A., Suyenobu, B., Derbyshire, S., Naliboff, B., et al. (2003). Brain responses to visceral and somatic stimuli in patients with irritable bowel syndrome with and without fibromyalgia. *American Journal of Gastroenterology, 98*, 1354–1361.

Chang, L., & Heitkemper, M. M. (2003). Gender differences in irritable bowel syndrome. *Gastroenterology, 123*, 1686–1701.

Chase, T. N., Shoulson, I., & Carter, A. C. (1976). Serotonergic functions in man. *Monographs in Neural Science, 3*, 8–14.

Chaudhuri, A., & Behan, P. O. (2000). Fatigue and basal ganglia. *Journal of Neurological Sciences, 179*, 34–42.

Chen, M. (1986). The epidemiology of self-perceived fatigue among adults. *Preventive Medicine, 15*, 74–81.

Chesterton, L. S., Barlas, P., Foster, N. E., Baxter, G. D., & Wright, C. C. (2002). Gender differences in pressure pain threshold in healthy humans. *Pain, 101*, 259–266.

Chircop, A., & Keddy, B. (2003). Women living with environmental illness. *Health Care for Women International, 24*, 371–383.

Chrisler, J. C., & O'Hea, E. L. (2000). Gender, culture, and autoimmune disorders. In R. M. Eisler (Ed.), *Handbook of gender, culture, and health* (pp. 321–342). Mahwah, NJ: Erlbaum.

Christodoulou, C., DeLuca, J., Lange, G., Johnson, S. K., Sisto, S. A., Korn, L., & Natelson, B. H. (1998). Relation between neuropsychological impairment and functional disability in patients with chronic fatigue syndrome. *Journal of Neurology, Neurosurgery, and Psychiatry, 64*, 431–434.

Ciccone, D. S., Busichio, K., Vickroy, M., & Natelson, B. H. (2003). Psychiatric morbidity in the chronic fatigue syndrome: Are patients with personality disorder more physically impaired? *Journal of Psychosomatic Research, 54*, 445–452.

Ciccone, D. S., Elliott, D. K., Chandler, H. K., Nayak, S., & Raphael, K. G. (2005). Sexual and physical abuse in women with fibromyalgia syndrome: A test of the trauma hypothesis. *Clinical Journal of Pain, 21*, 378–386.

Ciccone, D. S., & Natelson, B. (2003). Comorbid illness in women with chronic fatigue syndrome: A test of the single syndrome hypothesis. *Psychosomatic Medicine, 65*, 268–275.

Clark, J. N. (1999). Chronic fatigue syndrome: Gender differences in the search for legitimacy. *Australian and New Zealand Journal of Mental Health Nursing, 8*, 123–133.

Clark, M. R., Katon, W., Russo, J., Kith, P., Sintay, M., & Buchwald, D (1995). Chronic fatigue: Risk factors for symptom persistence in a 2 1/2-year follow-up study. *American Journal of Medicine, 98*, 187–195.

Clauw, D. J. (1994). The pathogenesis of chronic pain and fatigue syndromes with special reference to fibromyalgia. *Medical Hypotheses, 44*, 369–378.

Clauw, D. J. (2001). Potential mechanisms in chemical intolerance and related conditions. In B. A. Sorg & I. R. Bell (Eds.), *Annals of the New York Academy of Sciences: Vol. 933. The role of neural plasticity in chemical intolerance* (pp. 235–253). New York: New York Academy of Sciences.

Clauw, D. J., & Chrousos, G. P. (1997). Chronic pain and fatigue syndromes: Overlapping clinical and neuroendocrine features and potential pathogenic mechanisms. *Neuroimmunomodulation, 4*, 134–153.

Clauw, D. J., & Crofford, L. J. (2003). Chronic widespread pain and fibromyalgia: What we know, and what we need to know. *Best Practice & Research. Clinical Rheumatology, 17*, 685–701.

Cleare, A. J. (2003). The neuroendocrinology of chronic fatigue syndrome. *Endocrine Reviews, 24*, 236–252.

Cleare, A. (2004). Stress and fibromyalgia: What is the link? *Journal of Psychosomatic Research, 57*, 423–425.

Cleare, A. J., Bearn, J., McGregor, A., Allain, T., Wessely, S., Murray, R. M., & O'Kane, V. O. (1995). Contrasting neuroendocrine responses in depression and chronic fatigue syndrome. *Journal of Affective Disorders, 35*, 283–289.

Cleare, A. J., Heap, E., Malhi, G. S., Wessely, S., O'Keane, V., & Miell, J. (1999). Low-dose hydrocortisone in chronic fatigue syndrome: A randomized crossover trial. *The Lancet, 353*, 455–458.

Cleare, A. J., Miell, J., Heap, S., Sookdeo, L., Malhi, G. S., & O'Keane, V. (2001). Hypothalamo–pituitary–adrenal axis dysfunction in chronic fatigue syndrome, and the effects of low-dose hydrocortisone therapy. *Journal of Clinical Endocrinology and Metabolism, 86*, 3545–3554.

Cloninger, C. R. (1987). *The Tridimensional Personality Questionnaire, Version IV*. St. Louis, MO: Department of Psychiatry, Washington University School of Medicine.

Cloninger, C. R., Martin, R. L., Guze, S. B., & Clayton, P. J. (1986). A prospective follow-up and family study of somatization in men and women. *American Journal of Psychiatry, 143*, 873–878.

Clouse, R. E., & Lustman, P. J. (2005). Use of pharmacological agents for functional gastrointestinal disorders. *Gut, 54*, 1332–1341.

Comer, R. J. (2005). *Stress disorders. Fundamentals of abnormal psychology* (4th ed.). New York: Worth.

Cook, D. B., Lange, G., DeLuca, J., & Natelson, B. H. (2001). Relationship of brain MRI abnormalities and physical functional status in CFS. *International Journal of Neuroscience, 107*, 1–6.

Cook, I. J., van Eeden, A., & Collins, S. M. (1987). Patients with irritable bowel syndrome have greater pain tolerance than normal subjects. *Gastroenterology, 93*, 727–733.

Cope, H. (1992). Fatigue: A non-specific complaint? *International Review of Psychiatry, 4*, 273–280.

Cope, H., Mann, A., Pelosi, A., & David, A. (1996). Psychosocial risk factors for chronic fatigue and chronic fatigue syndrome following presumed viral illness: A case-control study. *Psychological Medicine, 26*, 1197–1209.

Cope, H., Pernet, A., Kendall, B., & Davis, A. (1995). Cognitive functioning and magnetic resonance imaging in chronic fatigue syndrome. *British Journal of Psychiatry, 167*, 86–94.

Costa, D. C., Tannock, C., & Brostoff, J. (1995). Brainstem profusion is impaired in chronic fatigue syndrome. *Quarterly Journal of Medicine, 88*, 767–773.

Costa, P. T., & McCrae, R. R. (1987). Neuroticism, somatic complaints and disease: Is the bark worse than the bite? *Journal of Personality, 55*, 299–316.

Costa, P. T., & McCrae, R. R. (1992). *Revised NEO Personality Inventory (NEO-PI-R) and NEO Five Factor Personality Inventory (NEO-FFI) professional manual*. Odessa, FL: Psychological Assessment Resources.

Costa, P. T., Terracciano, A., & McCrae, R. R. (2001). Gender differences in personality traits across cultures: Robust and surprising findings. *Journal of Personality and Social Psychology, 81*, 322–331.

Cox, D. L., & Findley, L. J. (2000). Severe and very severe patients with chronic fatigue syndrome: Perceived outcome following an inpatient programme. *Journal of Chronic Fatigue Syndrome, 7*(3), 33–47.

Crane, C., & Martin, M. (2004). Risk perception in individuals with irritable bowel syndrome: Perceived susceptibility to health and non-health threats. *Journal of Social and Clinical Psychology, 23*, 219–239.

Creed, F., & Barsky, A. (2004). A systematic review of the epidemiology of somatisation disorder and hypochondriasis. *Journal of Psychosomatic Research, 56*, 391–408.

Creed, F., Fernandes, L., Guthrie, E., Palmer, S., Ratcliffe, J., Read, N., et al. (2003). The cost-effectiveness of psychotherapy and paroxetine for severe irritable bowel syndrome. *Gastroenterology, 124*, 303–317.

Creed, F., Guthrie, E., Ratcliffe, J., Fernandes, L., Rigby, C., Tomenson, B., et al. (2005). Reported sexual abuse predicts impaired functioning but a good response to psychological treatments in patients with severe irritable bowel syndrome. *Psychosomatic Medicine, 67*, 490–499.

Creed, F., Ratcliffe, J., Fernandes, L., Palmer, S., Rigby, C., Tomenson, B., et al. (2005). Outcome in severe irritable bowel syndrome with and without accompanying depressive, panic and neurasthenic disorders. *British Journal of Psychiatry, 186*, 507–515.

Creswell, C., & Chalder, T. (2001). Defensive coping styles in chronic fatigue syndrome. *Journal of Psychosomatic Research, 51*, 607–610.

Creswell, C., & Chalder, T. (2002). Underlying self-esteem in chronic fatigue syndrome. *Journal of Psychosomatic Research, 53*, 755–761.

Crofford, L. J., Young, E. A., Engleberg, N. C., Korszun, A., Brucksch, C. B., McClure, L. A., et al. (2004). Basal circadian and pulsatile ACTH and cortisol secretion in patients with fibromyalgia and/or chronic fatigue syndrome. *Brain, Behavior, and Immunity, 18*, 314–325.

Crombez, G., Van Damme, S. V., & Eccleston, C. (2005). Hypervigilance to pain: An experimental and clinical analysis. *Pain, 116*, 4–7.

Cullen, M. R. (1987). The worker with chemical sensitivity: A overview. In M. R. Cullen (Ed.), *Occupational medicine: State of the art reviews* (Vol. 2, pp. 655–662). Philadelphia: Hanley & Belfus.

DaCosta, J. M. (1871). On irritable heart: A clinical study of a form of functional cardiac disorder and its consequences. *American Journal of Medical Science, 61*, 17–52.

Dalton, P., Doolittle, N., & Breslin, P. A. (2002). Gender specific induction of enhanced sensitivity to odors. *Nature Neuroscience, 5*, 199–200.

D'Amato, M. Labum, R. V., & Whorwell, P. J. (1999). The CCKa receptor antagonist dexloxiglumide in the treatment of IBS. *Gastroenterology, 116*, A981.

Dancey, C. P., Hutton-Young, S. A., Moye, S., & Devins, G. M. (2002). Perceived stigma, illness intrusiveness and quality of life in men and women with irritable bowel syndrome. *Psychology, Health & Medicine, 7*, 382–395.

Daun, J. M., Ball, R. W., & Cannon, J. G. (2000). Glucocorticoid sensitivity of interleukin-1 agonist and antagonist secretion: The effects of age and gender. *American Journal of Physiology: Regulatory Integrative and Comparative Physiology, 278*, R855–R862.

Davis, M. C., Matthews, K. A., & Twamley, E. W. (1999). Is life more difficult on Mars or Venus? A meta-analytic review of sex differences in major and minor life events. *Annals of Behavioral Medicine, 21,* 83–97.

Davis, M. C., Zautra, A. J., & Reich, J. W. (2001). Vulnerability to stress among women in chronic pain from fibromyalgia and osteoarthritis. *Annals of Behavioral Medicine, 23,* 215–226.

Davis, M. C., Zautra, A. J., & Smith, B. W. (2004). Chronic pain, stress, and the dynamics of affective differentiation. *Journal of Personality, 72,* 1133–1159.

Deale, A., Chalder, T., Marks, I., & Wessely, S. (1997). Cognitive behavior therapy for chronic fatigue syndrome: A randomized controlled trial. *American Journal of Psychiatry, 154,* 408–414.

Deale, A., Kaneez, H., Chalder, T., & Wessely, S. (2001). Long-term outcome of cognitive behavior therapy versus relaxation therapy for chronic fatigue syndrome: A 5-year follow-up study. *American Journal of Psychiatry, 158,* 2038–2042.

Deary, I. J. (1999). A taxonomy of medically unexplained symptoms. *Journal of Psychosomatic Research, 47,* 51–59.

De Bellis, M., Keshavan, M., Clark, D., Casey, B. J., Giedd, J., Boring, A., et al. (1999). Developmental traumatology: Part II. Brain development. *Biological Psychiatry, 45,* 1271–1284.

De Leeuw, R., Albuquerque, R. J., Anderson, A. H., & Carlson, C. R. (2006). Influence of estrogen on brain activation during stimulation with painful heat. *Journal of Oral Maxillofacial Surgery, 64,* 158–166.

DeLuca, J. (2005). *Fatigue as a window to the brain.* Cambridge, MA: MIT Press.

DeLuca, J., Christodoulou, C., Diamond, B. J., Rosenstein, E. D., Kramer, N., & Natelson, B. H. (2004). Working memory deficits in chronic fatigue syndrome: Differentiating between speed and accuracy of information processing. *Journal of the International Neuropsychological Society, 10,* 101–119.

DeLuca, J., Johnson, S. K., Ellis, S. P., & Natelson, B. H. (1997). Cognitive functioning is impaired in patients with chronic fatigue syndrome devoid of psychiatric disease. *Journal of Neurology, Neurosurgery, and Psychiatry, 62,* 151–155.

DeLuca, J., Johnson, S. K., & Natelson, B. H. (1997). Sudden versus gradual onset of chronic fatigue syndrome differentiates individuals on cognitive and psychiatric measures. *Journal of Psychiatric Research, 31,* 81–90.

Demitrack, M. A., Dale, J. K., Straus, S. E., Laue, L., Listwak, S. J., Kruesi, M. J. P., et al. (1991). Evidence for the impaired activation of the hypothalamic–pituitary–adrenal axis in patients with chronic fatigue syndrome. *Journal of Clinical Endocrinology and Metabolism, 73,* 1–11.

Dendy, C., Cooper, M., & Sharpe, M. (2001). Interpretation of symptoms in chronic fatigue syndrome. *Behavior Research & Therapy, 39,* 1369–1380.

Dessein, P. H., Shipton, E. A., Stanwix, A. E., & Joffe, B. I. (2000). Neuroendocrine deficiency-mediated development and persistence of pain in fibromyalgia: A promising paradigm? *Pain, 86,* 213–215.

Diseth, T. H. (2005). Dissociation in children and adolescents as reaction to trauma— An overview of conceptual issues and neurobiological factors. *Nordic Journal of Psychiatry, 59*, 79–91.

Donnay, A., & Ziem, G. (1995). *Chemical injury and disorders of porphyrin metabolism: Protocol for diagnosing disorders of porphyrin metabolism in chemically sensitive patients.* Baltimore, MD: MCS Referral and Resources.

Drossman, D. A. (1998). Presidential address: Gastrointestinal illness and the biopsychosocial model. *Psychosomatic Medicine, 60*, 258–267.

Drossman, D. A. (1999). Do psychosocial factors define symptom severity and patient status in irritable bowel syndrome? *American Journal of Medicine, 107*(5A), 41S–50S.

Drossman, D. A., Camilleri, M., Mayer, E. A., & Whitehead, W. E. (2002). AGA technical review on irritable bowel syndrome. *Gastroenterology, 123,* 2108–2131.

Drossman, D. A., Corazziari, E., Talley, N. J., Thompson, W. G., & Whitehead, W. E. (Eds.). (2000). *Rome II: The functional gastrointestinal disorders.* McLean, VA: Degnon Associates.

Drossman, D. A., Leserman, J., Li, Z., Keefe, F., Hu, Y. J. B., & Toomey, T. C. (2000). Effects of coping on health outcome among women with gastrointestinal disorders. *Psychosomatic Medicine, 62,* 309–317.

Drossman, D. A., Leserman, J., Nachman, G., Zhiming, L., Gluck, H., Toomey, T., & Mitchell, M. (1990). Sexual and physical abuse in women with functional or organic gastrointestinal disorders. *Annals of Internal Medicine, 113,* 828–833.

Drossman, D. A., Li, Z., Leserman, J., Toomey, T. C., & Hu, Y. J. B. (1996). Health status by gastrointestinal diagnosis and abuse history. *Gastroenterology, 110,* 999–1007.

Drossman, D. A., McKee, D. C., Sandler, R. S., Mitchell, C. M., Cramer, E. M., Lowman, B. C., & Burger, A. L. (1988). Psychosocial factors in the irritable bowel syndrome: A multivariate study of patients and nonpatients with irritable bowel syndrome. *Gastroenterology, 95,* 709–714.

Drossman, D. A., Sandler, R. S., McKee, D. C., & Lovitz, A. J. (1982). Bowel patterns among subjects not seeking health care: Use of a questionnaire to identify a population with bowel dysfunction. *Gastroenterology, 83,* 529–534.

Drossman, D. A., Talley, N. J., Leserman, J., Olden, K. W., & Barreiro, M. A. (1995). Sexual and physical abuse and gastrointestinal illness: Review and recommendations. *Annals of Internal Medicine, 123,* 782–794.

Drossman, D. A., Toner, B. B., Whitehead, W. E., Diamant, D. E., Dalton, C. B., Duncan, S., et al. (2003). Cognitive–behavioral therapy versus education and desipramine versus placebo for moderate to severe functional bowel disorders. *Gastroenterology, 125,* 19–31.

Dumit, J. (2006). Illnesses you have to fight to get: Facts as forces in uncertain, emergent illnesses. *Social Science & Medicine, 62,* 577–590.

Dunne, F. J., & Dunne, C. A. (1995). Fibromyalgia syndrome and psychiatric disorder. *British Journal of Hospital Medicine, 54,* 194–197.

Dzurec, L. C. (2000). Fatigue and relatedness experiences of inordinately tired women. *Journal of Nursing Scholarship, 32*, 339–345.

Dzurec, L. C., Hoover, P. M., & Fields, J. (2002). Acknowledging unexplained fatigue of tired women. *Journal of Nursing Scholarship, 34*, 41.

Efskind, P. S., Bernklev, T., & Vatn, M. H. (1996). A double-blind placebo controlled trial with loperamide in irritable bowel syndrome. *Scandinavian Journal of Gastroenterology, 31*, 463–468.

Else-Quest, N. M., Shibley Hyde, J., Hill Goldsmith, H., & Van Hulle, C. (2006). Gender differences in temperament: A meta-analysis. *Psychological Bulletin, 132*, 33–72.

El-Serag, H. B., Olden, K., & Bjorkman, D. (2002). Health-related quality of life among persons with irritable bowel syndrome: A systematic review. *Alimentary Pharmacology & Therapy, 16*, 1171–1185.

Emmanuel, A. V., Mason, H. J., & Kamm, M. A. (2001). Relationship between psychological state and level of activity of extrinsic gut innervation in patients with a functional gut disorder. *Gut, 49*, 209–213.

Engel, G. (1977, April 8). The need for a new medical model: A challenge for biomedicine. *Science, 196*, 129–136.

Ennis, M., Kelly, K. S., & Lambert, P. L. (2001). Sex differences in cortisol excretion during anticipation of a psychological stressor: Possible support for the tend-and-befriend hypothesis. *Stress and Health, 17*, 253–261.

Epstein, R. M., Shields, C. G., Meldrum, S. C., Fiscella, K., Carroll, J., Carney, P. A., & Duberstein, P. R. (2006). Physicians' responses to patients' medically unexplained symptoms. *Psychosomatic Medicine, 68*, 269–276.

Epstein, S. A., Kay, G., Clauw, D., Heaton, R., Klein, D., Krupp, L., et al. (1999). Psychiatric disorders in patients with fibromyalgia: A multicenter investigation. *Psychosomatics, 40*, 57–63.

Eriksen, H. R., Hellesnes, B., Staff, P., & Ursin, H. (2004). Are subjective health complaints a result of modern civilization? *International Journal of Behavioral Medicine, 11*, 122–125.

Eriksen, H. R., & Ursin, H. (2004). Subjective health complaints, sensitization, and sustained cognitive activation (stress). *Journal of Psychosomatic Research, 56*, 445–448.

Escobar, J. I., Burnam, M. A., Karno, M., Forsythe, A., & Golding, J. M. (1987). Somatization in the community. *Archives of General Psychiatry, 44*, 713–718.

Escobar, J. I., Waitzkin, H., Silver, R. C., Gara, M., & Holman, A. (1998). Abridged somatization: A study in primary care. *Psychosomatic Medicine, 60*, 466–472.

Evans, D. L., Charney, D. S., Lewis, L., Golden, R. N., Gorman, J. M., Krishnan, K. R., et al. (2005). Mood disorders in the medically ill: Review and recommendations. *Biological Psychiatry, 58*, 175–189.

Evcik, D., Kizilay, B., & Gokcen, E. (2002). The effects of balneotherapy on fibromyalgia patients. *Rheumatology International, 22*, 56–59.

Evengard, B., Jacks, A., Pedersen, N. L., & Sullivan, P. F. (2005). The epidemiology of chronic fatigue in the Swedish Twin Registry. *Psychological Medicine, 35*, 1317–1326.

Fang, H., Xie, Q., Boneva, R., Fostel, J., Perkins, R., & Tong, W. (2006). Gene expression profile exploration of a large dataset on chronic fatigue syndrome. *Pharmacogenomics, 7*, 429–440.

Feinstein, A. R. (2001). The Blame-X syndrome: Problems and lessons in nosology, spectrum, and etiology. *Journal of Clinical Epidemiology, 54*, 433–439.

Fiddler, M., Jackson, J., Kapur, N., Wells, A., & Creed, F. (2004). Childhood adversity and frequent medical consultations. *General Hospital Psychiatry, 26*, 367–377.

Fiedler, N. (1996). An overview of the symptoms of multiple chemical sensitivities. *New Jersey Medicine, 93*, 39–43.

Fiedler, N. (2000). Controlled human exposure to methyl tertiary butyl ether in gasoline: Symptoms, psychophysiologic and neurobehavioral responses of self-reported sensitive persons. *Environmental Health Perspectives, 108*, 753–763.

Fiedler, N., Giardino, N., Natelson, B., Ottenweller, J., Weisel, C., Lioy, P., et al. (2004). Responses to controlled diesel vapor exposure among chemically sensitive Gulf War veterans. *Psychosomatic Medicine, 66*, 588–598.

Fiedler, N., & Kipen, H. (1997). Chemical sensitivity: The scientific literature. *Environmental Health Perspectives, 105*(Suppl. 2), 409–415.

Fiedler, N., & Kipen, H. (2001). Controlled exposures to volatile organic compounds in sensitive groups. In B. A. Sorg & I. R. Bell (Eds.), *Annals of the New York Academy of Sciences: Vol. 933. The role of neural plasticity in chemical intolerance* (pp. 24–37). New York: New York Academy of Sciences.

Fiedler, N., Kipen, H., DeLuca, J., Kelly-McNeil, K., & Natelson, B. (1996). A controlled comparison of multiple chemical sensitivities and chronic fatigue syndrome. *Psychosomatic Medicine, 58*, 38–49.

Fiedler, N., Lange, G., Tiersky, L., DeLuca, J., Policastro, T., Kelly-McNeil, K., et al. (2000). Stressors, personality traits, and coping of Gulf War veterans with chronic fatigue. *Journal of Psychosomatic Research, 48*, 525–535.

Fiedler, N., Maccia, C., & Kipen, H. (1992). Evaluation of chemically sensitive patients. *Journal of Medicine, 34*, 529–538.

Findlay, D. A., & Miller, L. J. (1994). Medical power and women's bodies. In B. S. Bolaria & R. Bolaria (Eds.), *Women, medicine and health* (pp. 115–139). Halifax, Nova Scotia, Canada: Fernwood.

Finestone, H., Stenn, P., Davies, F., Stalker, C., Fry, R., & Koumanis, J. (2000). Chronic pain and health care utilization in women with a history of childhood sexual abuse. *Child Abuse and Neglect, 24*, 547–556.

Fink, P. (1996). Somatization—Beyond symptom count. *Journal of Psychosomatic Research, 40*, 7–10.

Fink, P., Hansen, M., & Oxhoj, M. (2004). The prevalence of somatoform disorders among internal medical inpatients. *Journal of Psychosomatic Research, 56*, 413–418.

Fink, P., Rosendal, M., & Toft, T. (2002). Assessment and treatment of functional disorders in general practice: The extended reattribution and management model—An advanced educational program for nonpsychiatric doctors. *Psychosomatics, 43*, 93–129.

Finkelhor, D. (1990). Early and long-term effects of child sexual abuse: An update. *Professional Psychology: Research and Practice, 21*, 325–330.

Floch, M. H., & Narayan, R. (2002). Diet in the irritable bowel syndrome. *Journal of Clinical Gastroenterology, 35*, 545–552.

Ford, C. V. (1997). Somatization and fashionable diagnoses: Illness as a way of life. *Scandinavian Journal of Work, Environment and Health, 23*, 7–16.

Fostel, J., Boneva, R., & Lloyd, A. (2006). Exploration of the gene expression correlates of chronic unexplained fatigue using factor analysis. *Pharmacogenomics, 7*, 441–454.

Frank, R., Chaney, J., Clay, D., Shutty, M. S., Beck, N. C., Kay, D. R., et al. (1992). Dysphoria: A major symptom factor in persons with disability or chronic illness. *Psychiatry Research, 43*, 231–241.

Frankenhaeuser, M., Lundberg, U., & Forsman, L. (1980). Dissociation between sympathetic-adrenal and pituitary-advanced responses to an achievement situation characterized by high controllability: Comparison between Type A and Type B males and females. *Biological Psychology, 10*, 79–91.

Friedberg, F., & Krupp, L. B. (1994). A comparison of cognitive behavioral treatment for chronic fatigue syndrome and primary depression. *Clinical Infectious Diseases, 18*(Suppl. 1), S105–S110.

Friedman, M. J. (1994). Neurobiological sensitization models of post-traumatic stress disorder: Their possible relevance to multiple chemical sensitivity syndrome. *Toxicology and Industrial Health, 10*, 449–462.

Fries, E., Hesse, J., Hellhammer, J., & Hellhammer, D. H. (2005). A new view on hypocortisolism. *Psychoneuroendocrinology, 10*, 1010–1016.

Fuhrer, R., & Wessely, S. (1995). The epidemiology of fatigue and depression: A French primary care study. *Psychological Medicine, 25*, 895–905.

Fukuda, K., Straus, S. E., Hickie, I., Sharpe, M. C., Dobbins, J. G., & Komaroff, A. (1994). The chronic fatigue syndrome: A comprehensive approach to its definition and study. International Chronic Fatigue Syndrome Study Group. *Annals of Internal Medicine, 121*, 953–959.

Fulcher, K. Y., & White, P. D. (1997). Randomised controlled trial of graded exercise in patients with the chronic fatigue syndrome. *British Medical Journal, 314*, 1647–1652.

Gaab, J., Huster, D., Peisen, R., Engret, V., Heitz, V., Schad, T., et al. (2000). Hypothalamic–pituitary–adrenal axis reactivity in chronic fatigue syndrome and health under psychological, physiological, and pharmacological stimulation. *Psychosomatic Medicine, 64*, 951–962.

Gaab, J., Huster, D., Peisen, R., Engret, V., Schad, T., Schurmeyer, & Ehlert, U. (2002). Low dose dexamethasone suppression test in chronic fatigue syndrome and health. *Psychosomatic Medicine, 64*, 311–318.

Galovski, T., & Blanchard, E. (1998). The treatment of irritable bowel syndrome with hypnotherapy. *Applied Psychophysiology and Biofeedback, 23,* 219–232.

Garrison, R. L., & Breeding, P. C. (2003). A metabolic basis for fibromyalgia and its related disorders: The possible role of resistance to thyroid hormone. *Medical Hypotheses, 61,* 182–189.

Gaston-Johansson, F., Gustafsson, M., Felldin, R., & Sanne, H. (1990). A comparative study of feelings, attitudes, and behaviors of patients with fibromyalgia and rheumatoid arthritis. *Social Science & Medicine, 31,* 941–947.

Geisser, M. E., Casey, K. L., Brucksch, C. B., Ribbens, C. M., Appleton, B. B., & Crofford, L. J. (2003). Perception of noxious and innocuous heat stimulation among healthy women and women with fibromyalgia: Association with mood, somatic focus, and catastrophizing. *Pain, 102,* 243–250.

Gershon, M. D. (1999). Endothelin and the development of the enteric nervous system. *Clinical and Experimental Pharmacology and Physiology, 26,* 985–988.

Gibson, P. R., Placek, E., Lane, J., Brohimer, S. O., & Lovelace, A. C. E. (2005). Disability-induced changes in persons with multiple chemical sensitivity. *Qualitative Health Research, 15,* 502–524.

Gijsbers van Wijk, C. M., & Kolk, A. M. (1997). Sex differences in physical symptoms: The contribution of symptom perception theory. *Social Science & Medicine, 45,* 231–246.

Gillespie, N. A., Zhu, G., Heath, A. C., Hickie, I. B., & Martin, N. G. (2000). The genetic aetiology of somatic distress. *Psychological Medicine, 30,* 1051–1061.

Glaser, R., & Kiecolt-Glaser, J. K. (1998). Stress-associated immune modulation: Relevance to viral infections and chronic fatigue syndrome. *American Journal of Medicine, 105,* 35S–42S.

Glaser, R., Padgett, D. A., Litsky, M. L., Baiocchi, R. A., Yang, E. V., & Chen, M. (2005). Stress-associated changes in the steady-state expression of latent Epstein–Barr virus: Implications for chronic fatigue syndrome and cancer. *Brain, Behavior, and Immunity, 19,* 91–103.

Gleason, O. C., & Yates, W. (2002) Somatoform disorders. In S. G. Kornstein & A. H. Clayton (Eds.), *Women's mental health: A comprehensive textbook* (pp. 307–322). New York: Guilford Press.

Goertzel, B. N., Pennachin, C., de Souza Coehlo, L., Gurbaxani, B., Maloney, E. M., & Jones, J. F. (2006). Combinations of single nucleotide polymorphism in neuroendocrine effector and receptor genes predict chronic fatigue syndrome. *Pharmacogenomics, 7,* 475–483.

Goertzel, B. N., Pennachin, C., de Souza Coelho, L., Maloney, E. M., Jones, J. F., & Gurbaxani, B. M. (2006). Allostatic load is associated with symptoms in chronic fatigue syndrome patients. *Pharmacogenomics, 7,* 485–494.

Goldberg, R. T., & Goldstein, R. (2000). A comparison of chronic pain patients and controls on traumatic events in childhood. *Disability and Rehabilitation, 22,* 756–763.

Goldberg, R. T., Pachas, W. N., & Keith, D. (1999). Relationship between traumatic events in childhood and chronic pain. *Disability and Rehabilitation, 21*, 23–30.

Goldenberg, D. L. (1989a). Fibromyalgia and its relation to chronic fatigue syndrome, viral illness and immune abnormalities. *Journal of Rheumatology, 16*, 91–93.

Goldenberg, D. L. (1989b). Psychological symptoms and psychiatric diagnosis in patients with fibromyalgia. *Journal of Rheumatology, 16*(Suppl. 19), 127–130.

Goldenberg, D. L. (1995). Fibromyalgia: Why such controversy? *Annals of the Rheumatic Diseases, 54*, 3–5.

Goldenberg, D. L. (1999). Fibromyalgia syndrome a decade later: What have we learned? *Archives of Internal Medicine, 159*, 77–85.

Goldenberg, D. L., Burckhardt, C., & Crofford, L. (2004). Management of fibromyalgia syndrome. *Journal of the American Medical Association, 292*, 2388–2395.

Goldenberg, D. L., Mayskiy, M., Mossey, C. J., Ruthazer, R., & Schmid, C. (1996). A randomized, double-blind crossover trial of fluoxetine and amitriptyline in the treatment of fibromyalgia. *Arthritis and Rheumatism, 39*, 1852–1859.

Gomez, R. L., Schvaneveldt, R. W., & Staudenmayer, H. (1996). Assessing beliefs about "environmental illness/multiple chemical sensitivity." *Journal of Health Psychology, 1*, 107–123.

Gonsalkorale, W. M., Houghton, L. A., & Whorwell, P. J. (2002). Hypnotherapy in irritable bowel syndrome: A large scale audit of a clinical service with examination of factors influencing responsiveness. *American Journal of Gastroenterology, 97*, 954–961.

Gonsalkorale, W. M., Miller, V., Afzal, A., & Whorwell, P. J. (2003). Long term benefits of hypnotherapy in irritable bowel syndrome. *Gut, 52*, 1623–1629.

Gonsalkorale, W. M., Toner, B. B., & Whorwell, P. J. (2004). Cognitive change in patients undergoing hypnotherapy for irritable bowel syndrome. *Journal of Psychosomatic Research, 56*, 271–278.

Goodnick, P. J., & Sandoval, R. (1993). Psychotropic treatment of chronic fatigue syndrome and related disorders. *Journal of Clinical Psychiatry, 54*, 13–20.

Goosens, M. E., Vlaeyen, J. W., Hidding, A., Kele-Snijders, A., & Evers, S. M. (2005). Treatment expectancy affects the outcome of cognitive-behavioral interventions in chronic pain. *Clinical Journal of Pain, 21*, 18–26.

Gowans, S. E., & deHueck, A. (2004). Effectiveness of exercise in management of fibromyalgia. *Current Opinions in Rheumatology, 16*, 138–142.

Gowans, S., deHueck, A., Voss, S., Salij, A., Abbey, S., & Reynolds, W. (2001). Effects of randomized, controlled trial of exercise on mood and physical function in individuals with fibromyalgia. *Journal of Arthritis Care and Research, 45*, 519–529.

Gowers, W. R. (1904). A lecture on lumbago: Its lessons and analogues. *British Medical Journal, 1*, 117–121.

Gracely, R. H., Geisser, M. E., Giesecke, T., Grant, M. A., Petzke, F., Williams, D. A., et al. (2004). Pain catastrophizing and neural responses to pain among persons with fibromyalgia. *Brain, 127,* 835–843.

Gralnek, I. M., Hays, R. D., Kilbourne, A., Naliboff, B., & Mayer, E. A. (2000). The impact of irritable bowel syndrome on health-related quality of life. *Gastroenterology, 119,* 654–660.

Gran, J. T. (2003). The epidemiology of chronic generalized musculoskeletal pain. *Best Practice & Research. Clinical Rheumatology, 17,* 547–561.

Granges, G., Zilko, P., & Littlejohn, G. (1994). Fibromyalgia syndrome: Assessment of the severity of the condition 2 years after diagnosis. *Journal of Rheumatology, 21,* 523–529.

Graveling, R. A., Pilkington, A., George, J. P. K., Butler, M. P., & Tannahill, S. N. (1999). A review of multiple chemical sensitivity. *Occupational Environmental Medicine, 56,* 73–85.

Gray, G. C., Reed, R. J., Kaiser, K. S., Smith, T. C., & Gastanaga, V. M. (2002). Self-reported symptoms and medical conditions among 11,868 Gulf War-era veterans: The Seabee Health Study. *American Journal of Epidemiology, 155,* 1033–1044.

Greco, A., Tannock, C., Brostoff, J., & Costa, D. (1997). Brain MR in chronic fatigue syndrome. *American Journal of Neuroradiology, 18,* 1265–1269.

Greenberg, D. B. (1990). Neurasthenia in the 1980's: Chronic mononucleosis, chronic fatigue syndrome, and anxiety and depressive disorders. *Psychosomatics, 31,* 129–137.

Greene, B., & Blanchard, E. B. (1994). Cognitive therapy for irritable bowel syndrome. *Journal of Consulting and Clinical Psychology, 62,* 576–582.

Gruber, A. J., Hudson, J. I., & Pope, H. G. (1996). The management of treatment-resistant depression in disorders on the interface of psychiatry and medicine: Fibromyalgia, chronic fatigue syndrome, migraine, irritable bowel syndrome, atypical facial pain, and premenstrual dysphoric disorder. *Psychiatric Clinics of North America, 19,* 351–369.

Guglielmi, R. S., Cox, D. J., & Spyker, D. A. (1994). Behavioral treatment of phobic avoidance in multiple chemical sensitivity. *Journal of Behavior Therapy and Experimental Psychiatry, 25,* 197–205.

Gupta, K., & Horne, R. (2001). The influence of health beliefs on the presentation and consultation outcome in patients with chemical sensitivities. *Journal of Psychosomatic Research, 50,* 131–137.

Gur, A., Cevik, R., Sarac, A. J., Colpan, L., & Em, S. (2004). Hypothalamic pituitary gonadal axis and cortisol in young women with primary fibromyalgia: The potential roles of depression, fatigue, and sleep disturbance in the occurrence of hypocortisolism. *Annals of Rheumatologic Disorders, 63,* 1504–1506.

Gureje, O. (2004). What can we learn from a cross-national study of somatic distress? *Journal of Psychosomatic Research, 56,* 409–412.

Guthrie, E., Creed, F., Dawson, D., & Tomenson, B. (1993). A randomised controlled trial of psychotherapy in patients with refractory irritable bowel syndrome. *British Journal of Psychiatry, 163*, 315–321.

Guthrie, E., Creed, F., Fernandes, L., Ratcliffe, J., Van Der Jagt, J., Martin, J., et al. (2003). Cluster analysis of symptoms and health seeking behaviour differentiates subgroups of patients with severe irritable bowel syndrom. *Gut, 52*, 1616–1622.

Guze, S. B. (1975). The validity and significance of the clinical diagnosis of hysteria (Briquet's syndrome). *American Journal of Psychiatry, 132*, 138–141.

Guze, S. B., Cloninger, R. C., Martin, R. L., & Clayton, P. J. (1986). A follow up and family study of Briquet's syndrome. *British Journal of Psychiatry, 149*, 17–23.

Guze, S. B., Woodruff, R. A., & Clayton, P. J. (1971). Hysteria and antisocial behavior: Further evidence of an association. *American Journal of Psychiatry, 127*, 957–960.

Gwee, K. A., Leong, Y. L., Graham, C., McKendrick, M. W., Collins, S. M., Walters, S. J., et al. (1999). The role of psychological and biological factors in postinfective gut dysfunction. *Gut, 44*, 400–406.

Hadhazy, V. A., Bausell, B., Berman, B., Creamer, P., & Ezzo, J. (2005). Mind and body therapy for fibromyalgia. *Cochrane Database of Systematic Reviews, 4*. Available from http//www.cochrane.org

Hadhazy, V., Ezzo, J. M., Creamer, P., & Berman, B. M. (2000). Mind and body therapy for fibromyalgia. *Journal of Rheumatology, 27*, 2911–2918.

Hadler, N. M. (1996). If you have to prove you are ill, you can't get well: The object lesson of fibromyalgia. *Spine, 21*, 2397–2400.

Hadler, N. M. (2003). "Fibromyalgia" and the medicalization of misery. *Journal of Rheumatology, 30*, 1668–1670.

Hahn, B. A., Yan, S., & Strassels, S. (1999). Impact of irritable bowel syndrome on quality of life and resource use in the United States and United Kingdom. *Digestion, 60*, 77–81.

Hahn, M., & Bonkovsky, H. L. (1997). Multiple chemical sensitivity syndrome and porphyria. *Archives of Internal Medicine, 157*, 281–285.

Hakala, M., Karlsson, H., Ruotsalainen, U., Koponen, S., Bergman, J., Stenman, H., et al. (2002). Severe somatization in women is associated with altered cerebral glucose metabolism. *Psychological Medicine, 32*, 1379–1385.

Hakala, M., Vahlberg, T., Niemi, P. M., & Karlsson, H. (2006). Brain glucose metabolism and temperament in relation to severe somatization. *Psychiatry and Clinical Neurosciences, 60*, 669–675.

Haller, E. (1993). Successful management of patients with "multiple chemical sensitivities" on an inpatient psychiatric unit. *Journal of Clinical Psychiatry, 54*, 196–199.

Halpert, A., & Drossman, D. (2005). Biopsychosocial issues in irritable bowel syndrome. *Journal of Clinical Gastroenterology, 39*, 665–669.

Hamilton, J. A. (1994). Feminist theory and the health psychology: Tools for an egalitarian, women centered approach to women's health. In A. Dan (Ed.), *Reframing women's health: Multidisciplinary research and practice* (pp. 56–66). Thousand Oaks, CA: Sage.

Hamilton, J. A., & Gallant, S. (1993). Premenstrual syndromes: A health psychology critique of biomedically oriented research. In R. J. Gatchel & E. B. Blanchard (Eds.), *Psychophysiological disorders: Research and clinical applications* (pp. 383–438). Washington, DC: American Psychological Association.

Hamilton, W. T., Gallager, A. M., Thomas, J. M., & White, P. D. (2005). The prognosis of different fatigue diagnostic labels: A longitudinal survey. *Family Practice, 22,* 383–388.

Hammer, J., Eslick, G. D., Howell, S. C., Altiparmack, E., & Talley, N. J. (2004). Diagnostic yield of alarm features in irritable bowel syndrome and functional dyspepsia. *Gut, 53,* 666–672.

Hapidou, E., & Rollman, G. (1998). Menstrual cycle modulation of tender points. *Journal of Pain, 77,* 151–161.

Hart, R. P., Wade, J. B., & Martelli, M. F. (2003). Cognitive impairment in patients with chronic pain: The significance of chronic stress. *Current Pain and Headache Reports, 7,* 116–226.

Hartz, A. J., Kuhn, E. M., Bentler, S. E., Levine, P. H., & London, R. (1999). Prognostic factors for persons with idiopathic chronic fatigue. *Archives of Family Medicine, 8,* 495–501.

Hartz, A. J., Kuhn, E. M., & Levine, P. (1998). Characteristics of fatigued persons associated with features of chronic fatigue syndrome. *Journal of Chronic Fatigue Syndrome, 4*(3), 71–97.

Haug, T. T., Mykletun, A., & Dahl, A. A. (2004). The association between anxiety, depression, and somatic symptoms in a large population: The HUNT-II Study. *Psychosomatic Medicine, 66,* 845–851.

Hawley, D. J., & Wolfe, F. (1993). Depression is not more common in rheumatoid arthritis: A 10-year longitudinal study of 6,153 patients with rheumatic disease. *Journal of Rheumatology, 20,* 2025–2031.

Hayes, S. C., Luoma, J. B., Bond, F. W., Masuda, A., & Lillis, J. (2006). Acceptance and commitment therapy: Model, processes and outcomes. *Behavior, Research and Therapy, 44,* 1–25.

Hazlett, R. L., & Haynes, S. N. (1992). Fibromyalgia: A time-series analysis of the stressor–physical symptom association. *Journal of Behavioral Medicine, 15,* 541–557.

Hazlett-Stevens, H., Craske, M., Mayer, E., Chang, L., & Naliboff, B. (2003). Prevalence of irritable bowel syndrome among university students: The roles of worry, neuroticism, anxiety sensitivity and visceral anxiety. *Journal of Psychosomatic Research, 55,* 501–505.

Heath, I. (1999). Commentary: There must be limits to the medicalisation of human distress. *British Medical Journal, 318,* 439–440.

Heim, C., Ehlert, U., & Hellhammer, D. H. (2000). The potential role of hypocortisolism in the pathophysiology of stress-related bodily disorders. *Psychoneuroendocrinology, 25*, 1–35.

Helgeson, V. S. (2005). *Psychology of gender* (2nd ed.). Upper Saddle River, NJ: Pearson Prentice Hall.

Hellstrom, O., Bullington, J., Karlsson, G., Lindqvist, P., & Mattsson, B. (1999). A phenomenological study of fibromyalgia: Patient perspectives. *Scandinavian Journal of Primary Health Care, 17*, 11–16.

Henderson, M., & Tannock, C. (2004). Objective assessment of personality disorder in chronic fatigue syndrome. *Journal of Psychosomatic Research, 56*, 251–254.

Henningsen, P., Zimmerman, T., & Sattel, H. (2003). Medically unexplained symptoms, anxiety and depression: A meta-analytic review. *Psychosomatic Medicine, 65*, 528–533.

Hersbach, P., Henrich, G., & von Rad, M. (1999). Psychological factors in functional gastrointestinal disorder: Characteristics of the disorder or of the illness behavior? *Psychosomatic Medicine, 61*, 148–153.

Heymann-Monnikes, I., Arnold, R., Florin, I., Herda, C., Melfsen, S., & Monnikes, H. (2000). The combination of medical treatment plus multicomponent behavioral therapy is superior to medical treatment alone in the therapy of irritable bowel syndrome. *American Journal of Gastroenterology, 95*, 981–994.

Hibbard, J. H., & Pope, C. R. (1983). Gender role, illness orientation, and the use of medical services. *Social Science & Medicine, 17*, 129–137.

Hickie, I., Hadzi-Pavlovic D., & Ricci, C. (1997). Reviving the diagnosis of neurasthenia. *Psychological Medicine, 27*, 989–994.

Hickie, I., Kirk, K., & Martin, N. (1999). Unique genetic and environmental determinants of prolonged fatigue: A twin study. *Psychological Medicine, 29*, 259–268.

Hickie, I., Lloyd, A., Hadzi-Pavlovic, D., Parker, G., Bird, K., & Wakefield, D. (1995). Can chronic fatigue syndrome be defined by distinct clinical features? *Psychological Medicine, 25*, 925–935.

Hill, A. B. (1965). The environmental disease: Association or causation? (president's address). *Proceedings of the Royal Society of Medicine, 9*, 295–300.

Hiller, W., & Fichter, M. M. (2004). High utilizers of medical care: A crucial subgroup among somatizing patients. *Journal of Psychosomatic Research, 56*, 437–443.

Hohmann, A. A. (1989). Gender bias in psychotropic prescribing in primary care. *Medical Care, 27*, 478–490.

Holdcraft, L. C., Assefi, N., & Buchwald, D. (2003). Complementary and alternative medicine in fibromyalgia and related syndromes. *Best Practice & Research. Clinical Rheumatology, 17*, 667–683.

Holmes, G. P., Kaplan, J. E., Gantz, N. M., Komaroff, A. L., Schonberger, L. B., Straus, S. E., et al. (1988). Chronic fatigue syndrome: A working case definition. *Annals of Internal Medicine, 108*, 387–389.

Horwitz, B. J., & Fisher, R. S. (2001). The irritable bowel syndrome. *The New England Journal of Medicine, 334*, 1846–1850.

Hotopf, M., Wadsworth, M., & Wessely, S. (2001). Is "somatisation" a defense against the acknowledgment of psychiatric disorder? *Journal of Psychosomatic Research, 50*, 119–124.

Houghton, L. A., Jackson, N. A., Whorwell, P. J., & Morris, J. (2000). Do male sex hormones protect from irritable bowel syndrome? *American Journal of Gastroenterology, 95*, 2296–2300.

Houghton, L. A., Lea, R., Jackson, N., & Whorwell, P. J. (2002). The menstrual cycle affects rectal sensitivity in patients with irritable bowel syndrome but not healthy volunteers. *Gut, 50*, 471–474.

Hudson, J. I., Arnold, L. M., Keck, P. E., Auchenbah, M. B., & Pope, H. G. (2004). Family study of fibromyalgia and affective spectrum disorder. *Biological Psychiatry, 56*, 884–891.

Hudson, J. I., Goldenberg, D. L., Pope, H. G., Keck, P. E., & Schlesinger, L. (1992). Comorbidity of fibromyalgia with medical and psychiatric disorders. *American Journal of Medicine, 92*, 363–367.

Hudson, J. I., Hudson, M. S., Pliner, L. F., Goldenberg, D. L., & Pope, H. G. (1985). Fibromyalgia and major affective disorder: A controlled phenomenology and family history study. *American Journal of Psychiatry, 142*, 441–446.

Hudson, J. I., Mangweth, B., Pope, H. G., Jr., DeCol, C., Hausmann, A., Gutweniger, S., et al. (2003). Family study of affective spectrum disorder. *Archives of General Psychiatry, 60*, 170–177.

Hudson, J. I., & Pope, H. G. (1989). Fibromyalgia and psychopathology: Is fibromyalgia a form of "affective spectrum disorder?" *Journal of Rheumatology, 16*, 15–22.

Ichise, M., Salit, I. E., Abbey, S. E., Chung, D. G., Gray, B., Kirsch, J. C., & Freedman, M. (1992). Assessment of regional cerebral perfusion by 99Tcm-HMPAO SPECT in chronic fatigue syndrome. *Nuclear Medicine Communications, 13*, 767–772.

Jackson, T., Iezzi, T., Gunderson, J., Nagasaka, T., & Fritch, A. (2002). Gender differences in pain perception: The mediating role of self-efficacy beliefs. *Sex Roles, 47*, 561–568.

Jacobson, D. L., Gange, S. J., Rose, N. R., & Graham, N. M. (1997). Epidemiology and estimated population burden of selected autoimmune diseases in the United States. *Clinical Immunology and Immunopathology, 84*, 223–243.

Jailwala, J., Imperiale, T., & Kroenke, K. (2000). Pharmacologic management of IBS: A systematic review of randomized controlled trials. *Annals of Internal Medicine, 133*, 136–147.

Jain, A. P., Gupta, O. P., Jajoo, U. N., & Sidhwa, H. K. (1991). Clinical profile of irritable bowel syndrome at a rural based teaching hospital in central India. *Journal of the Association of Physicians in India, 39*, 385–386.

Jason, L. A., Corradi, K., Torres-Harding, S., Taylor, R. R., & King, C. (2005). Chronic fatigue syndrome: The need for subtypes. *Neuropsychology Review, 15,* 29–58.

Jason, L. A., Holbert, C., Torres-Harding, S., & Taylor, R. R. (2004). Stigma and chronic fatigue syndrome: Surveying a name change. *Journal of Disability Policy Studies, 14,* 222–228.

Jason, L. A., Holbert, C., Torres-Harding, S., Taylor, R. R., Le Vassuer, J. J., Breitinger, P., et al. (2004). Chronic fatigue syndrome versus chronic neuroendocrine immune dysfunction syndrome: Differential attributions. *Journal of Health and Social Policy, 18,* 43–55.

Jason, L. A., Jordan, K. M., Richman, J. A., Rademaker, A. W., Huang, C., McCready, W., et al. (1999). A community-based study of prolonged and chronic fatigue. *Journal of Health Psychology, 4,* 9–26.

Jason, L. A., Richman, J. A., Freidberg, F., Wagner, L., Taylor, R. R., & Jordan, K. M. (1997). Politics, science, and the emergence of a new disease: The case of chronic fatigue syndrome. *American Psychologist, 52,* 973–983.

Jason, L. A., Richman, J. A., Rademaker, A. W., Jordan, K. M., Plioplys, A. V., Taylor, R. R., et al. (1999). A community based study of chronic fatigue syndrome. *Archives of Internal Medicine, 159,* 2129–2137.

Jason, L. A ., Taylor, R. R., Kennedy, C. L., Jordan, K. M., Song, S., Johnson, D., et al. (2003). Chronic fatigue syndrome: Symptom subtypes in a community based sample. *Women and Health, 37,* 1–13.

Jason, L. A., Taylor, R. R., Song, S., Kennedy, C., & Johnson, D. (1999). Functional somatic syndromes. *The Lancet, 354,* 2079.

Jensen, I., Bergstrom, G., Ljungquist, T., Bodin, L., & Nygren, A. L. (2001). A randomized controlled component analysis of a behavioral medicine rehabilitation program for chronic spinal pain: Are the effects dependent on gender? *Pain, 91,* 65–78.

Jensen, I., Nygren, A., Gamberale, F., Goldie, I., & Westerholm, P. (1994). Coping with long term musculoskeletal pain and its consequences: Is gender a factor? *Pain, 57,* 167–172.

Jensen, R. Rasmussen, B. K., Pedersen, B., Lous, I., & Olesen, J. (1992). Cephalic muscle tenderness and pressure pain threshold in a general population. *Pain, 48,* 197–203.

Jerjes, W. K., Peters, J., Taylor, N. F., Wood, P. J., Wessely, S., & Cleare, A. J. (2006). Diurnal excretion of urinary cortisol, cortisone, and cortisol metabolites in chronic fatigue syndrome. *Journal of Psychosomatic Research, 60,* 145–153.

Johns, K. R., & Littlejohn, G. O. (1999). The role of sex hormones in pain response. *Pain, 87,* 109–111.

Johnson, L. M., Zautra, A. J., & Davis, M. C. (2006). The role of illness uncertainty on coping with fibromyalgia symptoms. *Health Psychology, 25,* 696–703.

Johnson, S. K., & Blanchard, A. (2006). Alternative medicine and herbal use among university students. *Journal of American College Health, 55,* 163–168.

Johnson, S. K., & DeLuca, J. (2005). Chronic fatigue syndrome and the brain. In J. DeLuca (Ed.), *Fatigue: A window to the brain* (pp. 137–156). Cambridge, MA: MIT Press.

Johnson, S. K., DeLuca, J., & Natelson, B. H. (1996a). Assessing somatization disorder in chronic fatigue syndrome. *Psychosomatic Medicine, 58,* 50–57.

Johnson, S. K., DeLuca, J., & Natelson, B. H. (1996b). Depression in fatiguing illness: Comparing patients with chronic fatigue syndrome, multiple sclerosis and depression. *Journal of Affective Disorders, 39,* 21–30.

Johnson, S. K., DeLuca, J., & Natelson, B. H. (1996c). Personality dimensions in the chronic fatigue syndrome: A comparison with multiple sclerosis and depression. *Journal of Psychiatric Research, 30,* 9–20.

Johnson, S. K., DeLuca, J., & Natelson, B. H. (1999). Chronic fatigue syndrome: Reviewing the research findings. *Annals of Behavioral Medicine, 21,* 258–271.

Johnson, S. K., Gil-Rivas, V., & Schmaling, K. (2006, May). *Personality and coping variables on outcomes in chronic fatigue syndrome.* Paper presented at the 18th Annual Convention of the Association for Psychological Science, New York.

Johnson, S. K., Lange, G., DeLuca, J., Korn, L. R., & Natelson, B. H. (1997). Effects of fatigue on neuropsychological performance on patients with chronic fatigue syndrome, multiple sclerosis and depression. *Applied Neuropsychology, 4,* 145–153.

Johnson, S. K., Lange, G., Tiersky, L., DeLuca, J., & Natelson, B. H. (2001). Health-related personality factors in chronic fatigue syndrome and multiple sclerosis. *Journal of Chronic Fatigue Syndrome, 8,* 41–52.

Jones, A., & Zachariae, R. (2004). Investigation of the interactive effects of gender and psychological factors on pain response. *British Journal of Health Psychology, 9,* 405–418.

Kandrick, M. A., Grant, K. R., & Segall, A. (1991). Gender differences in health related behavior: Some unanswered questions. *Social Science & Medicine, 32,* 579–590.

Kaptein, A. A., Helder, D. I., Kleijn, W. C., Reif, W., Moss-Morris, R., & Petrie, K. J. (2005). Modern health worries in medical students. *Journal of Psychosomatic Research, 58,* 453–457.

Karjalainen, K., Malmivaara, A., van Tulder, M., Roine, R., Jauhiainen, M., Hurri, H., & Koes, B. (2000). Multidisciplinary rehabilitation for fibromyalgia and musculoskeletal pain in working age adults. *Cochrane Database of Systematic Reviews, 2,* CD001984. Available from http//www.cochrane.org

Karst, M., Rahe-Meyer, N., Gueduek, A., Hoy, L., Borsutzky, M., & Passie, T. (2005). Abnormality in the self-monitoring mechanism in patients with fibromyalgia and somatoform pain disorder. *Psychosomatic Medicine, 67,* 111–115.

Kashikar-Zuch, S., Graham, T., Huenefeld, M., & Powers, S. (2000). A review of biobehavioral research in juvenile primary fibromyalgia syndrome [Electronic version]. *Arthritis Care and Research, 13,* 388–397.

Kato, K., Sullivan, P. F., Evengard, B., & Pedersen, N. L. (2006). Premorbid predictors of chronic fatigue. *Archives of General Psychiatry, 63,* 1267–1272.

Katon, W., Lin, E., Von Korff, M., Russo, J., Lipscomb, P., & Bush, T. (1991). Somatization: A spectrum of severity. *American Journal of Psychiatry, 148,* 34–40.

Katon, W., Sullivan, M., & Walker, E. (2001). Medical symptoms without identified pathology: Relationship to psychiatric disorders, childhood and adult trauma, and personality traits. *Annals of Internal Medicine, 134,* 917–925.

Keefe, F., Lumley, M., Anderson, T., Lynch, T., & Carson, K. (2001). Pain and emotion: New research directions. *Journal of Clinical Psychology, 57,* 587–607.

Keefer, L., & Blanchard, E. B. (2001). The effects of relaxation response meditation on the symptoms of irritable bowel syndrome: Results of a controlled treatment study. *Behavior Research and Therapy, 39,* 801–811.

Kennedy, T. M., & Jones, R. H. (2000). Epidemiology of cholecystectomy and irritable bowel syndrome in a UK population. *British Journal of Surgery, 87,* 1658–1663.

Kennedy, T. M., Chalder, T., McCrone, P., Darnley, S., Knapp, M., Jones, R. H., et al. (2006). Cognitive behavioural therapy in addition to antispasmodic treatment for irritable bowel syndrome in primary care: Randomised controlled trial. *Health Technology Assessment, 10,* iii–iv, ix–x, 1–67.

Keogh, E., & Herdenfeldt, M. (2002). Gender, coping and the perception of pain. *Pain, 97,* 195–201.

Keogh, E., McCracken, L. M., & Eccleston, C. (2006). Gender moderates the association between depression and disability in chronic pain patients. *European Journal of Pain, 206,* 413–422.

Kessler, D., Lloyd, K., Lewis, G., & Gray, D. P. (1999). Cross sectional study of symptom attribution and recognition of depression and anxiety in primary care. *British Medical Journal, 318,* 436–440.

Khan, A. A., Gardner, C. O., Prescott, C. A., & Kendler, K. S. (2002). Gender differences in the symptoms of major depression in opposite-sex dizygotic twin pairs. *American Journal of Psychiatry, 159,* 1427–1429.

Kiecolt-Glaser, J. K., Bane, C., Glaser, R., & Malarkey, W. B. (2003). Love, marriage, and divorce: Newlyweds' stress hormones foreshadow relationship changes. *Journal of Consulting and Clinical Psychology, 71,* 176–188.

Kiecolt-Glaser, J. K., McGuire, L., Robles, T. F., & Glaser, R. (2002). Emotions, morbidity, and mortality: New perspectives from psychoneuroimmunology. *Annual Review of Psychology, 53,* 83–107.

Kiecolt-Glaser, J. K., Page, G. G., Marucha, P. T., MacCallum, R. C., & Glaser, R. (1998). Psychological influences on surgical recovery: Perspectives from psychoneuroimmunology. *American Psychologist, 53,* 1209–1218.

King, C., & Jason, L. A. (2005). Improving the diagnostic criteria and procedures for chronic fatigue syndrome. *Biological Psychology, 68,* 87–106.

Kipen, H. M., & Fiedler, N. (2002). Environmental factors in medically unexplained symptoms and related syndromes: The evidence and the challenge. *Environmental Health Perspectives, 110*(Suppl. 4), 597–599.

Kipen, H. M., Hallman, W., Kang, H., Fiedler, N., & Natelson, B. H. (1999). Prevalence of chronic fatigue and chemical sensitivities in Gulf Registry veterans. *Archives of Environmental Health, 54,* 313–318.

Kirk, J., Douglass, R., Nelson, E., Jaffee, J., & Lopez, A. (1990). Chief complaint of chronic fatigue: A prospective study. *Journal of Family Practice, 30,* 33–41.

Kirmayer, L. J., Groleau, D., Looper, K. J., & Dao, M. D. (2004). Explaining medically unexplained symptoms. *Canadian Journal of Psychiatry, 49,* 663–671.

Kirmayer, L. J., Robbins, J. M., & Kapusta, M. A. (1988). Somatization and depression in fibromyalgia syndrome. *American Journal of Psychiatry, 145,* 950–954.

Kirmayer, L. J., Robbins, J. M., & Paris, J. (1994). Somatoform disorders: Personality and the social matrix of somatic distress. *Journal of Abnormal Psychology, 103,* 125–136.

Kivimaki, M., Leino-Arjas, P., Virtanen, M., Elovainio, M., Keltikangas-Jarvinen, L., Puttonen, S., et al. (2004). Work stress and incidence of newly diagnosed fibromyalgia. *Journal of Psychosomatic Research, 57,* 417–422.

Klonoff, E. A., Landrine, H., & Campbell, R. (2000). Sexist discrimination may account for the well-known gender differences in psychiatric symptoms. *Psychology of Women Quarterly, 24,* 93–99.

Kolk, A. M. M., Hanewald, G. J. F. P., Schagen, C. M. T., & Gijsbers van Wijk, C. M. (2002). Predicting medically unexplained physical symptoms and health care utilization: A symptoms perception approach. *Journal of Psychosomatic Research, 52,* 35–44.

Kolk, A. M. M., Schagen, S., & Hanewald, G. J. (2004). Multiple medically unexplained physical symptoms and health care utilization: Outcome of psychological intervention and patient-related predictors of change. *Journal of Psychosomatic Research, 57,* 379–389.

Koloski, N. A., Boyce, P. M., & Talley, N. J. (2005). Is health care seeking for irritable bowel syndrome and functional dyspepsia a socially learned response to illness? *Digestive Diseases and Sciences, 50,* 153–162.

Komaroff, A. L. (1994). Clinical presentation and evaluation of fatigue and chronic fatigue syndrome. In S. E. Straus (Ed.), *Chronic fatigue syndrome* (pp. 61–84). New York: Marcel Dekker.

Komaroff, A. J., & Buchwald, D. (1991). Symptoms and signs of chronic fatigue syndrome. *Review of Infectious Diseases, 13,* S8–S11.

Komiyama, O., & De Laat, A. (2005). Tactile and pain thresholds in the intra- and extra-oral regions of symptom-free subjects. *Pain, 115,* 308–315.

Krantz, G., Forsman, M., & Lundberg, U. (2004). Consistency in physiological stress responses and electromyographic activity during induced stress exposure in women and men. *Integrative Physiological and Behavioral Science, 39,* 105–118.

Kroenke, K. (2001a). Patients presenting with somatic complaints: Epidemiology, psychiatric co-morbidity and management. *International Journal of Methods in Psychiatric Research, 12,* 34–43.

Kroenke, K. (2001b). Studying symptoms: Sampling and measurement issues. *Annals of Internal Medicine, 134*, 844–853.

Kroenke, K., & Harris, L. (2001). Symptoms research: A fertile field. *Annals of Internal Medicine, 134*, 801–802.

Kroenke, K., & Mangelsdorff, A. D. (1989). Common symptoms in ambulatory care: Incidence, evaluation, therapy, and outcome. *American Journal of Medicine, 86*, 262–266.

Kroenke, K., & Price, R. (1993). Symptoms in the community: Prevalence, classification and psychiatric comorbidity. *Archives of Internal Medicine, 153*, 2474–2480.

Kroenke, K., & Spitzer, R. L. (1998). Gender differences in the reporting of physical and somatoform symptoms. *Psychosomatic Medicine, 60*, 150–155.

Kroenke, K., Spitzer, R. L., deGruy, F. V., Hahn, S. R., Linzer, M., Williams, J. B. W., et al. (1997). Multisomatoform disorder: An alternative to undifferentiated somatoform disorder for the somatizing patient in primary care. *Archives of General Psychiatry, 54*, 352–358.

Kroenke, K., Spitzer, R. L., Williams, J. B. W., Linzer, M., Hahn, S. R., deGruy, F. V., et al. (1994). Physical symptoms in primary care: Predictors of psychiatric disorders and functional impairment. *Archives of Family Medicine, 3*, 374–379.

Kroenke, K., Wood, D. R., Mangelsdorff, A. D., Meier, N. J., & Powell, J. B. (1988). Chronic fatigue in primary care: Prevalence, patient characteristics, and outcome. *JAMA, 260*, 929–934.

Kreutzer, R., Neutra, R. R., & Lashuay, N. (1999). Prevalence of people reporting sensitivities to chemicals in a population based survey. *American Journal of Epidemiology, 150*, 1–12.

Kroll-Smith, S., & Floyd, H. H. (1997). *Bodies in protest and the struggle over medical knowledge.* New York: New York University Press.

Kuratsune, H., Yamaguti, K., Lindh, G., Evengard, B., Hagberg, G., Matsumura, K., et al. (2002). Brain regions involved in fatigue sensation: Reduced acetylcarnitine uptake into the brain. *NeuroImage, 17*, 1256–1265.

Kuslys, T., Vishwanath, B. S., Frey, F. J., & Frey, B. M. (1996). Differences in phospholipase A2 activity between males and females and Asian Indians and Caucasians. *European Journal of Clinical Investigation, 26*, 310–315.

Lackner, J. M., Gudleski, G. D., & Blanchard, E. B. (2004). Beyond abuse: The association among parenting style, abdominal pain, and somatization in IBS patients. *Behaviour Research and Therapy, 42*, 41–56.

Lackner, J. M., Gudleski, G. D., Zack, M. M., Katz, L. A., Powell, C., Krasner, S., et al. (2006). Measuring health-related quality of life in patients with irritable bowel syndrome: Can less be more? *Psychosomatic Medicine, 68*, 312–320.

Lackner, J. M., Quigley, B. M., & Blanchard, E. B. (2004). Depression and abdominal pain in IBS patients: The mediating role of catastrophizing. *Psychosomatic Medicine, 66*, 435–441.

Lacour, M., Zunder, T., Schmidtke, K., Vaith, P., & Scheidt, C. (2005). Multiple chemical sensitivity syndrome (MCS)—Suggestions for an extension of the U.S.

MCS-case definition. *International Journal of Hygiene and Environmental Health*, 308, 141–151.

Landis, C. A., Lentz, M. J., Tsuji, J., Buchwald, D., & Shaver, J. L. (2004). Pain, psychological variables, sleep quality, and natural killer cell activity in midlife women with and without fibromyalgia. *Brain Behavior and Immunity*, 18, 304–313.

Lange, G., DeLuca, J., Maldjian, J. A., Lee, H.-J., Tiersky, L. A., & Natelson, B. H. (1999). Brain MRI abnormalities exist in a subset of patients with chronic fatigue syndrome. *Journal of the Neurological Sciences*, 171, 3–7.

Lange, G., Steffener, D. B., Cook, D. B., Bly, B. M., Christodoulou, C., Liu, W.-C., et al. (2005). Objective evidence of cognitive complaints in chronic fatigue syndrome: A BOLD fMRI study of verbal working memory. *NeuroImage*, 26, 513–524.

Lautenbacher, S., & Rollman, G. B. (1997). Possible deficiencies of pain modulation in fibromyalgia. *Clinical Journal of Pain*, 13, 189–196.

Lawrie, S. M., Manders, D. N., Geddes, J. R., & Pelosi, A. J. (1997). A population-based incidence study of chronic fatigue. *Psychological Medicine*, 27, 343–353.

Lax, M. B., & Henneberger, P. K. (1995). Patients with multiple chemical sensitivities in an occupational health clinic: Presentation and follow-up. *Archives of Environmental Health*, 50, 425–431.

Lee, O. Y., Mayer, E. A., Schmulson, M., Chang, L., & Naliboff, B. (2001) Gender-related differences in IBS symptoms. *American Journal of Gastroenterology*, 96, 2184–2193.

Lembo, T., Naliboff, B., Munakata, J., Fullerton, S., Saba, L., Jung, S., et al. (1999). Symptoms and visceral perception in patients with pain-predominant irritable bowel syndrome. *American Journal of Gastroenterology*, 94, 1320–1326.

Leserman, J., Li, Z., Drossman, D. A., & Hu, Y. J. B. (1998). Selected symptoms associated with sexual and physical abuse history among female patients with gastrointestinal disorders: The impact on subsequent health care visits. *Psychological Medicine*, 28, 417–425.

Levine, P. H. (1994). Epidemic neuromyasthenia and chronic fatigue syndrome: Epidemiological importance of a cluster definition. *Clinical Infectious Diseases*, 18(Suppl. 1), S16–S20.

Levy, R. L., Von Korff, M., Whitehead, W. E., Stang, P., Saunders, K., Jhingran, P., et al. (2001). Costs of care for irritable bowel syndrome patients in a health maintenance organization. *American Journal of Gastroenterology*, 96, 3122–3129.

Levy, R. L., Whitehead, W. E., VonKorff, M. R., & Feld, A. D. (2000). Intergenerational transmission of gastrointestinal illness behavior. *American Journal of Gastroenterology*, 95, 451–456.

Levy, R. L., Whitehead, W. E., Walker, L. S., Von Korff, M., Feld, A. D., Garner, M., & Christie, D. (2004). Increased somatic complaints and health-care utilization in children: Effects of parent IBS status and parent response to gastrointestinal symptoms. *American Journal of Gastroenterology*, 99, 2442–2451.

Lewis, D. H., Mayberg, H. S., Fischer, M. E., Goldberg, J., Ashton, S., Graham, M. M., & Buchwald, D. (2001). Monozygotic twins discordant for chronic fatigue syndrome: Regional cerebral blood flow SPECT. *Radiology, 219,* 766–773.

Lewis, T. (1940). *The soldier's heart and the effort syndrome* (2nd ed.). London: Shaw & Sons.

Lindal, E., Stefansson, J. G., & Bergmann, S. (2002). The prevalence of chronic fatigue syndrome in Iceland—A national comparison by gender drawing on four different criteria. *Nordic Journal of Psychiatry, 56,* 273–277.

Linder, R., Dinser, R., Wagner, M., Krueger, G. R., & Hoffman, A. (2002) Generation of classification criteria for chronic fatigue syndrome using an artificial neural network and traditional criteria set. *In Vivo, 16,* 37–43.

Linton, S. J. (2002). A prospective study of the effects of sexual or physical abuse on back pain. *Pain, 96,* 347–351.

Lipowski, Z. J. (1988). Somatization: The concept and its clinical application. *American Journal of Psychiatry, 145,* 1358–1368.

Lipson, J. G. (2004). Multiple chemical sensitivities: Stigma and social experiences. *Medical Anthropology Quarterly, 18,* 200–213.

Liskow, B., Othmer, E., Penick, E. C., DeSouza, C., & Gabrielli, W. (1986). Is Briquet's syndrome a heterogeneous disorder? *American Journal of Psychiatry, 143,* 626–629.

Lloyd, A., Hickie, I., Brockman, A., Hickie, C., Wilson, A., Dwyer, J., & Wakefield, D. (1993). Immunological and psychologic therapy for patients with chronic fatigue syndrome. *American Journal of Medicine, 94,* 197–203.

Lloyd, A. R., Wakefield, D., Boughton, C., & Dwyer, J. (1990). Prevalence of chronic fatigue syndrome in an Australian population. *Medical Journal of Australia, 153,* 522–528.

Loge, J. H., Ekeberg, O., & Kaasa, S. (1998). Fatigue in the general Norwegian population: Normative data and associations. *Journal of Psychosomatic Research, 45,* 53–65.

Longstreth, G. F., Thompson, W. G., Chey, W. D., Houghton, L. A., Mearin, F., & Spiller, R. C. (2006). Functional bowel disorders. *Gastroenterology, 130,* 1480–1491.

Longstreth, G. F., & Wolde-Tsadik, G. (1993). Irritable bowel-type symptoms in HMO examinees: Prevalence, demographics, and clinical correlates. *Digestive Diseases and Sciences, 38,* 1581–1589.

Longstreth, G. F., & Yao, J. F. (2004). Irritable bowel syndrome and surgery: A multivariate analysis. *Gastroenterology, 126,* 1665–1673.

Looper, K. J., & Kirmayer, L. J. (2004). Perceived stigma in functional somatic syndromes and comparable medical conditions. *Journal of Psychosomatic Research, 57,* 373–378.

Lundberg, U. (2005). Stress hormones in health and illness: The roles of work and gender. *Psychoneuroendocrinology, 30,* 1017–1021.

Lundberg, U., de Chateau, P., Winberg, J., & Frankenhaeuser, M. (1981). Catecholamine and cortisol excretion patterns in three-year-old children and their parents. *Journal of Human Stress, 7*(3), 3–11.

Lundberg, U., & Frankenhaeuser, M. (1999). Stress and workload of men and women in high-ranking positions. *Journal of Occupational Health Psychology, 4,* 142–151.

Lydiard, R. B., Fossey, M. D., Marsh, W., & Ballenger, J. C. (1993). Prevalence of psychiatric disorders in patients with irritable bowel syndrome. *Psychosomatics, 34,* 229–234.

Mace, C. J., & Trimble, M. R. (1996). Ten-year prognosis of conversion disorder. *British Journal of Psychiatry, 169,* 282–288.

Macfarlane, T. V., Blinkhorn, A., Worthington, H. V., Davies, R. M., & Macfarlane, G. J. (2002). *Rheumatology, 41,* 454–457.

Machale, S. M., Lawrie, S. M., Cavanagh, J. T. O., Glabus, M. F., Murray, C. L., Goodwin, G. M., & Ebmeier, K. P. (2000). Cerebral perfusion in chronic fatigue syndrome and depression. *British Journal of Psychiatry, 176,* 550–556.

Macmillan, M. B. (1976). Beard's concept of neurasthenia and Freud's concept of the actual neuroses. *Journal of the History of the Behavioral Sciences, 12,* 376–390.

Magill, M. K., & Surada, A. (1998). Multiple chemical sensitivity syndrome. *American Family Physician, 58,* 721–728.

Maier, W., Gansicke, M., Gater, R., Rezaki, M., Tiemens, B., & Florenzano Urzúa, R. R. (1999). Gender differences in the prevalence of depression: A survey in primary care. *Journal of Affective Disorders, 53,* 241–252.

Malleson, A. (2002). *Whiplash and other useful illnesses.* Montreal, Quebec, Canada: McGill–Queens University Press.

Maloney, E. M., Gurbaxani, B. M., Jones, J. F., de Souza Coelho, L., Pennachin, C., & Goertzel, B. N. (2006). Chronic fatigue syndrome and high allostatic load. *Pharmacogenomics, 7,* 467–473.

Malterud, K. (2000). Symptoms as a source of medical knowledge: Understanding medically unexplained disorders in women. *Family Medicine, 32,* 603–611.

Mannerkorpi, K., Ahlmen, M., & Ekdahl, C. (2002). Six- and 24-month follow-up of pool exercise therapy and education for patients with fibromyalgia. *Scandinavian Journal of Rheumatology, 31,* 306–310.

Mannerkorpi, K., & Daly Iverson, M. (2003). Physical exercise in fibromyalgia and related syndromes. *Best Practice & Research. Clinical Rheumatology, 17,* 629–647.

Mannerkorpi, K., Nyberg, B., & Ekdahl, C. (2000). Pool exercise combined with an education program for patients with fibromyalgia syndrome. A prospective, randomized study. *Journal of Rheumatology, 27,* 2473–2481.

Manu, P. (2004). *The psychopathology of functional somatic syndromes: Neurobiology and illness behavior in CFS, fibromyalgia, Gulf War illness, irritable bowel, and premenstrual dysphoria.* New York: Haworth Press.

Manu, P., Lane, T. J., & Matthews, D. A. (1992). Chronic fatigue syndromes in clinical practice. *Psychotherapy and Psychosomatics, 58,* 60–68.

Manu, P., Matthews, D. A., Lane, T. J., Tennen, H., Hesselbrock, V., Mendola, R., & Affleck, G. (1989). Depression among patients with a chief complaint of chronic fatigue. *Journal of Affective Disorders, 17,* 165–172.

Maquet, D., Croisier, J., Demoulin, C., & Creilaard, M. (2004). Pressure pain thresholds of tender point sites in patients with fibromyalgia and healthy controls. *European Journal of Pain, 8,* 111–117.

Martin, M., & Crane, C. (2003). Cognition and the body: Somatic attributions in irritable bowel syndrome. *Behavioural and Cognitive Psychotherapy, 31,* 13–31.

Martin, R., Barron, J. J., & Zacker, C. (2001). Irritable bowel syndrome: Toward a cost-effective management approach. *American Journal of Managed Care, 7*(Suppl. 8), S268–S275.

Masi, A. T., White, K. P., & Pilcher, J. J. (2002). Person-centered approach to care, teaching, and research in fibromyalgia syndrome: Justification from biopsychosocial perspectives in populations. *Seminars in Arthritis and Rheumatism, 32,* 71–93.

Masuda, A., Hayes, S. C., Sackett, C. F., & Twohig, M. P. (2004). Cognitive defusion and self-relevant negative thoughts: Examining the impact of a ninety year old technique. *Behaviour Research and Therapy, 42,* 477–485.

Mayer, E. A. (1999). Emerging disease model for functional gastrointestinal disorders. *American Journal of Medicine, 107,* 12S–19S.

Mayer, E. A. (2000). Review: The neurobiology of stress and gastrointestinal disease. *Gut, 47,* 861–869.

Mayer, E. A., Berman, S., Chang, L., & Naliboff, B. D. (2004) Sex-based differences in gastrointestinal pain. *European Journal of Pain, 8,* 451–463.

Mayer, E. A., Berman, S. T., Suyenobu, B., Labus, J., Mandelkern, M. A., Naliboff, B. D., & Chang, L. (2005). Differences in brain responses to visceral pain between patients with irritable bowel syndrome and ulcerative colitis. *Pain, 115,* 398–409.

Mayer, E. A., Fass, R., & Fullerton, S. (1998). Intestinal and extraintestinal symptoms in functional gastrointestinal disorders. *European Journal of Surgery. Supplement, 583,* 29–31.

Mayer, E. A., Naliboff, B., Lee, O., Munakata, J., & Chang, L. (1999). Review article: Gender-related differences in functional gastrointestinal disorders. *Alimentary Pharmacology and Therapeutics, 13*(Suppl. 2), 65–69.

Mayou, R., Kirmayer, L. J., Simon, G., Kroenke, K., & Sharpe, M. (2005). Somatoform disorders: Time for a new approach in *DSM–V. American Journal of Psychiatry, 162,* 847–855.

McBeth, J., Macfarlane, G., Benjamin, S., Morris, S., & Silman, A. (1999). The association between tender points, psychological distress, and adverse childhood experiences. *Arthritis and Rheumatism, 42,* 1397–1404.

McBeth, J., Morris, S., Benjamin, S., Silman, A. J., & Macfarlane, G. (2001). Associations between adverse events in childhood and chronic widespread pain in adulthood: Are they explained by differential recall? *Journal of Rheumatology, 28,* 2305–2309.

McCain, G. A., Bell, D. A., Mai, F. M., & Halliday, P. D. (1988). A controlled study of the effects of a supervised cardiovascular fitness training program on the manifestations of primary fibromyalgia. *Arthritis and Rheumatism, 31,* 1135–1141.

McCracken, L. M., Carson, J. W., Eccleston, C., & Keefe, F. J. (2004). Acceptance and change in the context of chronic pain. *Pain, 109,* 4–7.

McDonagh, A. F., & Bissell, M. (1998). Porphyria and porphyrinology—The past fifteen years. *Seminars in Liver Disease, 18,* 3–15.

McEwen, B., & Lasley, E. N. (2003). Allostatic load: When protection gives way to damage. *Advances, 19,* 39–44.

McGeary, D. D., Mayer, T. G., Gatchel, R. J., Anagnostis, C., & Proctor, T. J. (2003). Gender-related differences in treatment outcomes for patients with musculoskeletal disorders. *The Spine Journal, 3,* 197–203.

McKee, D. P., & Quigley, E. M. (1993). Intestinal motility in irritable bowel syndrome: Is IBS a motility disorder? II. Motility of the small bowel, esophagus, stomach, and gallbladder. *Digestive Disease Science, 38,* 1773–1782.

McKenzie, R., O'Fallon, A., Dale, J., Demitrack, M., Sharma, G., Deloria, M., et al. (1998). Low-dose hydrocortisone for treatment of chronic fatigue syndrome: A randomized controlled trial. *JAMA, 280,* 1061–1066.

McLean, S. A., & Clauw, D. J. (2004). Predicting chronic symptoms after an acute "stressor"—Lessons learned from three medical conditions. *Medical Hypotheses, 63,* 653–658.

McWhinney, I. R., Epstein, R. M., & Freeman, T. R. (1997). Rethinking somatization. *Annals of Internal Medicine, 126,* 747–750.

Mechanic, D. (1972). Social psychological factors affecting the presentation of bodily complaints. *New England Journal of Medicine, 286,* 1132–1139.

Meeus, M., & Nijs, J. (2007). Central sensitization: A biopsychosocial explanation for chronic widespread pain in patients with fibromyalgia and chronic fatigue syndrome. *Clinical Rheumatology, 26,* 465–473.

Meggs, W. J. (1995). Multiple chemical sensitivities—Chemical sensitivity as a symptom of airway inflammation. *Journal of Toxicology and Clinical Toxicology, 33,* 107–110.

Meggs, W. J. (1999). Mechanisms of allergy and chemical sensitivity. *Toxicology and Industrial Health, 15,* 331–338.

Meisler, J. G. (2000). Toward optimal health: The experts discuss fibromyalgia. *Journal of Women's Health and Gender-Based Medicine, 9,* 1055–1060.

Mellner, C., Krantz, G., & Lundberg, U. (2005). Medically unexplained symptoms in women as related to physiological stress responses. *Stress and Health, 21,* 45–52.

Melville, D. L. (1987). Descriptive clinical research and medically unexplained physical symptoms. *Journal of Psychosomatic Research, 31,* 359–365.

Mertz, H. (2002). Role of the brain and sensory pathways in gastrointestinal sensory disorders in humans. *Gut, 51*(Suppl. 1), 29–33.

Mertz, H. R. (2003). Irritable bowel syndrome. *New England Journal of Medicine, 349*, 2136–2146.

Mertz, H., Morgan, V., Tanner, G., Pickens, D., Price, R., Shyr, Y., & Kessler, R. (2000). Regional cerebral activation in irritable bowel syndrome and control subjects with painful and nonpainful rectal distention. *Gastroenterology, 118*, 842–848.

Mertz, H., Naliboff, B. D., Munakata, J., Niazi, N., & Mayer, E. A. (1995). Altered rectal perception is a biological marker of patients with irritable bowel syndrome. *Gastroenterology, 109*, 40–52.

Meyer-Lindenberg, A., & Gallhofer, B. (1998). Somatized depression as a subgroup of fibromyalgia syndrome. *Zeitschrift für Rheumatologie, 57*(Suppl. 2), 92–93.

Micale, M. (1995). *Approaching hysteria: Disease and its interpretations.* Princeton, NJ: Princeton University Press.

Michiels, V., & Cluydts, R. (2001). Neuropsychological functioning in the chronic fatigue syndrome: A review. *Acta Psychiatrica Scandinavica, 103*, 84–93.

Millea, P. J., & Holloway, R. L. (2000). Treating fibromyalgia. *American Family Physician, 62*, 1575–1587.

Miller, A. R., North, C. S., Clouse, R. E., Wetzel, R. D., Spitznagel, E. L., & Alpers, D. H. (2001). The association of irritable bowel syndrome and somatization disorder. *Annals of Clinical Psychiatry, 13*, 25–30.

Miller, C. S. (1999). Are we on the threshold of a new theory of disease? Toxicant-induced loss of tolerance and its relationship to addiction and abdiction. *Toxicology and Industrial Health, 15*, 284–294.

Millon, C., Salvato, F., Blaney, N., Morgan, R., Mantero-Atienza, E., Klimas, N., & Fletcher, M. A. (1989) A psychological assessment of chronic fatigue syndrome/chronic Epstein–Barr virus patients. *Psychology and Health, 3*, 131–141.

Mischel, M. H. (1999). Uncertainty in chronic illness. *Annual Review of Nursing Research, 17*, 269–294.

Mitchell, C. M., & Drossman, D. A. (1987). Survey of the AGA membership relating to patients with functional gastrointestinal disorders. *Gastroenterology, 92*, 1282–1284.

Moldofsky, H. (1993). A chronobiologic theory of fibromyalgia. *Journal of Musculoskeletal Pain, 1*, 49–53.

Moldofsky, H., Scarisbrick, P., England, R., & Smythe, H. (1975). Musculoskeletal symptoms and non-REM sleep disturbance in patients with "fibrositis syndrome" and healthy subjects. *Psychosomatic Medicine, 37*, 341–351.

Monnikes, H., Tebbe, J. J., Hildebrandt, M., Arck, P., Osmanoglou, E., Rose, M., et al. (2001). Role of stress in functional gastrointestinal disorders. Evidence for stress-induced alterations in gastrointestinal motility and sensitivity. *Digestive Diseases, 19*, 201–211.

Monsbakken, K. W., Vandvik, P. O., & Farup, P. G. (2005). The value of a general therapeutic approach in subjects with irritable bowel syndrome. *Alimentary Pharmacology & Therapeutics, 21,* 21–27.

Mooser, S. B. (1987). The epidemiology of multiple chemical sensitivities (MCS). *Occupational Medicine, 2,* 663–668.

Mor, V., Laliberte, L., Morris, J. N., & Weiman, M. (1984). The Karnofsky Performance Status Scale. An examination of its reliability and validity in a research setting. *Cancer, 53,* 2002–2007.

Moss-Morris, R., & Petrie, K. J. (2001). Discriminating between chronic fatigue syndrome and depression: A cognitive analysis. *Psychological Medicine, 31,* 469–479.

Moss-Morris, R., Sharon, C., Tobin, R., & Baldi, J. C. (2005). A randomized controlled graded exercise trial for chronic fatigue syndrome: Outcomes and mechanisms of change. *Journal of Health Psychology, 10,* 245–259.

Moss-Morris, R., & Spence, M. (2006). To "lump" or to "split" the functional somatic syndromes: Can infectious and emotional risk factors differentiate between the onset of chronic fatigue syndrome and irritable bowel syndrome? *Psychosomatic Medicine, 68,* 463–469.

Muller-Lissner, S., Fumagalli, I., Bardhan, K. D., Pace, F., Pecher, E., Nault, B., et al. (2001). Tegaserod, a 5-HT4 receptor partial agonist, relieves symptoms in irritable bowel syndrome patients with abdominal pain, bloating, and constipation. *Alimentary Pharmacology & Therapeutics, 15,* 1655–1666.

Naliboff, B. D., Chang, L., Munakata, J., & Mayer, E. A. (2000). In E. A. Mayer & C. B. Saper (Eds.), *Progress in brain research: Vol. 122. The biological basis for mind body interactions* (pp. 413–423). New York: Elsevier.

Naliboff, B. D., Derbyshire, W. G., Munakata, J., Berman, S., Mandelkern, M., Chang, L., & Mayer, E. A. (2001). Cerebral activation in patients with irritable bowel syndrome and control subjects during rectosigmoid stimulation. *Psychosomatic Medicine, 63,* 365–375.

Naliboff, B. D., Heitkemper, M. M., Chang, L., & Mayer, E. A. (2000). Sex and gender in IBS. In R. B. Fillingim (Ed.), *Progress in pain research and management* (Vol. 17, pp. 327–353). Seattle, WA: IASP Press.

Naliboff, B. D., Munakata, J., Fullerton, S., Gracely, R. H., Kodner, A., Harraf, F., et al. (1997). Evidence for two distinct perceptual alterations in irritable bowel syndrome. *Gut, 41,* 505–512.

Natelson, B. H., Cohen, J. M., Brassloff, I., & Lee, H. J. (1993). A controlled study of brain magnetic resonance imaging in patients with fatiguing illnesses. *Journal of the Neurological Sciences, 120,* 213–217.

Natelson, B. H., Johnson, S. K., DeLuca, J., Sisto, S., Ellis, S. P., Hill, N., & Bergen, M. T. (1995). Reducing heterogeneity in chronic fatigue syndrome: A comparison with depression and multiple sclerosis. *Clinical Infectious Diseases, 21,* 1204–1210.

Natelson, B. H., & Lange, G. (2002). A status report on chronic fatigue syndrome. *Environmental Health Perspectives, 110*(Suppl. 4), 673–677.

Neeck, G. (2002). Pathogenic mechanisms of fibromyalgia. *Ageing Research Reviews*, *1*, 243–255.

Neitzert, C. S., Davis, C., & Kennedy, S. H. (1997). Personality factors related to the prevalence of somatic symptoms and medical complaints in a healthy student population. *British Journal of Medical Psychology*, *70*, 93–101.

Nelson, E., Kirk, J., McHugo, G., Douglass, R., Ohler, J., Wasson, J., & Zubkoff, M. (1987). Chief complaint fatigue: A longitudinal study from the patient's perspective. *Family Practice Research Journal*, *6*, 175–188.

Nelson, S. (2002). Physical symptoms in sexually abused women: Somatization or undetected injury? *Child Abuse Review*, *11*, 51–64.

Nettleton, S. (2006). "I just want permission to be ill": Towards a sociology of medically unexplained symptoms. *Social Science & Medicine*, *62*, 1167–1178.

Nielson, W. R., & Jensen, M. P. (2004). Relationship between changes in coping and treatment outcome in patients with fibromyalgia syndrome. *Pain*, *109*, 233–241.

Nisenbaum, R., Reyes, M., Mawle, A. C., & Reeves, W. (1998). Factor analysis of unexplained severe fatigue and interrelated symptoms. *American Journal of Epidemiology*, *148*, 72–77.

Nishizawa, S., Benkelfat, S. N., Young, S. N., Leyton, M., Mzengeza, S., De Montigny, C., et al. (1997). Differences between males and females in rates of serotonin synthesis in the brain. *Proceedings of the National Academy of Sciences, USA*, *94*, 5308–5313.

Nolen-Hoeksema, S., Larson, J., & Grayson, C. (1999). Explaining the gender difference in depressive symptoms. *Journal of Personality and Social Psychology*, *77*, 1061–1072.

Noor, W., Small, P. K., Loudon, M.A., Hau, C., & Campbell, F. C. (1998). Effects of cisapride on symptoms and postcibal small-bowel motor function in patients with irritable bowel syndrome. *Scandinavian Journal of Gastroenterology*, *33*, 605–611.

Nyenhuis, D. L., Rao, S. M., Zajecka, J. M., Luchetta, T., Bernardin, L., & Garron, D. C. (1995). Mood disturbance versus other symptoms of depression in multiple sclerosis. *Journal of the International Neuropsychological Society*, *1*, 291–296.

Nykvist, K., Kjellberg, A., & Bildt, C. (2002). Causal explanations for common somatic symptoms among women and men. *International Journal of Behavioral Medicine*, *9*, 286–300.

Okifuji, A., Turk, D. C., & Sherman, J. J. (2000). Evaluation of the relationship between depression and fibromyalgia syndrome: Why aren't all patients depressed? *Journal of Rheumatology*, *27*, 212–219.

olde Hartman, T. C., Lucassen, P. L. B. J., van de Lisdonk, E. H., Bor, H. H. J., & van Weel, C. (2004). Chronic functional somatic syndromes: A single syndrome? *British Journal of General Practice*, *54*, 922–927.

Olden, K. W. (2002). Diagnosis of irritable bowel syndrome. *Gastroenterology*, *122*, 1701–1714.

O'Malley, P. G., Balden, E., Tom King, G., Santoro, J., Kroenke, K., & Jackson, J. L. (2000). Treatment of fibromyalgia with antidepressants: A meta-analysis. *Journal of General Internal Medicine, 15,* 659–666.

Oppenheim, J. (1991). *"Shattered nerves": Doctors, patients, and depression in Victorian England.* New York: Oxford University Press.

Orenstein, H. (1989). Briquet's syndrome in association with depression and panic: A reconceptualization of Briquet's syndrome. *American Journal of Psychiatry, 146,* 334–338.

Ostensen, M., Rugelsjoen, A., & Wigers, S. H. (1997). The effect of reproductive events and alterations of sex hormone levels on the symptoms of fibromyalgia. *Scandinavian Journal of Rheumatology, 26,* 355–360.

Ottenweller, J., LaManca, J. J., Sisto, S. A., Guo, W., & Natelson, B. (1997). Endocrine hyporesponsiveness to exercise in patients with chronic fatigue syndrome. *Integrative Physiological Behavioral Science, 32,* 189.

Page, J. G., & Dirnberger, G. M. (1981). Treatment of the irritable bowel syndrome with bentyl (dicyclomine hydrochloride). *Journal of Clinical Gastroenterology, 3,* 153–156.

Palsson, O. S., & Drossman, D. A. (2005). Psychiatric and psychological dysfunction in irritable bowel syndrome and the role of psychological treatments. *Gastroenterology Clinics of North America, 34,* 281–303.

Palsson, O. S., Turner, M. J., Johnson, D. A., Burnett, C. K., & Whitehead, W. E. (2002). Hypnosis treatment for severe irritable bowel syndrome: Investigation of mechanism and effects on symptoms. *Digestive Diseases and Sciences, 47,* 2605–2614.

Parisi, G., Bottona, E., Carrara, M., Cardin, F., Faedo, A., Goldin, D., et al. (2005). Treatment effects of partially hydrolyzed guar gum on symptoms and quality of life of patients with irritable bowel syndrome. A multicenter randomized open trial. *Digestive Diseases and Sciences, 50,* 1107–1112.

Parker, A. J. R., Wessely, S., & Cleare, A. J. (2001). The neuroendocrinology of chronic fatigue syndrome and fibromyalgia. *Psychological Medicine, 31,* 1331–1345.

Pawlikowska, T., Chalder, T., Hirsch, S. R., Wallace, P., Wright, D. J. M., & Wessely, S. C. (1994). Population based study of fatigue and psychological distress. *British Medical Journal, 308,* 763–766.

Payne, A., & Blanchard, E. (1995). A controlled comparison of cognitive therapy and self-help support groups in the treatment of irritable bowel syndrome. *Journal of Consulting and Clinical Psychology, 63,* 779–786.

Pennebaker, J. (1994). Psychological bases of symptom reporting: Perceptual and emotional aspects of chemical sensitivity. *Toxicology and Industrial Health, 10,* 497–511.

Pepper, C. M., Krupp, L. B., Friedberg, F., Doscher, C., & Coyle, P. K. (1993) A comparison of neuropsychiatric characteristics in chronic fatigue syndrome, multiple sclerosis, and major depression. *Journal of Neuropsychiatry and Clinical Neurosciences, 5,* 200–205.

Peres, M. F. P. (2003). Fibromyalgia, fatigue, and headache disorders. *Current Neurology and Neuroscience Reports, 3*, 97–103.

Perkins, S. J., Keville, S., Schmidt, U., & Chalder, T. (2005). Eating disorders and irritable bowel syndrome: Is there a link? *Journal of Psychosomatic Research, 59*, 57–64.

Peters, M. L., Vlaeyen, J. W. S., & van Drunen, C. (2000). Do fibromyalgia patients display hypervigilance for innocuous somatosensory stimuli? Application of a body scanning reaction time paradigm. *Pain, 86*, 283–292.

Petrie, K. J., Broadbent, E. A., Kley, N., Moss-Morros, R., Horne, R., & Rief, W. (2005). Worries about modernity predict symptom complaints after environmental pesticide spraying. *Psychosomatic Medicine, 67*, 778–782.

Petzke, F., Clauw, D., Ambrose, K., Khine, A., & Gracely, R. (2003). Increased pain sensitivity in fibromyalgia: Effects of stimulus type and mode of presentation. *Journal of Pain, 105*, 403–413.

Petzke, F., Harris, R. E., Williams, D. A., Clauw, D. J., & Gracely, R. H. (2005). Differences in unpleasantness induced by experimental pressure pain between patients with fibromyalgia and healthy controls. *European Journal of Pain, 9*, 325–335.

Pfeiffer, A., Thompson, J. M., Nelson, A., Tucker, S., Luedtle, C., Finnie, S., et al. (2003). Effects of a 1.5-day multidisciplinary outpatient treatment program for fibromyalgia: A pilot study. *American Journal of Physical Medicine and Rehabilitation, 82*, 186–191.

Piccinelli, M., & Wilkinson, G. (2000). Gender differences in depression. *British Journal of Psychiatry, 177*, 486–492.

Pilowsky, I. (1969). Abnormal illness behaviour. *British Journal of Medical Psychology, 42*, 347–351.

Plant, E. A., Shibley Hyde, J., Keltner, D., & Devine, P. G. (2000). The gender stereotyping of emotions. *Psychology of Women Quarterly, 24*, 81–92.

Plumb, M., & Holland, J. (1977) Comparative studies of psychological function in patients with advanced cancer—I. Self-report depressive symptoms. *Psychosomatic Medicine, 39*, 264–276.

Poonai, N., Anthony, M. M., Binkley, K. E., Stenn, P., Swinson, R. P., Corey, P., et al. (2000). Carbon dioxide inhalation challenges in idiopathic environmental intolerance. *Journal of Allergy and Clinical Immunology, 105*, 358–363.

Poonai, N., Anthony, M. M., Binkley, K. E., Stenn, P., Swinson, R. P., Corey, P., et al. (2001). Psychologic features of patients with idiopathic environmental intolerance. *Journal of Psychosomatic Research, 51*, 537–541.

Powell, L. H., Shahabi, L., & Thoresen, C. E. (2003). Religion and spirituality: Linkages to physical health. *American Psychologist, 58*, 36–52.

Powell, P., Bentall, R. P., Nye, F. J., & Edwards, R. H. (2004). Patient education to encourage graded exercise in chronic fatigue syndrome. 2 year follow-up of randomised controlled trial. *British Journal of Psychiatry, 184*, 142–146.

Powell, R., Dolan, R., & Wessely S. (1990). Attributions and self-esteem in depression and chronic fatigue syndromes. *Journal of Psychosomatic Research, 34*, 665–673.

Poynard, T., Regimbeau, C., & Benhamou, Y. (2001). Meta-analysis of smooth muscle relaxants in the treatment of irritable bowel syndrome. *Alimentary Pharmacology & Therapeutics, 15*, 355–361.

Price, D. D., & Staud, R. (2005). Neurobiology of fibromyalgia syndrome. *Journal of Rheumatology Supplement, 75*, 22–28.

Prins, J. B., Bleijenberg, G., Bazelmans, E., Elving, L. D., deBoo, T. M., Severens, J. L., et al. (2001). Cognitive behaviour therapy for chronic fatigue syndrome: A multicentre randomised controlled trial. *The Lancet, 357*, 841–847.

Prins, J. B., Bleijenberg, G., & van der Meer, J. W. (2002). Chronic fatigue syndrome and myalgic encephalomyelitis: Correspondence. *The Lancet, 359*, 1699.

Prins, J. B., van der Meer, J. W. M., & Bleijenberg, G. (2006). Chronic fatigue syndrome. *The Lancet, 367*, 346–355.

Pritchard, W. (1905). The American disease: An interpretation. *Canadian Journal of Medicine and Surgery, 18*, 10–22.

Puri, B. K., Counsell, S. J., Zaman, R., Main, J., Collins, A. G., Hajnal, J. V., & Davey, N. J. (2002). Relative increase in choline in the occipital cortex in chronic fatigue syndrome. *Acta Psychiatrica Scandinavica, 106*, 224–226.

Putnam, F. W., & Trickett, P. K. (1997). Psychobiological effects of sexual abuse. A longitudinal study. In R. Yehuda & A. C. McFarlane (Eds.), *Annals of the New York Academy of Sciences: Vol. 821. Psychobiology of posttraumatic stress disorder* (pp. 150–159). New York: New York Academy of Sciences.

Quisel, A., Gill, J., &Walters, G. (2004). Exercise and antidepressants improve fibromyalgia. *Journal of Family Practice, 53*, 280–291.

Racciatti, D., Guagnano, M. T., Vecchiet, J., De Remigis, P. L., Pizzigallo, E., Della Vecchia, R., et al. (2001). Chronic fatigue syndrome: Circadian rhythm and hypothalamic–pituitary–adrenal (HPA) axis impairment. *International Journal of Immunopathology and Pharmacology, 14*, 11–15.

Raine, R., Haines, A., Sensky, T., Hutchings, A., Larkin, K., & Black, N. (2002). Systematic review of mental health interventions for patients with common somatic symptoms: Can research evidence from secondary care be extrapolated to primary care? *British Medical Journal, 325*, 1–11.

Rangel, L., Garralda, E., Levin, M., & Roberts, H. (2000). Personality in adolescents with chronic fatigue syndrome. *European Child & Adolescent Psychiatry, 9*, 39–45.

Rao, S. G., & Bennett, R. M. (2003). Pharmacological therapies in fibromyalgia. *Best Practice & Research. Clinical Rheumatology, 17*, 611–627.

Raphael, K. G., Spatz Widom, C., & Lange, G. (2001). Childhood victimization and pain in adulthood: A prospective investigation. *Pain, 92*, 283–293.

Reeves, W. C., Lloyd, A., Vernon, S. D., Klimas, N., Jason, L., Bleijenberg, G., et al. (2003). Identification of ambiguities in the 1994 chronic fatigue syndrome research case definition and recommendations for resolution. *BMC Health Services Research, 3,* 25–34.

Reeves, W. C., Wagner, D., Nisenbaum, R., Jones, J. F., Gurbaxani, B., Solomon, L., et al. (2005). Chronic fatigue syndrome—A clinically empirical approach to its definition and study. *BMC Medicine, 3,* 19–28.

Reich, J. W., Olmsted, M. E., & van Puymbroeck, C. M. (2006). Illness uncertainty, partner caregiver burden and support, and relationship satisfaction in fibromyalgia and osteoarthritis patients. *Arthritis and Rheumatism, 55,* 86–93.

Reid, S., Hotopf, M., Hull, L., Ismail, K., Unwin, C., & Wessely, S. (2002). Reported chemical sensitivities in a health survey of United Kingdom military personnel. *Occupational Environmental Medicine, 59,* 196–198.

Reilly, J., Baker, G. A., Rhodes, J., & Salmon, P. (1999). The association of sexual and physical abuse with somatization: Characteristics of patients presenting with irritable bowel syndromes and non-epileptic attack disorder. *Psychological Medicine, 29,* 399–406.

Reppetti, R. L. (1998). The promise of a multiple roles paradigm for women's health research. *Women's Health: Research on Gender, Behavior, and Policy, 4,* 273–280.

Reynolds, K. J., Vernon, S. D., Bouchery, E., & Reeves, W. C. (2004). The economic impact of chronic fatigue syndrome. *Cost Effectiveness and Resource Allocation, 2,* 4–13.

Richman, J. A., Jason, L. A., Taylor, R. R., & Jaahn, S. C. (2000). Feminist perspectives on the social construction of chronic fatigue syndrome. *Health Care for Women International, 21,* 173–185.

Rief, W., & Auer, C. (2001). Is somatization a habituation disorder? Physiological reactivity in somatization syndrome. *Psychiatry Research, 101,* 63–74.

Rief, W., & Barsky, A. J. (2005). Psychobiological perspectives on somatoform disorders. *Psychoneuroendocrinology, 30,* 996–1002.

Rief, W., Ihle, D., & Pilger, F. (2003). A new approach to assess illness behavior. *Journal of Psychosomatic Research, 54,* 405–414.

Rief, W., Martin, A., Klaiberg, A., & Brahler, E. (2005). Specific effects of depression, panic, and somatic symptoms on illness behavior. *Psychosomatic Medicine, 67,* 596–601.

Rief, W., Pilger, F., Ihle, D., Bosmans, E., Egyed, B., & Maes, M. (2001). Immunological differences between patients with major depression and somatization syndrome. *Psychiatry Research, 105,* 165–174.

Rief, W., Pilger, F., Ihle, D., Verkerk, R., Scharpe, S., & Maes, M. (2004). Psychobiological aspects of somatoform disorders: Contributions of monoaminergic transmitter systems. *Neuropsychobiology, 49,* 24–29.

Rief, W., & Sharpe, M. (2004). Somatoform disorders—New approaches to classification, conceptualization, and treatment. *Journal of Psychosomatic Research, 56,* 387–390.

Rief, W., Shaw, R., & Fichter, M. M. (1998). Elevated levels of psychophysiological arousal and cortisol in patients with somatization syndrome. *Psychosomatic Medicine, 60,* 198–203.

Riley, R. L., Robinson, E. A., Wise, E. A., Myers, C. D., & Fillingam, R. B. (1998). Sex differences in the perception of noxious experimental stimuli: A meta-analysis. *Pain, 74,* 181–187.

Riley, R. L., Robinson, M. E., Wise, E. A., & Price, D. D. (1999). A meta-analytic review of pain perception across the menstrual cycle. *Pain, 81,* 225–235.

Ringel, Y., Whitehead, W. E., Toner, B. B., Diamant, N. E., Hu, Y., Jia, H., et al. (2004). Sexual and physical abuse are not associated with rectal hypersensitivity in patients with irritable bowel syndrome. *Gut, 53,* 838–842.

Risdale, L., Darbishire, L., & Seed, P. T. (2004). Is graded exercise better than cognitive therapy for fatigue? A UK randomized trial in primary care. *Psychological Medicine, 34,* 37–49.

Rizzi, M., Sarzi-Puttini, P., Atzeni, F., Capsoni, F., Andreoli, A., Pecis, M., et al. (2004). Cyclic alternating pattern: A new marker of sleep alteration in patients with fibromyalgia. *Journal of Rheumatology, 31,* 1193–1199.

Robbins, J. M., & Kirmayer, L. J. (1991). Attributions of common somatic symptoms. *Psychological Medicine, 21,* 1029–1045.

Robbins, J. M., Kirmayer, L. J., & Hemami, S. (1997). Latent variable models of functional somatic distress. *Journal of Nervous and Mental Disease, 185,* 606–615.

Robins, L., Cottler, L., & Keating, S. (1991). *Diagnostic Interview Schedule (DIS): Version III Revised.* St. Louis, MO: Department of Psychiatry, Washington University School of Medicine.

Robins, L. N., Helzer, J. E., Weissman, M. M., Orvaschel, H., Gruenberg, E., Burke, J. D., & Regier, D. A. (1984) Lifetime prevalence of specific psychiatric disorders in three sites. *Archives of General Psychiatry, 41,* 949–958.

Robinson, M. E., Riley, J. L., Myers, C. D., Papas, R., Wise, E., Waxenberg, L. B., et al. (2001). Gender role expectations of pain: relationship to sex differences in pain. *Journal of Pain, 2,* 251–257.

Rollnik, J. D., Karst, M., Piepenbrock, S., Gehrke, A., Dengler, R., & Fink, M. (2003). Gender differences in coping with tension-type headaches. *European Neurology, 50,* 73–77.

Rossy, L. A., Buckelew, S. P., Dorr, N., Hagglund, K. J., Thayer, J. F., McIntosh, M. J. et al. (1999). A meta-analysis of fibromyalgia treatment interventions. *Annals of Behavioral Medicine, 21,* 180–91.

Roy-Byrne, P., Afari, N., Ashton, S., Fischer, M., Goldberg, J., & Buchwald, D. (2002). Chronic fatigue and anxiety/depression: A twin study. *British Journal of Psychiatry, 180,* 29–34.

Russell, I. J. (1996). Neurochemical pathogenesis of fibromyalgia syndrome. *Journal of Musculoskeletal Pain, 4,* 61–92.

Russell, I. J. (1999). Is fibromyalgia a distinct clinical entity? The clinical investigator's evidence. *Balliére's Clinical Rheumatology, 13*, 445–454.

Russell, I. J., Orr, M. D., Littman, B., Vipraio, G. A., Albourek, D., Michalek, J. E., et al. (1994). Elevated cerebrospinal fluid levels of Substance P in patients with the fibromyalgia syndrome. *Arthritis and Rheumatism 37*, 1593–1601.

Russo, J., Katon, W., Clark, M., Kith, P., Sintay, M., & Buchwald, D. (1998). Longitudinal changes associated with improvement in chronic fatigue syndrome patients. *Journal of Psychosomatic Research, 45*, 67–76.

Russo, M. W., Gaynes, B. N., & Drossman, D. A. (1999). A national survey of practice patterns of gastroenterologists with comparison to the past two decades. *Journal of Clinical Gastroenterology, 29*, 339–343.

Sachs-Ericcson, N., Blazer, D., Plant, E. A., & Arnow, B. (2005). Childhood sexual and physical abuse and the 1-year prevalence of medical problems in the national comorbidity survey. *Health Psychology, 24*, 32–40.

Sagami, Y., Shimada, Y., Tayama, J., Nomura, T., Satake, M., Endo, Y. et al. (2004). Effect of a corticotrophin releasing hormone receptor antagonist on colonic sensory and motor function in patients with irritable bowel syndrome [Electronic version]. *Gut, 53*, 958–964.

Salmon, P., Skaife, K., & Rhodes, J. (2003). Abuse, dissociation, and somatization in irritable bowel syndrome: Towards an explanatory model. *Journal of Behavioral Medicine, 26*, 1–18.

Sandler, R. S., Drossman, D. A., Nathan, H. P., & McKee, D. C. (1984). Symptom complaints and health care seeking behavior in subjects with bowel dysfunction. *Gastroenterology, 87*, 314–318.

Sarlani, E., & Greenspan, J. D. (2002). Gender differences in temporal summation of mechanically evoked pain. *Pain, 97*, 163–169.

Sarlani, E., & Greenspan, J. D. (2005). Why look in the brain for answers to temporomandibular disorder pain? *Cells Tissues Organs, 180*, 69–75.

Scarinci, I. C., McDonald-Hale, J., Bradley, L. A., & Richter, J. E. (1994). Altered pain perception and psychosocial features among women with gastrointestinal disorders and history of abuse: A preliminary model. *American Journal of Medicine, 97*, 108–118.

Schluederberg, A., Straus, S. E., Peterson, P., Blumenthal, S., Komaroff, A. L., Spring, S. B., et al. (1992). Chronic fatigue syndrome research. Definition and medical outcome assessment. *Annals of Internal Medicine, 117*, 325–331.

Schmaling, K. B., Fiedelak, J. I., Katon, W. J., Bader, J. O., & Buchwald, D. S. (2003). Prospective study of the prognosis of unexplained chronic fatigue in a clinic-based cohort. *Psychosomatic Medicine, 65*, 1047–1054.

Schmaling, K. B., Lewis, D. H., Fiedelak, J. I., Mahurin, R., & Buchwald, D. S. (2003). Single-photon emission computerized tomography and neurocognitive function in patients with chronic fatigue syndrome. *Psychosomatic Medicine, 65*, 129–136.

Schnurr, P. P., Friedman, M. J., & Bernady, N. C. (2002). Research on posttraumatic stress disorder: Epidemiology, pathophysiology, and assessment. *Journal of Clinical Psychology, 58*, 877–889.

Schoenfeld, P. (2005). Efficacy of current drug therapies in irritable bowel syndrome: What works and does not work. *Gastroenterology Clinics of North America, 34*, 319–335.

Schottenfeld, R. S. (1987). Workers with multiple chemical sensitivities: A psychiatric approach to diagnosis and treatment. *Occupational Medicine, 2*, 739–753.

Schwartz, P. Y. (2002). Why is neurasthenia important in Asian cultures? *Western Journal of Medicine, 176*, 257–258.

Schwartz, R. B., Garada, B. M., Komaroff, A. L., Tice, H. M., Gleit, M., & Jolesz, F. A., et al. (1994). Detection of intracranial abnormalities in patients with chronic fatigue syndrome: Comparison of MRI imaging and SPECT. *American Journal of Roentgenology, 162*, 935–941.

Schwartz, R. B., Komaroff, A. L., Garada, B. M., Gleit, M., Doolittle, T. H., Bates, D. W., et al. (1994). SPECT imaging of the brain: Comparisons of findings in patients with chronic fatigue syndrome, AIDS dementia complex, and major unipolar depression. *American Journal of Roentgenology, 162*, 943–951.

Schweitzer, R., Robertson, D. L., Kelly, B., & Whiting, J. (1993). Illness behavior of patients with chronic fatigue syndrome. *Journal of Psychosomatic Research, 38*, 41–49.

Segal, Z. V., Teasdale, J. D., & Williams, J. M. G. (2004). Mindfulness-based cognitive therapy: Theoretical rationale and empirical status. In S. C. Hayes, V. M. Follette, & M. Linehan (Eds.), *Mindfulness and acceptance: Expanding the cognitive–behavioral tradition* (pp. 45–65). New York: Guilford Press.

Segerstrom, S. C., & Miller, G. E. (2004). Psychological stress and the human immune system. *Psychological Bulletin, 130*, 601–630.

Sharpe, M. (1996). Chronic fatigue syndrome. *Psychiatric Clinics of North America, 19*, 549–573.

Sharpe, M. C., Archard, L. C., Banatvala, J. E., Borysiewicz, L. K., Clare, A. W., David A., et al. (1991). A report—Chronic fatigue syndrome: Guidelines for research. *Journal of the Royal Society of Medicine, 84*, 118–121.

Sharpe, M., & Carson, A. (2001). "Unexplained" somatic symptoms, functional syndromes, and somatization: Do we need a paradigm shift? *Annals of Internal Medicine, 134*, 926–930.

Sharpe, M., Hawton, K., Seagross, V., & Pasvol, G. (1992). Follow up of patients presenting with fatigue to an infectious diseases clinic. *British Medical Journal, 305*, 147–152.

Sharpe, M., Hawton, K., Simkin, S., Surawy, C., Hackmann, A., Klimes, I., et al. (1996). Cognitive behaviour therapy for the chronic fatigue syndrome: A randomized controlled trial. *British Medical Journal, 312*, 22–26.

Sharpe, M., & Wessely, S. (1998). Putting the rest cure to rest—again. *British Medical Journal, 316*, 796–800.

Shaver, J. L. F., Lentz, M., Landis, C. A., Heitkemper, M. M., Buchwald, D., & Woods, N. (1997). Sleep, psychological distress and stress arousal in women with fibromyalgia. *Research in Nursing and Health, 20*, 247–257.

Shaver, J. L. F., Wilbur, J., Robinson, F. P., Wang, E., & Buntin, M. S. (2006). Women's health issues with fibromyalgia syndrome. *Journal of Women's Health, 15,* 1035–1045.

Shaw, G., Srivistava, E. D., Sadlier, M., Swann, P., James, J. Y., & Rhodes, J. (1991). Stress management for irritable bowel syndrome: A controlled trial. *Digestion, 50,* 36–42.

Sherman, J., Turk, D., & Okifuji, A. (2000). Prevalence and impact of posttraumatic stress disorder–like symptoms on patients with fibromyalgia syndrome. *Clinical Journal of Pain, 16,* 127–134.

Short, K., McCabe, M., & Tooley, G. (2002). Cognitive functioning in chronic fatigue syndrome and the role of depression, anxiety, and fatigue. *Journal of Psychosomatic Research, 52,* 475–483.

Shorter, E. (1992). *From paralysis to fatigue: A history of psychosomatic illness in the modern era.* New York: Free Press.

Shorter, E. (1993). Chronic fatigue in historical perspective. In G. R. Bock & J. Whelan (Eds.), *Chronic Fatigue Syndrome: CIBA Foundation Symposium* (pp. 6–22). Chichester, England: Wiley.

Shorter, E. (1997). Multiple chemical sensitivity: Pseudodisease in historical perspective. *Scandinavian Journal of Work and Environmental Health, 23*(Suppl. 3), 35–42.

Shorter, E. (2005). The diagnosis and treatment of fatigue in psychiatry: A historical overview. In J. DeLuca (Ed.), *Fatigue as a window to the brain* (pp. 127–136). Cambridge, MA: MIT Press.

Showalter, E. (1985). *The female malady: Women, madness, and English culture 1830–1980.* New York: Pantheon Books.

Showalter, E. (1997). *Hystories: Hysterical epidemics and modern culture.* New York: Columbia University Press.

Siessmeier, T., Nix, W. A., Hardt, J., Schreckenberger, M., Egle, U. T., & Bartenstein, P. (2003). Observer independent analysis of cerebral glucose metabolism in patients with chronic fatigue syndrome. *Journal of Neurology, Neurosurgery, and Psychiatry, 74,* 922–928.

Sigmon, S. T., Stanton, A. L., & Snyder, C. R. (1995). Gender differences in coping: A further test of socialization and role constraint theories. *Sex Role, 33,* 565–587.

Silverman, D. H. S., Munakata, J., Ennes, H., Mandelkern, M. A., Hoh, C. K., & Mayer, E. A. (1997). Regional cerebral activity in normal and pathological perception of visceral pain. *Gastroenterology, 112,* 64–72.

Silverstein, B. (2002). Gender differences in the prevalence of somatic versus pure depression: A replication. *American Journal of Psychiatry, 159,* 1051–1052.

Silverstein, B., & Blumenthal, E. (1997). Depression mixed with anxiety, somatization, and disordered eating: Relationship with gender role–related limitations experienced by females. *Sex Roles, 36,* 709–724.

Silverstein, B., Caceres, J., Perdue, L., & Cimarolli, V. (1995). Gender differences in depressive symptomatology: The role played by "anxious somatic depression" associated with gender-related achievement concerns. *Sex Roles, 33*, 621–636.

Silverstein, B., & Lynch, A. (1998). Gender differences in depression: The role played by paternal attitudes of male superiority and maternal modeling of gender-related limitations. *Sex Roles, 38*, 539–555.

Silverthorn, D. U. (2001). *Human physiology: An integrated approach* (2nd ed.). Upper Saddle River, NJ: Prentice Hall.

Sim, J., & Adams, N. (2002). Systematic review of randomized controlled trials of nonpharmacological interventions for fibromyalgia. *Clinical Journal of Pain, 18*, 324–336.

Simon, G. E. (1994). Psychiatric symptoms in multiple chemical sensitivity. *Toxicolology and Industrial Health, 10*, 487–496.

Simon, G. E., Daniell, W., Stockbridge, H., Claypoole, K., & Rosenstock, L. (1993). Immunologic, psychological, and neuropsychological factors in multiple chemical sensitivity. A controlled study. *Annals of Internal Medicine, 119*, 97–103.

Simon, G. E., Katon, W. J., & Sparks, P. J. (1990). Allergic to life: Psychological factors in environmental illness. *American Journal of Psychiatry, 147*, 901–905.

Simren, M., Abrahamsson, J., Svedlund, J., & Bjornsson, E. S. (2001). Quality of life in patients with irritable bowel syndrome seen in referral centers versus primary care: The impact of gender and predominant bowel pattern. *Scandinavian Journal of Gastroenterology, 5*, 545–552.

Sinaii, N., Cleary, S. D., Ballweg, M. L., Nieman, L. K., & Stratton, P. (2002). High rates of autoimmune and endocrine disorders, fibromyalgia, chronic fatigue syndrome and atopic disease among women with endometriosis: A survey analysis. *Human Reproduction, 17*, 2715–2724.

Skapinakas, P., Lewis, G., & Mavreas, V. (2003). Unexplained fatigue syndromes in a multinational primary care sample: Specificity of definition and prevalence and distinctiveness from depression and generalized anxiety. *American Journal of Psychiatry, 160*, 785–787.

Skapinakas, P., Lewis, G., & Meltzer, H. (2000). Clarifying the relationship between unexplained chronic fatigue and psychiatric morbidity: Results from a community survey in Great Britain. *American Journal of Psychiatry, 157*, 1492–1498.

Slater, E., & Glithero, E. (1965). A follow-up of patients diagnosed as suffering from "hysteria." *Journal of Psychosomatic Research, 9*, 9–13.

Smith, G. R., Monson, R. A., & Ray, D. C. (1986). Patients with multiple unexplained symptoms: Their characteristics, functional health, and health care utilization. *Archives of Internal Medicine, 146*, 69–72.

Smith, L. K., Pope, C., & Botha, J. L. (2005). Patients' help-seeking experiences and delay in cancer presentation: A qualitative synthesis. *The Lancet, 366*, 825–831.

Smith, R. C., Gardiner, J. C., Lyles, J. S., Sirbu, C., Dwanmena, F. C., Hodges, A., et al. (2005). Exploration of *DSM–IV* criteria in primary care patients with medically unexplained symptoms. *Psychosomatic Medicine, 6*, 123–129.

Smith, R. C., Greenbaum, D. S., Vancouver, J. B., Henry, R. C., Reinhart, M. A., Greenbaum, R. B., et al. (1991). Gender differences in Manning criteria in the irritable bowel syndrome. *Gastroenterology, 100,* 591–595.

Smith-Rosenberg, C. (1985). *Disorderly conduct: Visions of gender in Victorian America.* New York: Knopf.

Smythe, H. (1989). Fibrositis syndrome: A historical perspective. *Journal of Rheumatology, 16*(Suppl. 19), 2–6.

Snyder, H. (2000). *Sexual assault of young children as reported to law enforcement: Victim, incident, and offender characteristics* (NIBRS Statistical Report NCJ 182990). Washington, DC: Bureau of Justice Statistics.

Soderlund, A., & Malterud, K. (2005). Why did I get chronic fatigue syndrome? A qualitative interview study of causal attributions in women patients. *Scandinavian Journal of Primary Health Care, 23,* 242–247.

Song, S., Taylor, R. R., & Jason, L. A. (1999). The relationship between ethnicity and fatigue in a community-based sample. *Journal of Gender, Culture, and Health, 4,* 255–268.

Spence, J. T., Helmreich, R. L., & Stapp, J. C. (1974). The Personal Attributes Questionnaire: A measure of sex role stereotypes and masculinity–femininity. *JSAS Catalogue of Selected Documents in Psychology, 4,* 43–44.

Sperber, A. D., Carmel, S., Atzmon, Y., Weisberg, I., Shalit, Y., Neumann, L., et al. (2000). Use of the Functional Bowel Disorder Severity Index (FBDSI) in a study of patients with the irritable bowel syndrome and fibromyalgia. *American Journal of Gastroenterology, 95,* 995–998.

Spertus, I., Yehuda, R., Wong, C., Halligan, S., & Seremetis, S. (2003). Childhood emotional abuse and neglect as predictors of psychological and physical symptoms in women presenting to a primary care practice. *Child Abuse and Neglect, 27,* 1247–1258.

Spitzer, R. L., Williams, J. B. W., Kroenke, K., Linzer, M., deGruy, F. V., Hahn, S. R., et al. (1994). Utility of a new procedure for diagnosing mental disorders in primary care. The PRIME-MD 1000 Study. *JAMA, 272,* 1749–1756.

Staud, R. (2005). Predictors of clinical pain intensity in patients with fibromyalgia syndrome. *Current Pain and Headache Reports, 9,* 316–321.

Staud, R., Robinson, M., Vierck, C., & Price, D. (2003). Diffuse noxious inhibitory controls (DNIC) attenuate temporal summation of second pain in normal males but not in normal females or fibromyalgia patients. *Journal of Pain, 101,* 167–174.

Staudenmayer, H. (2000). Psychological treatment of psychogenic idiopathic environmental intolerance. *Occupational Medicine, 15,* 627–646.

Staudenmayer, H., Binkley, K. E., Leznoff, A., & Phillips, S. (2000). Idiopathic environmental intolerance: Part 1. Causation analysis applying Bradford Hill's criteria to the toxicogenic theory. *Toxicology Review, 22,* 235–246.

Steele, L., Dobbins, J. G., Fukuda, K., Reyes, M., Randall, B., Koppelman, M., & Reeves, W. C. (1998). The epidemiology of chronic fatigue in San Francisco. *American Journal of Medicine, 105,* 835–905.

Stein, M., Lang, A., Laffaye, C., Satz, L., Lenox, R., & Dressellhaus, T. (2004). Relationship of sexual assault history to somatic symptoms and health anxiety in women. *General Hospital Psychiatry, 26,* 178–183.

Stone, J., Smyth, R., Carson, A., Lewis, S., Prescott, R., Warlow, C., & Sharpe, M. (2005, October 13). Systematic review of misdiagnosis of conversion symptoms and "hysteria" [DOI:10.1136/bmj.38628.466898.55]. *British Medical Journal.* Retrieved March 1, 2007, from http://www.bmj.com/cgi/content/full/331/7523/989

Stone, J., Wojcik, W., Durrance, D., Carson, A., Lewis, S., MacKenzie, L., et al. (2002). What should we say to patients with symptoms unexplained by disease? The "number needed to offend." *British Medical Journal, 325,* 1449–1450.

Strayer, D. R., Carter, W. A., Brodsky, I., Cheney, P., Peterson, D., Salvato, P., et al. (1994). A controlled clinical trial with a specifically configured RNA drug, Poly(I):Poly(C12U), in chronic fatigue syndrome. *Clinical Infectious Diseases, 18*(Suppl. 1), S88–S95.

Stricklin, A., Sewell, M., & Austad, C. (1988) Objective measurement of personality variables in epidemic neuromyesthenia patients. *South African Medical Journal, 77,* 31–34.

Sullivan, M. J. L., Bishop, S. R., & Pivik, J. (1995). The Pain Catastrophizing Scale: Development and validation. *Psychological Assessment, 7,* 524–532.

Sullivan, M., Haythornthwaite, J., Keefe, F., Martin, M., Bradley, L., & Lefebvre, J. (2001). Theoretical perspectives on the relation between catastrophizing and pain. *Clinical Journal of Pain, 17,* 52–64.

Sullivan, M. J. L., Tripp, D. A., & Santor, D. (2000). Gender differences in pain and pain behavior: The role of catastrophizing. *Cognitive Therapy and Research, 24,* 121–134.

Sullivan, P. F., Evengard, B., Jacks, A., & Pedersen, N. L. (2005). Twin analyses of chronic fatigue in a Swedish national sample. *Psychological Medicine, 35,* 1327–1336.

Surawy, C., Hackman, A., Hawton, K., & Sharpe, M. (1995). Chronic fatigue syndrome: A cognitive approach. *Behavior Research Therapy, 33,* 535–544.

Swartz, M., Blazer, D., George, L., & Landerman, R. (1986). Somatization disorder in a community population. *American Journal of Psychiatry, 143,* 1403–1408.

Taillefer, S. S., Kirmayer, L. J., Robbins, J. M., & Lasry, J. C. (2002). Psychological correlates of functional status in chronic fatigue syndrome. *Journal of Psychosomatic Research, 53,* 1097–1106.

Taillefer, S. S., Kirmayer, L. J., Robbins, J. M., & Lasry, J. C. (2003). Correlates of illness worry in chronic fatigue syndrome. *Journal of Psychosomatic Research, 54,* 331–337.

Talley, N. J. (1992). Review article: 5-Hydroxytryptamine agonists and antagonists in the modulation of gastrointestinal motility and sensation: Clinical implications. *Alimentary Pharmacology & Therapeutics, 6,* 273–289.

Talley, N. J. (2003). Pharmacologic therapy for the irritable bowel syndrome. *American Journal of Gastroenterology, 98,* 750–758.

Talley, N. J., & Boyce, P. (1996). Abuse and functional gastrointestinal disorders: What is the link and should we care? *Gastroenterology, 110,* 1301–1313.

Talley, N. J., Boyce, P. M., & Jones, M. (1997). Predictors of health care seeking for irritable bowel syndrome: A population based study. *Gut, 41,* 394–398.

Talley, N. J., Boyce, P. M., & Jones, M. (1998). Is the association between irritable bowel syndrome and abuse explained by neuroticism? A population based study. *Gut, 42,* 47–53.

Talley, N. J., Howell, S., & Poulton, R. (2001). The irritable bowel syndrome and psychiatric disorders in the community: Is there a link? *American Journal of Gastroenterology, 96,* 1072–1079.

Talley, N. J., Phillips, S. F., Melton, L. J., Mulvihill, C., Wiltgen, C., & Zinsmeister, A. R. (1990). Diagnostic value of the Manning criteria in irritable bowel syndrome. *Gut, 31,* 77–81.

Talley, N. J., & Spiller, R. (2002). Irritable bowel syndrome: A little understood organic bowel disease? *The Lancet, 360,* 555–564.

Talley, N. J., Zinsmeister, A. R., & Melton, L. J. (1995). Irritable bowel syndrome in a community: Symptom subgroups, risk factors, and health care utilization. *American Journal of Epidemiology, 142,* 76–83.

Tan, G., Corydon Hammond, D., & Gurrala, J. (2005). Hypnosis and irritable bowel syndrome: A review of efficacy and mechanism of action. *American Journal of Clinical Hypnosis, 47,* 161–178.

Tanaka, H., Matsushima, R., Tamai, H., & Kajumoto, Y. (2002). Impaired postural cerebral hemodynamics in young patients with chronic fatigue with and without orthostatic intolerance. *Journal of Pediatrics, 140,* 412–417.

Tarlo, S. M., Poonai, N., Binkley, K., Antony, M. M., & Swinson, R. P. (2002). Responses to panic induction procedures in subjects with multiple chemical sensitivity/idiopathic environmental intolerance: Understanding the relationship with panic disorder. *Environmental Health Perspectives, 110*(Suppl. 4), 669–671.

Taylor, M. L., Trotter, D. R., & Csuka, M. E. (1995). The prevalence of sexual abuse in women with fibromyalgia. *Arthritis and Rheumatism, 2,* 229–234.

Taylor, R. (2001). Death of neurasthenia and its psychological reincarnation: A study of neurasthenia at the National Hospital for the Relief and Cure of the Paralysed and Epileptic, Queen Square, London, 1870–1932. *British Journal of Psychiatry, 179,* 550–557.

Taylor, R. R., & Jason, L. A. (2001). Sexual abuse, physical abuse, chronic fatigue and chronic fatigue syndrome: A community based study. *Journal of Nervous and Mental Disease, 189,* 709–715.

Taylor, R. R., Jason, L. A., & Curie, C. J. (2002). Prognosis of chronic fatigue in a community-based sample. *Psychosomatic Medicine, 64,* 319–327.

Taylor, R. R., Jason, L. A., & Schoeny, M. E. (2001). Evaluating latent variable models of functional somatic distress in a community-based sample. *Journal of Mental Health, 10,* 335–349.

Taylor, S. E., Klein, L. C., Lewis, B., Gruenewald, T. L., Gurung, R. A. R., & Updegraff, J. A. (2000). Biobehavioral responses to stress in females: Tend and befriend, not fight or flight. *Psychological Review, 107*, 411–429.

Thieme, K., Turk, D. C., & Flor, H. (2004). Comorbid depression and anxiety in fibromyalgia syndrome: Relationship to somatic and psychosocial variables. *Psychosomatic Medicine, 66*, 837–844.

Thompson, W. G. (1997). Gender differences in irritable bowel symptoms. *European Journal of Gastroenterology & Hepatology, 9*, 299–302.

Thompson, W. G., & Heaton, K. W. (1980). Functional bowel disorders in apparently healthy people. *Gastroenterology, 79*, 283–288.

Thompson, W. G., Heaton, K. W., Smyth, G. T., & Smyth, C. (2000). Irritable bowel syndrome in general practice: Prevalence, characteristics, and referral. *Gut, 46*, 78–82.

Thompson, W. G., Longstreth, G. F., Drossman, D. A., Heaton, K. W., Irvin, E. J., & Muller-Lissner, S. A. (2000). Functional bowel disorders and functional abdominal pain. In D. A. Drossman, E. Corazziari, N. J. Talley, W. G. Thompson, & W. E. Whitehead (Eds.), *Rome II: The functional gastrointestinal disorders* (pp. 352–396). McLean, VA: Degnon Associates.

Tibblin, G., Bengstsson, C., Furunes, B., & Lapidus, L. (1990). Symptoms by age and sex. *Scandinavian Journal of Primary Health Care, 8*, 9–17.

Tiersky, L. A., DeLuca, J., Hill, N., Dhar, S. K., Johnson, S. K., Lange, G., et al. (2001). Longitudinal assessment of neuropsychological functioning, psychiatric status, functional disability and employment status in chronic fatigue syndrome. *Applied Neuropsychology, 8*, 41–50.

Tiersky, L. A., Johnson, S. K., Lange, G., Natelson, B. H., & DeLuca, J. (1997). Neuropsychology of chronic fatigue syndrome: A critical review. *Journal of Clinical and Experimental Neuropsychology, 19*, 560–586.

Tikiz, C., Muezzinoglu, T., Pirildar, T., Taskn, E. O., Frat, A., & Tuzun, C. (2005). Sexual dysfunction in female subjects with fibromyalgia. *Journal of Urology, 174*, 620–623.

Tirelli, U., Chierichetti, F., Tavio, M., Simonelli, C., Bianchin, G., Zanco, P., & Ferlin, G. (1998). Brain positron emission tomography (PET) in chronic fatigue syndrome: Preliminary data. *American Journal of Medicine, 105*, 54S–58S.

Toner, B. B. (1994). Cognitive–behavioral treatment of functional somatic syndromes: Integrating gender issues. *Cognitive and Behavioral Practice, 1*, 157–178.

Toner, B. B. (1995). Gender differences in somatoform disorders. In M. V. Seeman (Ed.), *Gender and psychopathology* (pp. 287–309). Washington, DC: American Psychiatric Association.

Toner, B. B., & Akman, D. (2000). Gender role and irritable bowel syndrome: Literature review and hypothesis. *American Journal of Gastroenterology, 95*, 11–16.

Toner, B. B., Koyama, E., Garfinkel, P. E., Jeejeebhoy, K. N., & Gasbarro, I. D. (1992). Social desirability and irritable bowel syndrome. *International Journal of Psychiatry in Medicine, 22*, 99–103.

Toner, B. B., Segal, Z. V., Emmott, S., Myran, D., Ali, A., DiGasbarro, I., & Stuckless, N. (1998). Cognitive–behavioral group therapy for patients with irritable bowel syndrome. *International Journal of Group Psychotherapy, 48,* 215–234.

Toner, B. B., Stuckless, N., Ali, A., Downie, F., Emmott, S., & Akman, D. (1998). The development of a cognitive scale for functional bowel disorders. *Psychosomatic Medicine, 60,* 492–497.

Tonori, H., Aizawa, Y., Ojima, M., Miyata, M., Ishikawa, S., & Sakabe, K. (2001). Anxiety and depressive states in multiple chemical sensitivity. *Tokuku Journal of Experimental Medicine, 193,* 115–126.

Torpy, D. J., Papanicolaou, D. A., Lotsikas, A. J., Wilder, R. L., Chrousos, G. P., & Pillemer, S. (2000). Responses of the sympathetic nervous system and the hypothalamic–pituitary–adrenal axis to interleukin-6. *Arthritis and Rheumatism, 43,* 872–880.

Torres-Harding, S., & Jason, L. A. (2005). What is fatigue? History and epidemiology. In J. DeLuca (Ed.), *Fatigue as a window to the brain* (pp. 3–18). Cambridge, MA: MIT Press.

Trimble, M. (2004). *Somatoform disorders: A medicolegal guide.* Cambridge, England: Cambridge University Press.

Tseng, C. L., & Natelson, B. H. (2004). Few gender differences exist between men and women with chronic fatigue syndrome. *Journal of Clinical Psychology in Medical Settings, 11,* 55–62.

Turk, D. C. (2003). Cognitive–behavioral approach to the treatment of chronic pain patients. *Regional Anesthesia and Pain Medicine, 28,* 573–579.

Turk, D. C., Okifuji, A., Sinclair, J. D., & Starz, T. W (1996). Pain, disability and physical functioning in subgroups of patients with fibromyalgia. *Journal of Rheumatology, 23,* 1255–1262.

Turk, D. C., Okifuji, A., Sinclair, J. D., & Starz, T. W. (1998). Differential responses by psychosocial subgroups of fibromyalgia syndrome patients to an interdisciplinary treatment. *American College of Rheumatology, 11,* 397–404.

Turk, D. C., Okifuji, A., Starz, T. W., & Sinclair, J. D. (1996). Effects of type of symptom onset on psychological distress and disability in fibromyalgia syndrome patients. *Pain, 68,* 423–430.

Ullman, S., & Brecklin, L. (2003). Sexual assault history and health-related outcomes in a national sample of women. *Psychology of Women Quarterly, 27,* 46–57.

Unruh, A. M. (1996). Gender variations in clinical pain experience. *Pain, 65,* 123–167.

Van der Werf, S. P., de Vree, B., Alberts, M., van der Meer, J. W. M., & Bleijenberg, G. (2002). Natural course and predicting self-reported improvement in patients with chronic fatigue syndrome with a relatively short illness duration. *Journal of Psychosomatic Research, 53,* 749–753.

Van Hoof, E., Cluydts, R., & De Meirleir, K. (2003). Atypical depression as a secondary symptom in chronic fatigue syndrome. *Medical Hypotheses, 61,* 52–55.

Van Houdenhove, B., & Egle, U. T. (2004). Fibromyalgia: A stress disorder? *Psychotherapy and Psychosomatics, 73,* 267–275.

Van Houdenhove, B., Egle, U., & Luyten, P. (2005). The role of life stress in fibromyalgia. *Current Rheumatology Reports, 7,* 365–370.

Van Houdenhove, B., Neerinckx, E., Lysens, R., Vertommen, H., Van Houdenhove, L., Onghena, P., et al. (2001). Victimization in chronic fatigue syndrome and fibromyalgia in tertiary care: A controlled study on prevalence and characteristics. *Psychosomatics, 42,* 21–28.

Van Houdenhove, B., Onghena, P., Neerinckx, E., & Hellin, J. (1995) Does high "action-proneness" make people more vulnerable to chronic fatigue syndrome? A controlled psychometric study. *Journal of Psychosomatic Research, 39,* 633–640.

Vandvik, P. O., Wilhemsen, I., Ihlebaek, C., & Farup, P. G. (2004). Comorbidity of irritable bowel syndrome in general practice: A striking feature with clinical implications. *Alimentary Pharmacology & Therapeutics, 20,* 1195–1203.

Vanner, S. J., Depew, W. T., Paterson, W. G., DaCosta, L. R., Groll, A. G., Simon, J. B., & Djurfeldt, M. (1999). Predictive value of the Rome criteria for diagnosing the irritable bowel syndrome. *American Journal of Gastroenterology, 94,* 2912–2917.

Van Santen, M., Bolwijn, P., Verstappen, F., Bakker, C., Hidding, A., Houben, H., et al. (2002). A randomized clinical trial comparing fitness and biofeedback training versus basic treatment in patients with fibromyalgia. *Journal of Rheumatology, 29,* 575–581.

Vassallo, C. M., Feldman, E., Peto, T., Castell, L., Sharpley, A. L., Cowen, P. J., et al. (2001). Decreased tryptophan availability but normal post-synaptic 5-HT receptor sensitivity in chronic fatigue syndrome. *Psychological Medicine, 31,* 585–591.

Veale, D., Kavanagh, G., Fielding, J. F., & Fitzgerald, O. (1991). Primary fibromyalgia and the irritable bowel syndrome: Different expressions of a common pathogenetic process. *British Journal of Rheumatology, 30,* 220–222.

Verbrugge, L. (1985). Gender and health: An update on hypotheses and evidence. *Journal of Health and Social Behavior, 26,* 156–182.

Verbrugge, L. (1989). The twain meet: Empirical explanation of sex differences in health and mortality. *Journal of Health and Social Behavior, 30,* 282–304.

Vercoulen, J. H., Hommes, O. R., Swanink, C. M., Jongen, P. J., Fennis, J. F., Galama, J. M., et al. (1998). The persistence of fatigue in chronic fatigue syndrome and multiple sclerosis: Development of a model. *Journal of Psychosomatic Research, 45,* 507–517.

Vercoulen, J. H., Swanink, C. M. A., Zitman, F. G., Vreden, S. G. S., Hoofs, M. P. H., Fennis, J. F. M., et al. (1996). Randomized, double-blind, placebo-controlled study of fluoxetine in chronic fatigue syndrome. *The Lancet, 347,* 858–861.

Verhaak, P. F. M., Meijer, S. A., Visser, A. P., & Wolters, G. (2006). Persistent presentation of medically unexplained symptoms in general practice. *Family Practice, 23*, 414–420.

Vermetten, E., & Bremner, J. D. (2002). Circuits and systems in stress: II. Applications to neurobiology and treatment in posttraumatic stress disorder. *Depression and Anxiety, 16*, 14–38.

Viramontes, B. E., Camilleri, M., McKinzie, S., Pardi, D. S., Burton, D., & Thomforde, G. M. (2001). Gender-related differences in slowing colonic transit by a 5-HT3 antagonist in subjects with diarrhea-predominant IBS. *American Journal of Gastroenterology, 96*, 2671–2676.

Walen, H. R., Cronan, T. A., Serber, E. R., Groessl, E., & Oliver, K. (2002). Subgroups of fibromyalgia patients: Evidence for heterogeneity and an examination of differential effects following a community-based intervention. *Journal of Musculoskeletal Pain, 10*(3), 9–32.

Walker, E. A., Gelfand, A., Katon, W. J., Koss, M. P., Von Korff, M., Bernstein, D., & Russo, J. (1999). Adult health status of women with histories of childhood abuse and neglect. *American Journal of Medicine, 107*, 332–339.

Walker, E. A., Gelfand, A. N., Gelfand, M. D., Green, C., & Katon, W. J. (1996). Chronic pelvic pain and gynecological symptoms in women with irritable bowel syndrome. *Journal of Psychosomatics, Obstetrics and Gynecology, 17*, 39–46.

Walker, E. A., Katon, W. J., Roy-Byrne, P. P., Jemelka, R. P., & Russo, J. (1993). Histories of sexual victimization in patients with IBS or inflammatory bowel disease. *American Journal of Psychiatry, 150*, 1502–1506.

Walker, E. A., Katon, W. J., Roy-Byrne, P. P., Katon, W. J., Li, L., Amos, D., & Jiranek, G. (1990). Psychiatric illness and irritable bowel syndrome: A comparison with inflammatory bowel disease. *American Journal of Psychiatry, 147*, 1656–1661.

Walker, E., Keegan, D., Gardner, G., Sullivan, M., Bernstein, D., & Katon, W. (1997). Psychosocial factors in fibromyalgia compared with rheumatoid arthritis: II. Sexual, physical, and emotional abuse and neglect. *Psychosomatic Medicine, 59*, 572–577.

Walker, E., Keegan, D., Gardner, G., Sullivan, M., Katon, W., & Bernstein, D. (1997). Psychosocial factors in fibromyalgia compared with rheumatoid arthritis: I. Psychiatric diagnoses and functional disability. *Journal of Psychosomatic Medicine, 59*, 565–571.

Walker, E. A., Unutzer, J., Rutter, C., Gelfand, A., Saunders, K., VonKorff, M., et al. (1999). Costs of health care use by women HMO members with a history of childhood abuse and neglect. *Archives of General Psychiatry, 56*, 609–613.

Wallman, K. E., Morton, A. R., Goodman, C., Grove, R., & Guilfoyle, A. M. (2004). Randomised controlled trial of graded exercise in chronic fatigue syndrome. *Medical Journal of Australia, 180*, 444–448.

Walsh, S. J., & Rau, L. M. (2000). Autoimmune diseases: A leading cause of death among young and middle-aged women in the United States. *American Journal of Public Health, 90*, 1463–1466.

Ware, N. C., & Kleinman, A. (1992). Culture and somatic experience: The social cause of illness in neurasthenia and chronic fatigue syndrome. *Psychosomatic Medicine, 54,* 546–560.

Wearden, A. J., & Appleby, L. (1996). Research on cognitive complaints and cognitive functioning in patients with chronic fatigue syndrome: What conclusions can we draw? *Journal of Psychosomatic Research, 41,* 197–211.

Wearden, A. J., Morriss, R. K., Mullis, R., Strickland, P. L., Pearson, D. J., Appleby, L., et al. (1998). Randomised, double-blind, placebo-controlled treatment trial of fluoxetine and graded exercise for chronic fatigue syndrome. *British Journal of Psychiatry, 172,* 485–490.

We Are FMily. (2002). *Diagnosing fibromyalgia syndrome.* Retrieved May 22, 2007, from http://wearefmily.com/diagnosis.htm

Weber, D. A., & Reynolds, C. R. (2004). Clinical perspectives on neurobiological effects of trauma. *Neuropsychology Review, 14,* 115–129.

Webster, R. (1995). *Why Freud was wrong.* New York: Basic Books.

Weir, P. T., Harlan, G. A., Nkoy, F. L., Jones, S. S., Hegman, K. T., Gren, L. H. et al. (2006). The incidence of fibromyalgia and its associated comorbidities: A population based retrospective cohort study based on the International Classification of Diseases, 9th Revision codes. *Journal of Clinical Rheumatology, 12,* 124–128.

Weisenberg, M., Tepper, I., & Schwarzwald, J. (1995). Humor as a cognitive technique for increasing pain tolerance. *Pain, 63,* 202–212.

Weiss, E. L., Longhurst, J. G., & Mazure, C. M. (1999). Childhood sexual abuse as a risk factor for depression in women: Psychosocial and neurobiological correlates. *American Journal of Psychiatry, 156,* 816–828.

Werner, A., Isaksen, L. W., & Malterud, K. (2004). "I am not the kind of woman who complains of everything": Illness stories on self and shame in women with chronic pain. *Social Science & Medicine, 59,* 1035–1045.

Wessely, S. (1990). Old wine in new bottles: Neurasthenia and "ME." *Psychological Medicine, 20,* 35–53.

Wessely, S. (1991). History of postviral fatigue syndrome. *British Medical Bulletin, 47,* 919–941.

Wessely, S. (1996a). Chronic fatigue syndrome. Summary of a report of a joint committee of the Royal Colleges of Physicians, Psychiatrists and General Practitioners. *Journal of the Royal College of Physicians of London, 30,* 497–504.

Wessely, S. (1996b). Neurasthenia and fatigue syndromes, Part 3. In R. Porter & G. E. Berrios (Eds.), *A history of clinical psychiatry* (pp. 509–532). London: Athlone.

Wessely, S., Chadler, T., Hirsch, S., Wallace, P., & Wright, D. (1997). The prevalence and morbidity of chronic fatigue and chronic fatigue syndrome: A prospective primary care study. *American Journal of Public Health, 87,* 1449–1455.

Wessely, S., Nimnuan, C., & Sharpe, M. (1999). Functional somatic syndromes: One or many? *The Lancet, 354,* 936–939.

Wetzel, R. D., Guze, S. B., Cloninger, C. R., Martin, R. L., & Clayton, P. J. (1994). Briquet's syndrome (hysteria) is both a somatoform and a "psychoform" illness: A Minnesota Multiphasic Personality Inventory study. *Psychosomatic Medicine, 56,* 564–569.

White, C., & Schweitzer, R. (2000). The role of personality in the development and perpetuation of chronic fatigue syndrome. *Journal of Psychosomatic Research, 48,* 515–524.

White, K. P., Nielson, W. R., Harth, M., Ostbye, T., & Speechley, M. (2002). Does the label "fibromyalgia" alter health status, function, and health service utilization? A prospective, within-group comparison in a community cohort of adults with chronic widespread pain. *Arthritis and Rheumatism, 47,* 260–265.

Whitehead, W. E. (1999). Patient subgroups in irritable bowel syndrome that can be defined by symptom evaluation and physical examination. *American Journal of Medicine, 107,* 33S–40S.

Whitehead, W. E., Bosmajian, L., Zonderman, A. B., Costa, P. T., & Schuster, M. M. (1988). Symptoms of psychologic distress associated with irritable bowel syndrome. Comparison of community and medical clinic samples. *Gastroenterology, 95,* 709–714.

Whitehead, W. E., Cheskin, L. J., Heller, B. R., Robinson, J. C., Crowell, M. D., Benjamin, C., & Schuster, M. M. (1990). Evidence for exacerbation of irritable bowel syndrome during menses. *Gastroenterology, 98,* 1485–1489.

Whitehead, W. E., Crowell, M. D., Davidoff, A. L., Palsson, O. S., & Schuster, M. M. (1997). Pain from rectal distension in women with irritable bowel syndrome: Relationship to sexual abuse. *Digestive Diseases and Sciences, 42,* 796–804.

Whitehead, W. E., Crowell, M. D., Robinson, J. C., Heller, B. R., & Schuster, M. M. (1992). Effects of stressful life events on bowel symptoms: Subjects with irritable bowel syndrome compared with subjects without bowel dysfunction. *Gut, 33,* 825–830.

Whitehead, W. E., Holtkotter, B., Enck, P., Hoelzl, R., Holmes, K. D., Anthony, J., et al. (1990). Tolerance for rectosigmoid distention in irritable bowel syndrome. *Gastroenterology, 98,* 1187–1192.

Whitehead, W. E., & Palsson, O. S. (1998). Is rectal pain sensitivity a biological marker for irritable bowel syndrome: Psychological influences on pain perception. *Gastroenterology, 115,* 1263–1271.

Whitehead, W. E., Palsson, O., & Jones, K. R. (2002). Systematic review of the comorbidity of irritable bowel syndrome with other disorders: What are the causes and implications? *Gastroenterology, 122,* 1140–1156.

Whitehead, W. E., Palsson, O. S., Levy, R. L., Von Korff, M., Feld, A. D., & Turner, M. J. (2003). Comorbid psychiatric disorders in irritable bowel syndrome (IBS) and inflammatory bowel disease (IBD). *Gastroenterology, 124,* A398.

Whitehead, W. E., Winget, C., Fedoravicius, A. S., Wooley, S., & Blackwell, B. (1982). Learned illness behavior in patients with irritable bowel syndrome and peptic ulcer. *Digestive Diseases Science, 27,* 202–208.

Widiger, T. A., & Samuel, D. B. (2005). Diagnostic categories or dimensions? A question for the *Diagnostic and Statistical Manual of Mental Disorders—Fifth Edition. Journal of Abnormal Psychology, 114,* 494–504.

Wiesmuller, G. A., Ebel, H., Hornberg, C., Kwan, O., & Friel, J. (2003). Are syndromes in environmental medicine variants of somatoform disorders? *Medical Hypotheses, 61,* 419–430.

Wilhelmsen, I. (2005). Biological sensitization and psychological amplification: Gateways to subjective health complaints and somatoform disorders. *Psychoneuroendocrinology, 30,* 990–995.

Williams, A., & Richardson, P. (1993). What does the BDI measure in chronic pain? *Pain, 55,* 259–266.

Williams, D. A. (2003). Psychological and behavioural therapies in fibromyalgia and related syndromes. *Best Practice & Research. Clinical Rheumatology, 17,* 649–665.

Wilson, A., Hickie, I., Lloyd, A., Hadzi-Pavlovic, D., Boughton, C., Dwyer, J., & Wakefield, D. (1994). Longitudinal study of outcome of chronic fatigue syndrome. *British Medical Journal, 208,* 756–759.

Winters, W., Devriese, S., Van Deist, I., Nemery, B., Veulemans, H., Elen, P., et al. (2003). Media warnings about environmental pollution facilitate the acquisition of symptoms in response to chemical substances. *Psychosomatic Medicine, 65,* 332–338.

Wise, E. A., Price, D. D., Myers, C. D., Heft, M. W., & Robinson, M. E. (2002). Gender role expectations of pain: Relationship to experimental pain perception. *Pain, 96,* 335–342.

Wolfe, F., Anderson, J., Harkness, D., Bennet, R. M., Caro, X. J., Goldenberg, D. C., et al. (1997a). Health status and disease severity in fibromyalgia: Results of a six-center longitudinal study. *Arthritis and Rheumatism, 40,* 1571–1579.

Wolfe, F., Ross, K., Anderson, J., & Russell, I. J. (1995). Aspects of fibromyalgia in the general population: Sex, pain threshold, and fibromyalgia symptoms. *Journal of Rheumatology, 22,* 151–156.

Wolfe, F., Ross, K., Anderson, J., Russell, I. J., & Herbert, L. (1995). The prevalence and characteristics of fibromyalgia in the general population. *Arthritis and Rheumatism, 38,* 19–28.

Wolfe, F., Smythe, H. A., Yunus, M. B., Bennett, R. M., Bombardier, C., Goldenberg, D. L., et al. (1990). The American College of Rheumatology 1990 criteria for the classification of fibromyalgia: Report of the Multicenter Criteria Committee. *Arthritis and Rheumatism, 33,* 160–172.

Wolkowitz, O. M., & Reus, V. I. (1999). Treatment of depression with antiglucocorticoid drugs. *Psychosomatic Medicine, 61,* 698–711.

Wood, B., & Wessely, S. (1999) Personality and social attitudes in chronic fatigue syndrome. *Journal of Psychosomatic Research*, 385–397.

Woodman, C. L., Breen, K., Noyes, R. J., Moss, C., Fagerholm, R., Yagla, S. J., et al. (1998). The relationship between irritable bowel syndrome and psychiatric illness: A family study. *Psychosomatics, 39*, 45–54.

Wool, C. A., & Barsky, A. J. (1994). Do women somatize more than men? Gender differences in somatization. *Psychosomatics, 35*, 445–452.

World Health Organization. (1992). *International classification of diseases and related health problems, 10th revision.* Albany, NY: WHO Publications Center USA.

World Health Organization. (2007). *Gender and women's mental health.* Retrieved March 1, 2007, from http://www.who.int/mental_health/prevention/genderwomen/

Yoder, J. D., & Kahn, A. S. (2003). Making gender comparisons meaningful: A call for more attention to social context. *Psychology of Women Quarterly, 27*, 281–290.

Yunus, M. B. (1992). Towards a model of pathophysiology of fibromyalgia: Aberrant central pain mechanisms with peripheral modulation. *Journal of Rheumatology, 19*, 846–850.

Yunus, M. B. (2001). The role of gender in fibromyalgia syndrome. *Current Rheumatology Reports, 3*, 128–134.

Yunus, M. B. (2002). Gender differences in fibromyalgia and other related syndromes. *Journal of Gender-Specific Medicine, 5*, 42–47.

Yunus, M. B., Ahles, T. A., Aldag, J. C., & Masi, A. T. (1991). Relationship of clinical features with psychological status in primary fibromyalgia. *Arthritis and Rheumatism, 34*, 15–21.

Yunus, M. B., Celiker, R., & Aldag, J. C. (2004). Fibromyalgia in men: Comparison of psychological features with women. *Journal of Rheumatology, 31*, 2464–2467.

Yunus, M. B., Inanici, F., Aldag, J. C., & Mangold, J. C. (2000). Fibromyalgia in men: Comparison of clinical features with women. *Journal of Rheumatology, 27*, 485–490.

Zar, S., Kumar, D., & Benson, M. J. (2001). Review article: Food hypersensitivity and irritable bowel syndrome. *Aliment Pharmacology Therapy, 15*, 439–449.

Zautra, A. J., Fasman, R., Reich, J. W., Harakas, P., Johnson, L. M., Olmsted, M. E., & Davis, M. C. (2005). Fibromyalgia: Evidence for deficits in positive affect regulation. *Psychosomatic Medicine, 67*, 147–155.

Zautra, A., Johnson, L., & Davis, M. (2005). Positive affect as a source of resilience for women in chronic pain. *Journal of Consulting and Clinical Psychology, 73*, 212–220.

Zavestoski, S., Brown, P., McCormick, S., Mayer, B., D'Ottavi, M., & Lucove, J. C. (2004). Patient activism and the struggle for diagnosis: Gulf War illnesses and other medically unexplained physical symptoms in the U.S. *Social Science & Medicine, 58*, 161–175.

Ziem, G., & McTamney, J. (1997). Profiles of patients with chemical injury and sensitivity. *Environmental Health Perspectives, 105,* 417–436.

Zigmond, A. S., & Snaith, R. P. (1983). The Hospital Anxiety and Depression Scale. *Acta Psychiatrica Scandinavica, 67,* 370–371.

Zurowski, M., & Shapiro, C. (2004). Stress, fibromyalgia, and sleep. *Journal of Psychosomatic Research, 57,* 415–416.

AUTHOR INDEX

Gaston-Johansson, F., 110, 167
Gatchel, R. J., 45
Gaynes, B. N., 70
Geddes, J. R., 118
Geisser, M. E., 59, 96–97
Gelfand, A., 41
Gelfand, A. N., 72
George, J. P. K., 131
George, L., 15, 24
Gershon, M. D., 80
Gibson, P. R., 144
Gijsbers van Wijk, C. M., 25, 33, 36, 39
Gilchrist, J., 155
Gill, J., 167
Gillespie, N. A., 50
Gil-Rivas, V., 127, 174
Glaser, R., 54, 55, 120
Gleason, O. C., 23, 25
Glithero, E., 19
Goertzel, B. N., 55, 120, 122
Gokcen, E., 167
Goldberg, D. L., 108
Goldberg, R. T., 107
Goldenberg, D. L., 62, 92–93, 95, 108, 116, 164, 165
Goldie, I., 45
Golding, J. M., 24
Goldstein, R., 107
Gomez, R. L., 181
Gonsalkorale, W. M., 155, 159, 160
Goodman, C., 178
Goodnick, P. J., 90, 108
Goosens, M. E., 167
Gowans, S. E., 166, 167
Gowers, W. R., 18
Gracely, R. H., 95, 98
Graham, N. M., 56
Graham, T., 92, 103
Gralnek, I. M., 74
Gran, J. T., 4, 89, 99
Granges, G., 93
Grant, K. R., 32
Graveling, R. A., 131, 133, 138
Gray, C. E., 121
Gray, D. P., 40
Gray, G. C., 61
Grayson, C., 28
Greco, A., 122
Green, C., 72
Greenberg, D. B., 116
Greene, B., 154, 155
Greenspan, J. D., 58

Groessl, E., 112
Groleau, D., 146
Grove, R., 178
Gruber, A. J., 62
Gudleski, G. D., 43, 87
Guerriero, R. C., 167
Guglielmi, R. S., 182
Guilfoyle, A. M., 178
Gunderson, J., 59
Guo, W., 120
Gupta, K., 142
Gupta, O. P., 75
Gur, A., 104
Gurbaxani, B., 120
Gureje, O., 20
Gurrala, J., 151
Gustafsson, M., 110
Guthrie, E., 147, 149, 160, 161
Guze, S. B., 16, 17, 24
Gwee, K. A., 69

Hackman, A., 128, 174
Hadhazy, V., 165, 167
Hadler, N. M., 37, 46, 92, 111
Hadzi-Pavlovic, D., 18
Hafizi, S., 54
Hahn, B. A., 74
Hahn, M., 139
Hakala, M., 50
Hallberg, I. R., 33
Haller, E., 182
Halliday, P. D., 166
Halligan, S., 42
Hallman, J., 101
Hallman, W., 136
Halpert, A., 81, 154
Hamilton, J. A., 7, 38, 39, 187
Hamilton, W. T., 94
Hammer, J., 68
Hanewald, G. J. F. P., 24, 39
Hanno, P. M., 72
Hansen, M., 24
Hapidou, E., 100
Harris, L., 21
Harris, R. E., 97
Hart, R. P., 59
Harth, M., 92
Hartz, A. J., 63, 118
Haug, T. T., 27, 33, 34
Hausteiner, C., 23, 142
Hawley, D. J., 108–109
Hawton, K., 128, 174

Hayes, S. C., 148
Haynes, S. N., 90, 110, 167
Hays, R. D., 74
Hayton, B. C., 115
Hazlett, R. L., 90, 110, 167
Hazlett-Stevens, H., 82
Heath, A. C., 50
Heath, I., 186
Heaton, K. W., 70, 71
Hedenberg, L., 166
Heft, M. W., 59
Heim, C., 54
Heist, V., 121
Heitkemper, M. M., 36, 72, 76, 77
Helgeson, V. S., 45
Hellesnes, B., 47
Hellhammer, D. H., 53, 54
Hellhammer, J., 53
Hellstrom, O., 111
Helmreich, R. L., 77
Hemami, S., 64
Henderson, M., 127
Henneberger, P. K., 136
Henningsen, P., 26, 127
Henrich, G., 83
Herbert, L., 109
Herdenfeldt, M., 59
Hersbach, P., 83
Hesse, J., 53
Heymann-Monnikes, I., 155
Hibbard, J. H., 34
Hickie, I. B., 18, 50, 65
Hidding, A., 167
Hill, A. B., 140
Hiller, W., 24
Hill Goldsmith, H., 35
Hirsch, S., 119
Hoffman, A., 64
Hohmann, A. A., 29
Holbert, C., 39
Holdcraft, L. C., 165
Holland, J., 29
Holloway, R. L., 163
Holman, A., 24
Holmes, G. P., 116, 117
Holtkotter, B., 79
Hommes, O. R., 147
Hoover, P. M., 127, 174
Hornberg, C., 131
Horne, R., 142
Horwitz, B. J., 67, 70
Hotopf, M., 25, 117

Houghton, L. A., 76, 77, 159
Howell, S. C., 68, 82
Hu, Y. J. B., 54, 84, 85
Hudson, J. I., 30, 62, 95, 108–109
Hudson, M. S., 108
Huenefeld, M., 92, 103
Huster, D., 121
Hutton-Young, S. A., 78

Ichise, M., 122
Iezzi, T., 59
Ihle, D., 30, 50
Ihlebaek, C., 72
Imperiale, T., 150
Inanici, F., 61, 99
Isaksen, L. W., 37

Jacks, A., 4, 118, 124
Jackson, J., 42
Jackson, N. A., 76, 77
Jackson, T., 59
Jacobson, D. L., 56
Jaffee, J., 124
Jahn, S. C., 46
Jailwala, J., 150, 152
Jain, A. P., 75
Jajoo, U. N., 75
Jakobsson, U., 33
Jason, L. A., 4, 14, 15, 18, 39, 46, 64, 115,
    116, 118, 119, 124, 125, 179
Jeejeebhoy, K. N., 147, 158
Jemelka, R. P., 84
Jensen, I., 45, 167, 168
Jensen, M. P., 168
Jensen, R., 58
Jerjes, W. K., 54, 121
Joffe, B. I., 98
Johns, K. R., 58, 100
Johnson, D., 4, 64
Johnson, D. A., 159
Johnson, L. M., 37, 43, 112
Johnson, S. K., 19, 22, 29, 36, 39, 47, 65,
    116, 119, 126–128, 137, 141, 174
Jones, A., 59
Jones, K. R., 4, 30, 63, 72
Jones, M., 71, 85
Jones, R. H., 73, 75
Jordan, K. M., 115, 124
Junghaenel, D. U., 168

Kaasa, S., 124
Kael, A., 103

Ron, M., 176
Rose, D., 155
Rose, N. R., 56
Rosendal, M., 21
Rosenstock, L., 138
Ross, K., 92, 109
Rossy, L. A., 164, 165
Roy-Byrne, P., 50, 84
Rugelsjoen, A., 102
Russell, I. J., 89, 92, 99, 109
Russo, J., 84, 118
Russo, M. W., 70

Sachs-Ericsson, N., 42
Sackett, C. F., 148
Sagami, Y., 81, 152
Saisto, S. A., 120
Salmon, P., 85, 87
Samuel, D. B., 10
Sandler, R. S., 70, 71
Sandoval, R., 90, 108
Sanne, H., 110
Santor, D., 44
Sarac, A. J., 104
Sarlani, E., 58
Sattel, H., 26, 127
Scarinci, I. C., 85, 86
Scarisbrick, P., 105
Schacter, C. L., 166
Schad, T., 121
Schagen, C. M. T., 39
Schagen, S., 24
Scheidt, C., 133
Schlesinger, L., 62, 108
Schlosser, S., 135
Schluederberg, A., 116
Schmaling, K. B., 61, 118, 119, 123, 124,
        126, 127, 174
Schmidt, U., 73
Schmidtke, K., 133
Schmulson, M., 57, 76
Schnurr, P. P., 54
Schoenfeld, P., 151
Schoeny, M. E., 64
Schottenfeld, R. S., 143
Schuster, M. M., 71, 86, 146, 152
Schvaneveldt, R. W., 181
Schwartz, G. E., 136, 138, 141
Schwartz, J. E., 168
Schwartz, P. Y., 16
Schwartz, R. B., 122
Schwarz, S. P., 153

Schwarzwald, J., 58
Schweitzer, R., 174
Seed, P. T., 179
Segal, Z. V., 148, 157, 158
Segall, A., 32
Segerstrom, S. C., 55
Serber, E. R., 112
Seremetis, S., 42
Sewell, M., 127
Shafran, S. D., 173
Shahabi, L., 175
Shapiro, C., 107
Sharon, C., 178
Sharpe, M., 4, 17, 25, 26, 62, 116, 118, 119,
        126, 128, 174, 175, 177, 186
Shaver, J. L. F., 102, 106, 113
Shaw, G., 153
Shaw, R., 50
Sherman, J. J., 108–110
Shibley Hyde, J., 35, 45
Shipton, E. A., 98
Short, K., 119
Shorter, E., 14–19
Shoulson, I., 99
Showalter, E., 13–15, 19
Sidhwa, H. K., 75
Siessmeier, T, 123
Sigmon, S. T., 44
Silman, A. J., 90, 104
Silver, R. C., 24
Silverman, D. H. S., 80
Silverstein, B., 27, 28
Silverthorn, D. U., 51, 55
Sim, J., 165, 167
Simon, C., 25
Simon, G. E., 131, 138, 140, 142
Simren, M., 75
Sinaii, N., 56
Sinclair, J. D., 112, 169
Skaife, K., 87
Skapinakas, P., 127
Slade, D., 72
Slater, E., 19
Smith, B. W., 113
Smith, G. R., 24
Smith, L. K., 36
Smith, R. C., 26, 68
Smith, T. C., 61
Smith, W. R., 37
Smith-Rosenberg, C., 13, 15
Smyth, C., 71
Smyth, G. T., 71

Uslan, D., 37

Vahlberg, T., 50
Vaith, P., 133
Van Damme, S. V., 44
van der Meer, J. W. M., 115, 118, 175
Van der Werf, S. P., 118
van Drunen, C., 44, 96
Vandvik, P. O., 72, 152
Van Hoof, E., 121
Van Houdenhove, B., 7, 105, 128, 146, 147, 187
Van Houdenhove, L., 128
Van Hulle, C., 35
Vanner, S. J., 68
van Puymbroeck, C. M., 37
Van Santen, M., 166
van Weel, C., 62
Vassallo, C. M., 121
Vatn, M. H., 150
Veale, D., 93
Verbrugge, L., 4, 33, 36, 46
Vercoulen, J. H., 147, 174
Vercoulen, J. W., 119, 127
Verhaak, P. F. M., 21
Vermetten, E., 54
Vernon, S. D., 119
Vertommen, H., 128
Vickroy, M., 118
Vierck, C., 97
Viramontes, B. E., 150
Vishwanath, B. S., 56
Visser, A. P., 21
Vlaeyen, J. W. S., 44, 96, 167
Von Korff, M. R., 74
von Rad, M., 83
Vythilingam, M., 54

Wade, J. B., 59
Wadsworth, M., 25
Wagner, M., 64
Waitzkin, H., 24
Wakefield, D., 116
Walen, H. R., 112
Walker, E. A., 20, 26, 41, 42, 63, 72, 73, 81, 84, 107, 109
Wallace, P., 119
Wallman, K. E., 178
Walsh, S. J., 56
Walters, G., 167
Wang, E., 102
Ware, N. C., 46

Wearden, A. J., 119, 178
We Are FMily, 91
Weber, D. A., 53
Webster, R., 19
Weiman, M., 177n
Weir, P. T., 92
Weisenberg, M., 58
Weiss, E. L., 28, 54
Wells, A., 42
Werner, A., 37
Wessely, S., 4, 9, 14–16, 18, 19, 25, 26, 30, 62, 103, 115, 118, 119, 128, 174, 176, 177
Westerholm, P., 45
Wetzel, R. D., 17
White, C., 128
White, K. P., 9, 92, 113
White, P. D., 94, 178
Whitehead, W. E., 4, 23, 30, 32, 63, 65, 69, 71, 72, 74–76, 79, 82, 83, 86, 88, 146, 149, 152, 159
Whiting, J., 174
Whorwell, P. J., 76, 77, 80, 155, 159, 160
Widiger, T. A., 10
Wiesmuller, G. A., 131, 132
Wigers, S. H., 102
Wilbur, J., 102
Wilhelmsen, I., 57, 72, 185, 186
Wilkinson, G., 27, 28
Williams, A., 29
Williams, D. A., 97, 146, 147
Williams, J. M. G., 148
Wilson, A., 118
Wilson, R. J., 143
Winberg, J., 51
Winget, C., 32
Winters, W., 143
Wise, E. A., 58, 59
Witter, E. A., 119
Witthöft, M., 142
Wolde-Tsadik, G., 70
Wolfe, F., 89, 92–94, 96, 99, 108–109
Wolters, G., 21
Wong, C., 42
Wood, D. R., 115
Woodman, C. L., 81
Woodruff, R. A., 16
Wool, C. A., 4, 23, 27, 35, 57
Wooley, S., 32
World Health Organization, 16, 24, 26
Worthington, H. V., 101
Wright, C. C., 57
Wright, D., 119

Wyshak, G., 22, 23

Yan, S., 74
Yao, J. F., 73
Yates, W., 23, 25
Yehuda, R., 42
Yoder, J. D., 46
Yunus, M. B., 4, 61, 62, 95, 99–100, 108–109

Zachariae, R., 59
Zacker, C., 73
Zar, S., 70, 151

Zautra, A. J., 37, 43, 111, 112, 113
Zavestoski, S., 20, 37, 132
Zhu, G., 50
Ziem, G., 132, 139
Zigmond, A. S., 65
Zilker, T., 23, 142
Zilko, P., 93
Zimmerman, T., 26, 127
Zinsmeister, A. R., 67, 70
Zonderman, A. B., 71, 146, 152
Zunder, T., 133
Zurowski, M., 107

SUBJECT INDEX

Cognitive therapy, 154–155
Colpermin, 153
Communication, 44
Comorbidity, 61–63
Complementary and alternative medicine (CAM) treatments, 165
Contact thermal heat, 96–97
Conversion disorder, 16
Coping/coping styles
    and CFS, 174
    and FMS, 111–113
    and gender, 43–44
    and pain, 59
Coproporhyrin levels, 139
Corticosteroids
    for FMS, 164
    and SD, 51
Corticotropin-releasing hormone (CRH)
    and CFS, 120, 121
    and IBS, 81
    and SD, 51, 52
    and stress, 55
Cortisol
    and CFS, 120, 121, 174
    and FMS, 103–105
    and MUIs, 53–55
    and SD, 51, 53
CRH. See Corticotropin-releasing hormone
CRH antagonist, 81
CRH injections, 103
Cross-sensitization, 138
Cultural context, 18–19, 125
Culture-driven disorders, 38

Deep sleep, 105
Deep vein thrombosis, 38
Defensiveness, 128–129
Dehydroepiandrosterone sulphate (DHEAS), 99
Dependent personality disorder, 17
Depression
    and CFS, 65, 126–127, 178
    and childhood sexual abuse, 42
    and FMS, 102, 108–109
    and gender, 46
    and health care seeking, 36
    and IBS, 78, 81, 83, 161
    and MCS, 140–142
    as overlapping symptom, 64
    and physical exercise, 166
    and somatization, 25–26
    and symptom perception, 35

Desensitization training, 182
Desipramine, 150, 157
Dexamethosone, 121
DHEAS (dehydroepiandrosterone sulphate), 99
Diagnosis, psychiatric vs. medical, 38
Diagnostic and Statistical Manual of Mental Disorders (DSM), 10, 16, 17, 24, 25
Diary keeping, 171
Diet, 151–152
Diffuse noxious inhibitory control (DNIC) system, 97
Disability, 37, 74–75
Disclosure writing, 168–169
Disease conviction beliefs, 37–43
    and CFS, 174–175
    and childhood maltreatment, 41–43
    and disability, 37
    and FMS, 167–168
    and IBS, 154, 156–157
    and legitimization of symptoms, 37–39
    and MCS, 181–182
    and somatic attribution, 39–41
Dissociation, 38, 87
DNIC (diffuse noxious inhibitory control) system, 97
Doctor shopping, 6
    and legitimization of symptoms, 38
    and MCS, 133
Dolorimetry, 90, 91
DSM. See Diagnostic and Statistical Manual of Mental Disorders
Dual etiology hypothesis, 65
Dualism, 25
Dysfunctional copers, 112
Dyspareria, 72

Eating disorders, 73
Ecologic illness, 131
Economic impact
    of CFS, 119
    of IBS, 73–74
    of MCS, 132
Education
    about IBS, 163
    about MCS, 147
Education level, 34
Effort syndrome, 18
Emotion
    and FMS, 98, 110
    and IBS, 154
Emotional abuse

and health care utilization, 42
and IBS, 78
Emotional flexibility, 148
Employment, 37
Empowerment, 148
Endometriosis, 56
Engel, George, x
Enteric nervous system, 80
Environmental cues, 35
Environmental illness, 131
Environmental medicine physicians, 133
Epinephrine
    and SD, 51, 52
    and stress, 55
Epstein–Barr virus, 18, 116, 120
Estrogen
    and FMS, 99
    and MCS, 137
    and pain perception, 58
Exercise, physical. *See* Physical exercise
Expressiveness, 45, 46

Fact-based medicine, ix
Familial aggregation, 94–95
Family social climate, 87
Fatigue. *See also* Chronic fatigue syndrome
    as common symptom of MUIs, 17–18
    as comorbid symptom, 63
    and neurasthenia, 14
Fearfulness, 35
Female body, medicalization of, 39
Feminine gender role, 77–78
Fiber, 151–152, 156
Fibromyalgia syndrome (FMS), 3, 5, 89–113
    ACR criteria, 90
    and anxiety, 27
    and childhood sexual abuse, 41
    and childhood trauma, 107–108
    comorbid conditions, 92
    and coping, 111–113
    diagnosis, 89–91
    and disease conviction beliefs, 37, 38
    and emotional flexibility, 148
    and emotion/pain, 98
    etiology, 94–113
    gender disparity in, 4, 99–103
    genetic contributions to, 94–95
    and health care seeking, 37
    history of, 18
    and IBS, 72
    and immunological changes, 106–107
    juvenile primary, 92

and legitimization of symptoms, 38
and MCS, 136
and modern social strains, 46
and neuroendocrine system, 98–99
nonrheumatic symptoms, 90
overlap with other MUIs, 92–93
and pain hypersensitivity/central sensitivity, 95–97
prevalence, 91–92
prognosis, 93–94
and psychiatric disorders, 108–111
and psychosocial issues, 107–113
and sensitization, 57
and sleep disturbance, 105–106
and stress, 103–105
and suggestibility, 23
treatments. *See* FMS treatments
Fibrositis, 18, 89
Filter model, 57
5-HT$_3$ receptors, 150
5-HT$_4$ receptors, 151
Florence Nightingale disease, 39
Fluoxetine, 178
fMRI (functional MRI), 123
FMS. *See* Fibromyalgia syndrome
FMS treatments, 163–172
    case study, 169–172
    cognitive–behavioral therapy, 167–169
    drugs, 164
    physical exercise, 166–167
    studies of, 164–165
Food allergies, 18, 137, 151
Food hypersensitivity, 70
Freud, Sigmund, 14
Functional dyspepsia, 71–72
Functional MRI (fMRI), 123

Gastroenteritis, 65, 69–70
Gender. *See also* Women
    and autoimmune disease, 56
    and catastrophizing, 43–45
    and CFS, 123–125
    and depression/anxiety, 25–26
    and FMS, 99–103
    and health care seeking, 36–37
    and IBS, 75–77
    and MCS, 136–137, 140
    and mood/anxiety disorders, 27–28
    and MUIs, 4–5, 65, 186
    and pain, 28–29
    and sensitivity, 56–59
    and somatic attribution, 39–41

and somatization, 23–25
and stress, 46–47, 51–53
and symptom perception, 34–36
and symptom report, 22, 33–34
Gender-related medically unexplained
    illness(es), 13–17
    Briquet's syndrome as, 16–17
    chronic fatigue syndrome as, 15
    and *DSM*, 16
    hysteria as, 13–14
    neurasthenia, 14–15
Gender-related social roles, 47
Gender role
    catastrophizing and expectations of, 45–
        46
    and IBS, 77–79
    and pain, 59
    and symptom perception, 35
    and treatment, 147–148
Gender Role Expectations of Pain (GREP),
    59
Genetic factors
    of CFS, 120–122
    of FMS, 94–95
    of MUIs, 49–50
Glucose, 51
Gonadal function, 103
Graded exercise, 177–179
GREP (Gender Role Expectations of Pain),
    59
Group therapy
    for CFS, 177
    for IBS, 157–158
Guar gum, 152
Gulf War illness/syndrome, 3, 136
Gulf War veterans
    with CFS, 174
    and MCS, 135, 140
Gut motility, 69
Gut transit times, 75

Hamlet (William Shakespeare), 63
Harm avoidance, 36
Hazards, 47
Headaches
    FMS overlap with, 93
    tension, 4, 44
Health beliefs, 36
Health care utilization
    and childhood sexual abuse, 41–42
    and illness behavior, 36–37
    and somatic attributions, 40

and symptom perception, 35
Heat, 96–97
Helplessness, 44
Heme, 139
Histrionic personality disorder, 16, 127
Hormones
    and FMS, 100–102
    and IBS, 76–77
    and MCS, 137
    and stress, 51–53
HPA. *See* Hypothalamic–pituitary–adrenal
    axis
Hydrocortisone, 174
Hyperalgesia, 63, 89
Hyperventilation syndrome, 4
Hypervigilance
    and catastrophizing, 44–45
    and IBS, 85
    and pain, 59
Hypnotherapy, 159–160
Hypochondriasis, 25
Hypocortisolism, 174
Hypothalamic–pituitary–adrenal (HPA) axis
    and CFS, 120–122
    and FMS, 93, 103–104
    and MUIs, 53–55
    and SD, 51–52
Hysterectomy, 73
Hysteria, 13–18
Hysterical personality, 16

IBS. *See* Irritable bowel syndrome
IBS treatments, 149–161
    and diet, 151–152
    drugs, 150–151
    hypnotherapy, 159–160
    psychological, 153–159
    psychotherapy, 160–161
    stress reduction, 152–153
Idiopathic environmental intolerance (IEI),
    131, 142, 143
Illness behavior, 32–37
    abnormal, 32
    characteristics of, 32
    and health care seeking, 36–37
    and IBS, 82–84
    learned, 32–33
    and symptom perception, 34–36
    and symptom reporting, 33–34
Illness uncertainty, 36–37
Immune system
    and autoimmune disease, 56

and FMS, 106–107
and MCS, 138
and SD, 51–52
and stress, 55–56
Inflammatory bowel disease, 72
Injections, 164
Insula, 76
Interleukin-1-receptor-II, 56
International Classification of Diseases (WHO), 16, 24
Interpersonally distressed copers, 112
Interstitital cystitis, 72, 93
Irritable bowel syndrome (IBS), 3, 5, 67–88
    and biopsychosocial model, 20
    and childhood sexual abuse, 41, 84–87
    diagnosis, 68–69
    and disability/quality of life, 74–75
    and disease conviction beliefs, 38
    dual etiology hypothesis of, 65
    economic impact, 73–74
    etiology, 69–70
    female gender as risk factor for, 65
    FMS overlap with, 93
    and gender, 4, 75–77
    and gender role, 77–79
    and illness behavior, 83–84
    and learned illness behavior, 32–33
    overlap with other MUIs, 71–73
    and pain hypersensitivity, 96
    pathophysiology, 79–81
    prevalence, 70–71
    and psychiatric disorders, 81–83
    and sensitization, 57
    and somatic attributions, 40–41
    subgroups of, 67
    subtypes of, 68
    treatments. *See* IBS treatments

Journal of the American Medical Association, 131–132
Juvenile primary fibromyalgia syndrome, 92

Karnofsky Performance Status Scale, 177

Lactose malabsorption, 71
Learned illness behavior, 32–33
Learning, associative, 143–144
Legitimization of symptoms
    and disease conviction beliefs, 37–39
    of MCS, 182
Lifelong victimization, 126
Limbic system, 81

Limit setting, 171
Local anesthetics, 164
Loperamide, 150
Luteinizing hormone, 77

Magnetic resonance imaging (MRI), 122
Major depressive disorder (MDD), 108
Manning criteria, 68
MCS. *See* Multiple chemical sensitivities
MCS treatments, 181–183
MDD (major depressive disorder), 108
Mebeverine, 157
Media coverage
    and disease conviction beliefs, 37, 38
    and MCS, 132
Medical diagnosis
    and mood/anxiety disorders, 29–30
    psychiatric vs., 38
Medicalization of female body, 39
Medically unexplained illnesses (MUIs), 3–7, 9–11
    biopsychosocial factors influencing, 10, 11
    biopsychosocial model for understanding, 5
    common factors among, 4
    comorbidity among, 61–63
    cultural context of, 19–20
    defined, 3
    difficulties presented with, 6–7
    as distinct disorders, 63–66
    and *DSM*, 10
    fatigue as, 17–18
    gender disparity in, 4–5
    illnesses classified as, 3–4
    MCS as, 18
    misdiagnosis of, 18–19
    and sensitization, 56–59
    shared factors of, 38
    treatments, 6, 145–148
    women with, 6
Medically unexplained symptoms (MUS), 21, 26
Medical utilization. *See* Health care utilization
Menstrual cycle
    and FMS, 99, 100–102
    and pain perception, 58
Methyl tertiary butyl ether (MTBE), 139
Mind–body interactions, 148
Mind–body therapies, 165
Mindfulness-based cognitive therapy, 148

Modern social strains, 45–46
Mononucleosis, 65
Mood disorders, 26–30
    and gender, 27–28
    and medical illness, 29–30
    and pain, 28–29
Morbidity, 4, 29
Mortality, 40
MRI (magnetic resonance imaging), 122
MTBE (methyl tertiary butyl ether), 139
MUIs. See Medically unexplained illnesses
Multiple chemical sensitivities (MCS), 3, 5,
        9, 131–144
    and associative learning, 143–144
    defining, 132–134
    etiology, 138–144
    FMS overlap with, 93
    and gender, 136–137
    gender disparity in, 4
    history of, 18
    and legitimization of symptoms, 38
    overlap with other MUIs, 136
    prevalence, 134–135
    prognosis, 135–136
    and psychological factors, 140–143
    and sensitization, 56
    treatments. See MCS treatments
Multiple sclerosis, 36
Muscular pain, fibromyalgia as. See
        Fibromyalgia syndrome
MUS. See Medically unexplained symptoms
Myalgic encephalitis, 94
Myalgic encephalomyelitis, 39, 116
Myelasthenia, 15

Negative affect
    and somatic attributions, 40
    and symptom perception, 35
Negative-thought restructuring, 171
Neurasthenia, 14–17, 65
Neurasthenic neurosis, 17
Neuroendocrine system, 98–99, 103
Neurogenic mechanism, 138–139
Neuroimaging, 122–123
Neuropeptide Y, 101
Neuropsychological performance, 119
Neuroticism
    and CFS, 128
    and symptom perception, 35
New England Journal of Medicine, 132
Nociceptin, 101
Nociceptive processing, 58

Noncardiac chest pain, 4
Norepinephrine
    and FMS, 99, 103
    and SD, 51
Normalizing attributions, 39, 40

Obsessive–compulsive personality disorder,
        127
Olfactory sensitivity, 137

Paced Auditory Serial Addition Test (PASAT),
        123
Pain
    catastrophizing of, 98
    and gender, 57–59
    and mood/anxiety disorders, 28–29
    perception of, 58–59
    sensitivity to, 57–58, 95–97
Pain Catastrophizing Scale, 44
Panic attacks/disorder, 30
    and IBS, 161
    and MCS, 141–142
Parasympathetic response
    and IBS, 80
    and SD, 53
Parenting style, 87
Paroxetine, 150
Partially hydrolyzed guar gum, 152
PASAT (Paced Auditory Serial Addition
        Test), 123
Patient activism, 37
Patient education
    about FMS, 163
    about MCS, 147
Pelvic pain. See Chronic pelvic pain
Pelvic symptoms, FMS and, 102
Perfectionism
    and CFS, 128
    and FMS, 111
    and IBS, 73, 158
Peripheral–visceral mechanism, 79
Personality factors
    and CFS, 127–129
    and symptom perception, 35
Pesticides, 134, 137
Pharmacotherapy
    for CFS, 173–175
    for FMS, 164
    for IBS, 150–151
Phospholipase A2, 56
Physical abuse
    and IBS, 87

and pain reports, 43
and unexplained pain, 107
Physical exercise, 63
    for CFS, 177–179
    and deep sleep, 105
    for FMS, 94, 165–167
Physiological cues, 35
Pleasurable activities, seeking out, 171
Porphyrias, 139
Postinfectious neuromyasthenia, 116
Postpartum period, 102
Posttraumatic stress disorder (PTSD)
    and abuse, 108
    and cortisol, 54
    and FMS, 110
Postviral fatigue syndrome, 94, 116
Pregnancy, 102
Premenstrual dysphoric disorder, 101
Premenstrual syndrome, 3
Pressure algometer, 90, 91
Prioritizing, 171
Progesterone, 99
Psychiatric diagnosis, medical vs., 38
Psychiatric disorders, 21–30
    and CFS, 126–127
    and FMS, 108–111
    and IBS, 81–83
    and MCS, 140–143
    mood/anxiety disorders, 26–30
    MUIs comorbid with, 21–23
    as overlapping symptom, 64
    somatoform disorders/somatization, 23–
    26
Psychiatric morbidity, 29
Psychoeducational treatment, 154
Psychological attributions, 39, 40, 146
Psychological treatment, 153–159
Psychosocial factor(s), 31–47
    catastrophizing as, 43–47
    disease conviction beliefs as, 37–43
    illness behavior as, 32–37
Psychosocial issues, 107–113
    childhood trauma, 107–108
    coping, 111–113
    psychiatric disorders, 108–111
Psychotherapy, 160–161
Psyllium husk, 156
PTSD. See Posttraumatic stress disorder

Quality of life, 74–75

Rape

and FMS, 108
and IBS, 86, 161
and PTSD, 54
Relaxation training
    for CFS, 176–177
    for FMS, 171
    for IBS, 153, 156, 158
Religious involvement, 175
Rome I criteria, 68
Rome II criteria, 68, 69
Rome III criteria, 68
Rumination, 28, 44

SD. See Somatization/somatoform disorder
Secondary gains
    and learned illness behavior, 32–33
    and trauma history, 43
Selective serotonin reuptake inhibitors
    (SSRIs)
    for FMS, 164
    for IBS, 150
Self-assessed health, 40
Self-blame, 86
Self-help groups, 174–175
Self-monitoring, 98
Sensitivity
    and childhood sexual abuse, 41, 42
    and FMS, 89, 95–97
    and IBS, 79–80
    and MCS. See Multiple chemical sensi-
    tivities
    to pain, 57–58, 95–97
    and symptom perception, 35
Sensitization
    as MCS stage, 133
    and MUIs, 56–59
Serotonin
    and CFS, 121
    and FMS, 99
    and IBS, 80
    and stress, 55–56
Sexual abuse. See also Rape
    in childhood. See Childhood sexual
    abuse
    and health care utilization, 42
    and IBS, 84–85, 87
Sexual dysfunction
    and FMS, 102
    and IBS, 72
Sick building syndrome, 19, 133
Sick role
    concept, 32

and health care seeking, 36
and legitimization of symptoms, 38
and symptom perception, 35
Single photon emission computed tomography (SPECT), 122–123
Situational cues, 35
Sleep disturbance, 105–106
Sleep-spindle, 106
Social involvement, 46
Sociocultural trends, 23
Soldiers, 18
Solvent exposure, 134
Somatic attribution, 39–41
Somatization/somatoform disorder (SD), 23–26
    abridged, 24–26
    and CFS, 22
    characteristic of, 22
    classification of, 16
    and depression/anxiety, 25–26
    as DSM classification, 24, 25
    and dualism, 25
    and gender, 23–25
    hysteria as, 17
    and IBS, 82
    and MCS, 142
    and medical illness, 30
    physiology of, 50–56
    and treatment issues, 145–146
Somatosensory cortex, 81
Specificity, fibromyalgia and, 89, 90
SPECT. See Single photon emission computed tomography
Spinal disorders, 45
SSRIs. See Selective serotonin reuptake inhibitors
Stigma
    with MCS, 144, 182
    with MUIs, 38–39
    of psychiatric labels, 146
Stress
    accumulation of, 28
    and FMS, 103–105
    and gender, 46–47
    and IBS, 83, 154
    and immune system, 55–56
    and MCS, 137
    and SD, 51–53
    and treatment issues, 146
    workplace, 108
Stress reduction, 149, 152–153
Substance abuse

and IBS, 82
and MCS, 137
Substance P, 98, 99
Suggestibility, 23
Support groups, 155
Sympathetic nervous system
    and IBS, 80
    and SD, 51–53
Symptom perception, 34–36
Symptom report
    cognitive traits related to, 23
    and gender, 22
    and illness behavior, 33–34
    and somatization, 23

TDS (time-dependent sensitization), 138
Tegaserod, 151
Temperature, FMS and, 96–97
Temporomandibular joint dysfunction (TMD), 3
    FMS overlap with, 93
    and IBS, 72
Tend-and-befriend response, 52–53
Tender points
    and FMS, 89–91, 100
    injections into, 164
    and overlap of MUIs, 93
Tension headaches, 4, 44
Testosterone, 77
Thermal heat, 96–97
Time-dependent sensitization (TDS), 138
TMD. See Temporomandibular joint dysfunction
Total allergy syndrome, 131
Toxic agoraphobia, 142
Toxicant induced loss of tolerance, 139
Trauma
    childhood, 54, 107–108
    and FMS, 107
    symptom reports and undisclosed, 43
Treatment issues, 145–148
Treatments. See specific treatment, e.g.: CFS treatment
Tricyclic antidepressants
    for FMS, 164, 165
    IBS, 149
Triggering, 133, 139
Triggers
    of IBS, 151
    of MCS, 133, 139
20th century disease, 131

ABOUT THE AUTHOR

Susan K. Johnson received her MA in general psychology from New York University in 1986 and her PhD in behavioral neuroscience from Rutgers University in 1991. She was a neuropsychology fellow and research scientist at the University of Medicine and Dentistry of New Jersey from 1992 through 1996. She joined the faculty of the Department of Psychology at the University of North Carolina at Charlotte, in 1996, where she is currently an associate professor. She has published extensively in the fields of neuropsychology and health psychology. She lives with her husband and two daughters in Davidson, North Carolina.